Register Now for Online Access to Your Book!

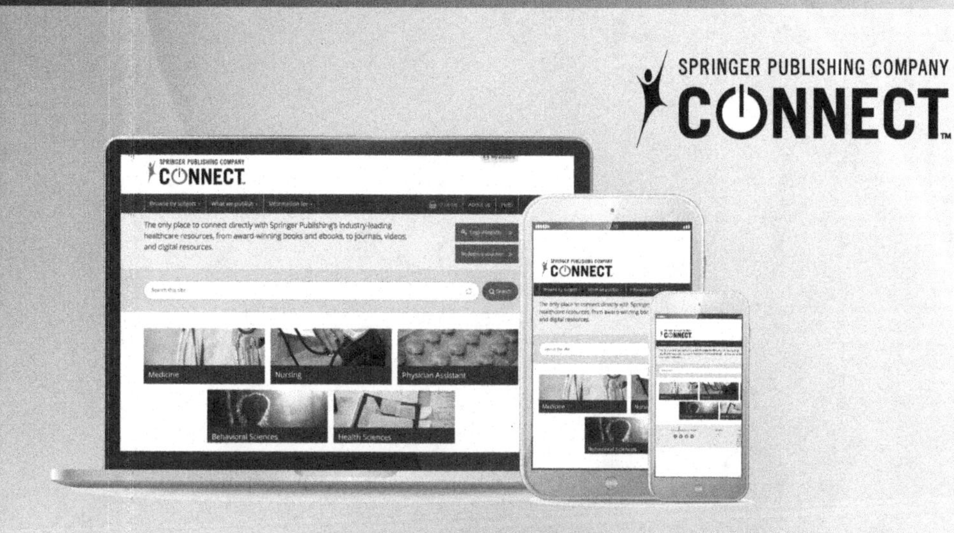

Your print purchase of *Leadership and Management Competence in Nursing Practice* **includes online access to the contents of your book**—increasing accessibility, portability, and searchability!

Access today at:

http://connect.springerpub.com/content/book/978-0-8261-2534-7 or scan the QR code at the right with your smartphone and enter the access code below.

5MUPR5L7

Scan here for quick access.

If you are experiencing problems accessing the digital component of this product, please contact our customer service department at cs@springerpub.com

The online access with your print purchase is available at the publisher's discretion and may be removed at any time without notice.

Publisher's Note: New and used products purchased from third-party sellers are not guaranteed for quality, authenticity, or access to any included digital components.

Leadership and Management Competence in Nursing Practice

Audrey Marie Beauvais, DNP, MSN, MBA, RN, is the associate dean for undergraduate programs in the Marion Peckham Egan School of Nursing and Health Studies at Fairfield University, Connecticut. She has experience in academic and hospital settings as well as in the insurance industry. Immediately prior to Fairfield, Dr. Beauvais was an assistant professor, director of the undergraduate nursing program, and coordinator of the patient care services administrative track at Sacred Heart University's School of Nursing in Fairfield. For the 11 years prior to her employment at Sacred Heart University, Dr. Beauvais worked in various leadership positions at Stamford Hospital including nurse manager of the pediatric and psychiatric units, case manager, and performance improvement coordinator. Dr. Beauvais was the Magnet® coordinator who successfully led Stamford Hospital to be recognized as a Magnet hospital. The Magnet Recognition Program is a prestigious designation administered by the American Nurses Credentialing Center for excellence in nursing practice. Dr. Beauvais has earned a range of formal certifications in the areas of psychiatric and mental health nursing, nurse case management, clinical nurse leader, emotional intelligence, and trauma nursing. She has been the recipient of several honors and distinctions including the Connecticut Nurses Association Diamond Jubilee Josephine A. Dolan Award for Outstanding Contribution to Nursing Education, the Connecticut League for Nursing Ruth M. Olson Excellence in Nurse Education Award, and Sacred Heart University's Dean's Leadership Award. Dr. Beauvais holds a BSN from Fairfield University, an MSN and MBA from Sacred Heart University, and a DNP from Case Western Reserve University in Cleveland, Ohio.

Leadership and Management Competence in Nursing Practice

Competencies, Skills, Decision-Making

Audrey Marie Beauvais, DNP, MSN, MBA, RN

EDITOR

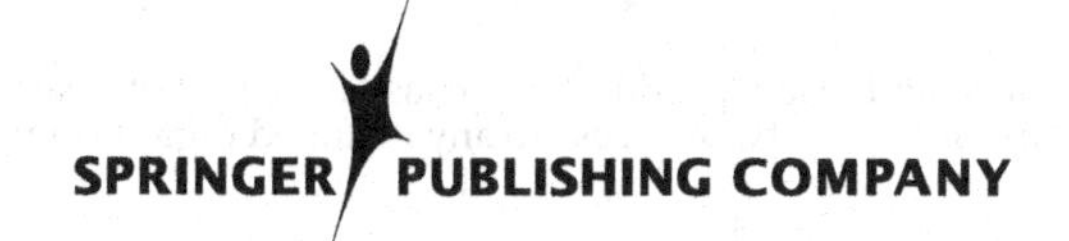

Springer Publishing Company, LLC
11 West 42nd Street
New York, NY 10036
www.springerpub.com

Acquisitions Editor: Elizabeth Nieginski
Production Manager: Kris Parrish
Compositor: Graphic World

ISBN: 978-0-8261-2524-8
ebook ISBN: 978-0-8261-2534-7
Instructor's Manual ISBN: 978-0-8261-2619-1

Instructors Materials: Qualified instructors may request supplements by emailing textbook@springerpub.com.

19 20 21 22 23 / 5 4 3 2 1

The author and the publisher of this Work have made every effort to use sources believed to be reliable to provide information that is accurate and compatible with the standards generally accepted at the time of publication. The author and publisher shall not be liable for any special, consequential, or exemplary damages resulting, in whole or in part, from the readers' use of, or reliance on, the information contained in this book. The publisher has no responsibility for the persistence or accuracy of URLs for external or third-party Internet websites referred to in this publication and does not guarantee that any content on such websites is, or will remain, accurate or appropriate.

Library of Congress Cataloging-in-Publication Data

Names: Beauvais, Audrey Marie, editor.
Title: Leadership and management competence in nursing practice : competencies, skills, decision-making / [edited by] Audrey Marie Beauvais.
Description: New York, NY : Springer Publishing Company, [2019] | Includes bibliographical references and index.
Identifiers: LCCN 2018032247 (print) | LCCN 2018033043 (ebook) | ISBN 9780826125347 (ebook) | ISBN 9780826125248 (pbk.) | ISBN 9780826126191 (Instructors manual)
Subjects: | MESH: Nursing | Leadership | Nurse's Role | Decision Making, Organizational
Classification: LCC RT89 (ebook) | LCC RT89 (print) | NLM WY 105 | DDC 362.17/3--dc23
LC record available at https://lccn.loc.gov/2018032247

Publisher's Note: New and used products purchased from third-party sellers are not guaranteed for quality, authenticity, or access to any included digital components.

Printed in the United States of America.

This book is dedicated to my family:
To my husband, John, whose support helped make this possible.
To my children, Jeffrey and Rebecca, who fill my heart with joy.
To my mom and dad, who have always been my biggest fans.

CONTENTS

V. INTEGRATING LEADERSHIP AND MANAGEMENT COMPETENCIES INTO NURSING PRACTICE—YOUR EVOLUTION AS A PROFESSIONAL

CONTRIBUTORS

Audrey Marie Beauvais, DNP, MSN, MBA, RN
Associate Dean and Associate Professor
Marion Peckham Egan School of Nursing and Health Studies
Fairfield University
Fairfield, Connecticut

Karen Burrows, DNP, MAHSM, RN, C-EFM
Professor of the Practice
Marion Peckham Egan School of Nursing and Health Studies
Fairfield University
Fairfield, Connecticut

James Cyrus, MSN, RN-BC
Nurse Manager, Medical Step-Down Unit
U.S. Department of Veterans Affairs (VA)
VA Connecticut Healthcare System
West Haven, Connecticut

Karri Davis, DNP, RN, NE-BC
Critical Care Clinical Nurse Educator
Lahey Hospital and Medical Center
Merrimac, Massachusetts

Susan DeNisco, DNP, APRN, FNP-BC, CNE, CNL
Professor of Nursing
Sacred Heart University
Fairfield, Connecticut

David M. Depukat, PhD, RN-BC, CNE
Nursing Outcomes Specialist and Policy Lead
Office of Nursing Excellence
Yale New Haven Hospital
New Haven, Connecticut

Jean Marie DiNapoli, DNP, RN
Associate Director
Institute for Advanced Medicine
Mount Sinai Health System
New York, New York

Susan A. Goncalves, DNP, MS, RN-BC
Assistant Professor
College of Nursing
Sacred Heart University
Fairfield, Connecticut

Kelly Hancock, DNP, RN, NE-BC
Executive Chief Nursing Officer, Cleveland Clinic Health System, and
Chief Nursing Officer—Main Campus
Nursing Institute
Cleveland, Ohio

Bonnie Haupt, DNP, RN, CNL, CHSE
Clinical Nurse Leader
South Texas Veterans Healthcare Systems
San Antonio, Texas

Robin S. Krinsky, DNP, RN-BC, CCRN
Adjunct Assistant Professor
Department of Nursing
Lehman College
Bronx, New York;
Clinical Nurse
Electrophysiology Lab
Mount Sinai Medical Center
New York, New York

Deirdre O'Flaherty, DNP, APRN-BC, NE-BC, ONC
Senior Administrative Director, Patient Care Services
Surgical Nursing
Orthopaedic Program Coordinator
Lenox Hill Hospital
New York, New York

Mary E. Quinn, DNP, RN
Director of Nursing Quality and Improvement Initiatives
New York-Presbyterian Hospital
New York, New York

Mary T. Quinn Griffin, PhD, RN, FAAN
Assistant Provost for Outcome Assessment and Accreditation Professor
Case Western Reserve University, Frances Payne Bolton School of Nursing
Cleveland, Ohio

Lisa M. Rebeschi, PhD, MSN, RN, CNE
Chairperson and Associate Professor
Department of Nursing
Southern Connecticut State University
New Haven, Connecticut

Linda Roney, EdD, RN-BC, CPEN, CNE
Assistant Professor
Marion Peckham Egan School of Nursing and Health Studies
Fairfield University
Fairfield, Connecticut

Kimberly Spahn, MSN, FNP-BC, RN
Nurse Consultant
The Vitality Method
Louisville, Kentucky

Kristy Dixon Stinger, DNP, RN, NEA-BC
Clinical Nurse Specialist, Nursing Education
Department of Nursing
Western Connecticut Health Network
Danbury, Connecticut

Sherylyn M. Watson, PhD, MSN, RN, CNE
Associate Dean and Assistant Professor
College of Nursing
Sacred Heart University
Fairfield, Connecticut

SUPERVISORY EDITOR

Janet Weber, PhD
Professor Emerita in Nursing
Southeast Missouri State University
Cape Girardeau, Missouri

FOREWORD

This book, *Leadership and Management Competence in Nursing Practice: Competencies, Skills, Decision-Making,* is a very welcome addition to the nursing leadership and management literature. Geared toward RNs enrolled in RN-to-BSN programs, it is concise, straightforward, and engaging. The academic standards for baccalaureate nursing programs promulgated by the American Association of Colleges of Nursing in the *Essentials of Baccalaureate Nursing Programs* provides the rationale for leadership and management content as core components of all BSN curricula.

This new book on leadership and management includes all of the basic content that RN-to-BSN students need. Personal attributes of leaders are addressed so that students can develop their self-awareness regarding their own leadership and management styles. Leadership skills such as effective communication, priority and time management, accountability, teamwork, decision-making, conflict management, and stress management are all important topics that are thoroughly addressed in the chapters.

Each chapter begins with learning objectives for the student. The format is useful to students who are often expert clinicians but have not previously been introduced to the key concepts central to leadership and management in nursing and healthcare. Chapters also include a case scenario demonstrating the specific topic of the chapter and self-assessment tools that will help students discover their learning needs, strengths, and weaknesses in the important content areas.

Another important section of the book is focused on preparing nurses to lead change. Basic components of organizational analysis are addressed as important to understanding the systems in which nurses work. Managing quality and safety, and managing resources are dimensions that are addressed in the section of the book on developing management skills. These are significant issues in care delivery today, and nurses who are in management and leadership positions, or those who aspire to be in these positions, must have the necessary skills in the ever-changing healthcare arena. This book includes the basic content in a user-friendly format. The structured chapter format is particularly useful to faculty new to teaching these students as well as to faculty who have large classes of RN-to-BSN students, including virtual and in-person classes. As the external pressures increase for RNs without BSN degrees to return to school for the BSN degree, we can expect that the class sizes will further increase, particularly in core-required courses such as leadership and management.

The chapter contributors have a wealth of experience and expertise in their content areas. Many of the authors have held or currently hold leadership positions in healthcare delivery organizations and academic nursing. Their real-life leadership experiences enhance the basic content in the chapters, particularly in the case scenarios included.

The book editor, Dr. Audrey Beauvais, has gathered the necessary content experts and structured the content to be included in each chapter. She has authored the first two chapters of the book. Both of these introductory chapters set the tone for the students, introducing core content in ways that help students relate to the learning objectives. The depth of Dr. Beauvais's leadership in both content and style of the book will make it easy for both faculty and students to follow her lead.

Joyce J. Fitzpatrick, PhD, MBA, RN, FAAN, FNAP
Elizabeth Brooks Ford Professor of Nursing
Frances Payne Bolton School of Nursing
Case Western Reserve University
Cleveland, Ohio

PREFACE

This leadership and management textbook is part of a series of concise, interactive, and engaging textbooks geared toward nurses enrolled in RN-to-BSN or RN-to-MSN completion programs. Leadership and management skills are necessary at all levels and roles of nursing practice. The American Association of Colleges of Nursing's *Essentials of Baccalaureate Education for Professional Nursing Practice* states that baccalaureate-prepared nurses need beginning leadership and management skills to effectively practice professional nursing. The content in this book directly relates to the associate degree nurse's practice and assists the nurse in developing a higher level of self-awareness and skill to be able to function effectively in a leadership and management role. There are currently no books specifically designed for RN-to-BSN or RN-to-MSN students on this topic. Many of the current leadership textbooks are designed primarily for BSN students who are not yet licensed and have not worked as practicing nurses. As a result, many of the books have a focus on preparing them for the National Council Licensure Examination (NCLEX-RN® exam) which is not necessary or relevant for students in the RN-to-BSN and RN-to-MSN programs.

Each chapter of the book contains essential information that acknowledges the prior learning experience of the practicing nurse who is now an RN-to-BSN or RN-to-MSN student. It provides information needed for the associate's degree nurse to advance to the professionally prepared baccalaureate degree nurse. Each chapter begins with a brief overview of specific leadership and management topics. Case scenarios are woven throughout the chapters to help readers apply the information to practical situations. It provides concise and application-based examples that help promote self-growth as a professional. Self-assessment tools are included in most chapters for the reader to see where they are now on the topic and to what point they need to advance to obtain competence and confidence in the professional nursing role. The book provides application opportunities geared to one's own practice. Questions are posed throughout each chapter in an effort to promote discernment and reflection. Each chapter is built on the framework of the American Association of Colleges of Nursing's *Essentials of Baccalaureate Education for Professional Nursing Practice,* the National Academy of Medicine (formerly called the Institute of Medicine) competencies, and the Quality and

Safety Education for Nurses (QSEN) knowledge, skills, and attitudes (KSAs). Each chapter ends with critical thinking activities that are intended to promote reflection and application of the material presented in the chapter.

This textbook contains five parts. Part I provides introductory information such as leadership attributes, leadership and management roles in professional nursing, and foundational aspects of leadership. Part II discusses leadership skills that are essential to the practice of nursing. Those skills include handling stress, setting priorities, managing time, communication, accountability, delegation, teams, problem-solving, decision-making, and conflict resolution. Given the need for nurses to lead us to a preferred healthcare future, Part III focuses on leading change. Readers are introduced to the factors that influence organizational culture, innovation, change, power, politics, and managing quality and safety. Part IV concentrates on the business aspect of healthcare by reviewing how to manage human and fiscal resources. Finally, Part V of the book helps the reader to contemplate his or her evolution as a professional by discussing how to integrate leadership and management competencies into his or her nursing practice. Although one book cannot cover all aspects of leadership and management, our goal is to provide a core framework and useful skills and strategies to successfully lead nursing and healthcare forward.

ACKNOWLEDGMENTS

I would like to acknowledge Dr. Joyce Fitzpatrick, who provided my name to Springer Publishing for this opportunity: Dr. Fitzpatrick is an inspirational nursing leader and legend. I have had the good fortune to get to know her during my doctoral studies at Case Western Reserve University and have appreciated her support and mentorship ever since. I am honored and grateful that she wrote the Foreword to this book.

I would also like to acknowledge the support I had throughout the process from Dr. Meredith Wallace Kazer and my colleagues at Fairfield University. Their kind words, guidance, and encouragement were an enormous help to me as I worked on this project.

I thank my talented colleagues who contributed to the chapters: This project would not have been possible without their willingness to share their leadership and management expertise.

I am grateful to Elizabeth Nieginski, executive editor at Springer Publishing Company, and Rachel X. Landes, assistant editor for nursing, for their support, guidance, and encouragement throughout the publication process.

And last, but by no means the least, I would like to acknowledge Janet Weber, the supervising editor for her constructive critiques and skillful edits. I cannot thank her enough for all her time and effort. She was supportive and encouraging, a true joy to work with. She is a wonderful example of what mentorship is all about.

I

INTRODUCTION

1

TRANSITION TO THE PROFESSIONAL NURSE ROLE

AUDREY MARIE BEAUVAIS

LEARNING OBJECTIVES

After completion of this chapter, the reader will be able to

- Discuss the benefit of studying leadership.
- Identify the strengths of the associate's degree nurse.
- Identify the leadership expectations of the professional nurse in leading others.
- Assess his or her own current leadership abilities and roles.

Leaders have influence and inspire desired outcomes. As a nurse in direct patient care, you are a leader! You may not see yourself as one, but hopefully by the end of this book you will see the valuable role you play. You have significant influence within the interdisciplinary team, over patient safety issues, over care decisions, and on patient satisfaction (Duffy & Smith, 2013). Your leadership will help influence desired patient outcomes as well as organizational outcomes.

In this chapter, we discuss why it is important for nurses to learn about leadership. We review the strengths of the associate's degree nurse and how you can build upon that as you evolve in your professional development. Finally, we discuss leadership expectations and differentiate leadership skills from management skills.

In the case scenario (Box 1.1), Mary is an example of a nurse leader who is influencing change, guiding practice development, and assuming accountability for improving standards of care while containing costs (Taylor & Martindale, 2013). Mary is trying to enhance the quality of care while keeping her patient, Mrs. Smith, at the center of care. She is trying to work strategically and with a vision for better practice across the healthcare team. In addition, Mary has established her credibility by continuing her education

BOX 1.1 CASE SCENARIO

As you read the following case scenario, ask yourself:

- Can staff nurses (like Mary in this case scenario) be considered leaders? Do you need to be in an appointed position of power and authority (i.e., nurse manager or nurse administrator) to be considered a leader?
- If you consider Mary to be a leader, what evidence supports your decision?

Mary has an associate's degree and recently returned to school to obtain a baccalaureate degree in nursing. She is a staff nurse who has worked for the past 7 years on the medical–surgical unit of a 350-bed community hospital. Mary was recently awarded the American Nurses Credentialing Center (ANCC) Medical-Surgical Nursing board certification. The past few days, Mary took care of Mrs. Smith who was admitted with pneumonia. When Mary was tending to another patient, Mrs. Smith fell while going to the bathroom and broke her hip. Mary was devastated to learn that her patient experienced harm while on her watch. Mary wondered if she had been there earlier to offer toileting perhaps this would not have happened. Mary decided to complete a literature search on preventing patient falls. She learned that the evidence suggests hourly rounds may help reduce the incidents of falls in her unit. Mary talked with her peers who said they are also concerned about the recent rise in the number of falls and think that it might be a great initiative to start on the floor. Mary decided to approach her manager with this idea.

and obtaining her certification in her specialty. She has found evidence in the literature to support her action plan. As registered nurses like Mary, we need to display appropriate leadership and communication skills because we work within interprofessional teams in various healthcare settings. We need to inspire others to achieve desired outcomes for our patients, families, and communities.

QUESTIONS TO CONSIDER BEFORE READING ON

Identify an effective leader in your organization. What is it about this person that makes an impression on you? What makes him or her successful in leading others? What appointed position or role does the person hold? Do you consider yourself to be a leader in your professional role at work? Explain.

When envisioning a leader, you might think of a visionary chief nursing officer at your organization. The chief nursing officer is a leader as he or she holds an appointed position of power and influence. However, leadership is not just about the position someone holds. Leadership is a process and relationship among individuals. Frontline nurses providing and coordinating direct patient care are also valuable leaders. Nurses lead in the many different roles they perform. Nurses lead as they integrate the plan of care in collaboration with patients and their families. In the acute care setting, nurses lead by functioning as charge nurses who coordinate the unit activities during a shift. During any given shift, nurses lead by managing patient flow, assigning human resources (nurses and nursing assistants) to match patient needs, and providing effective hand-off communication with the next leader (Feldman, 2012, p. 224).

WHY STUDY LEADERSHIP?

Nurses study leadership to prepare themselves for the essential expectations of the professional nurse. Leadership competencies are viewed as a fundamental human activity and a critical component of nursing (Glazer & Fitzpatrick, 2013). Nursing roles have expanded making leadership skills more important than ever. Leadership skills are needed because nurses work in intraprofessional teams to solve urgent issues at the individual (micro) level, and also at the greater systems (macro) level (Morton & Hyrkas, 2012).

Many nurses enter the profession given their desire to make a positive difference in the world. Leadership competencies help nurses make that difference because leadership skills are needed to facilitate and implement beneficial change. Nurses make a positive difference with patients because they lead the interdisciplinary team to help improve patient outcomes. Nursing leadership skills and abilities have been linked to many improved outcomes such as quality patient care, healthy workplaces, job satisfaction, and driving cultural change (Mannix, Wilkes, & Daly, 2013). Leadership skills enable nurses to become trailblazers among their colleagues because they help to lead change and inspire others within the organization.

WHAT ARE THE BENEFITS OF BEING A LEADER?

There are many benefits of being a leader. Some of the benefits impact the nurse personally. For example, nurse leaders working in direct patient care have reported improved job and personal satisfaction as well as increased opportunity for career advancement (Grindel, 2016). Nurse leaders who mentor others report the personal benefit of feeling a sense of pride and accomplishment. Other benefits of nurse leaders are related to patients and the organization. For example, nurse leaders benefit patients by improving patient care, safety, outcomes, and satisfaction (Grindel, 2016). In addition, effective nursing leaders benefit the organization by enhancing work processes, decreasing errors, and reducing waste, all of which help to support a healthy work environment (Downey, Parslow, & Smart, 2011; George et al., 2002).

WHAT IS LEADERSHIP?

There is no one universally accepted definition of "leadership." In fact, leadership may mean different things in different situations. Although definitions may differ, the overall sentiments are frequently similar. Leadership can be defined as the process by which one influences others to follow one's direction or to accomplish a goal (Huber, 2014; Mannix, Wilkes, & Daly, 2013). Leaders typically demonstrate integrity and have developed core values and a vision that inspires people.

Inherent in the definition of leadership is the notion that a leader has followers. Those followers are inspired to accomplish a goal. In the healthcare setting, those goals often revolve around improving care and achieving positive patient outcomes (Taylor & Martindale, 2013). Leaders help their followers feel empowered to solve problems and to be innovative and creative. Leaders provide the direction and use their management abilities to assist people in the proper path.

Leadership is not about authority or power, nor is it about the individual's position or title. Rather, leadership is derived from social influence. Leadership requires the assistance of other people who help you reach goals. Leadership is a learned skill achieved through developing a high level of self-awareness. Leaders can expand their knowledge and skills through education and practice.

STRENGTHS OF THE ASSOCIATE'S DEGREE NURSE

As an associate's degree nurse (ADN), you have been prepared with the knowledge and skills to be a nurse. You have been groomed to be a capable, caring, and dedicated healthcare professional who plays an important role in the care of patients in various communities (Mahaffey, 2002). Some would even argue that you may be more clinically prepared than new BSN graduates (Lauren1021, 2006). You have had the opportunity to have first-rate clinical experiences in many settings—acute as well as community based. You have undoubtedly worked with experienced faculty with a strong clinical focus. Your ADN education provides you a solid foundation to develop your leadership skills with your continued education.

BUILDING ON THE ASSOCIATE'S DEGREE FOUNDATION IN THE PROFESSIONAL NURSE ROLE EVOLUTION

The professional nurse role has evolved over the past decade with attention given to the differences among registered nurses educated at the associate's degree level from those who are educated at the baccalaureate level.

The American Association of Colleges of Nursing (AACN) states that the educational preparation of baccalaureate nurses should include leadership, an essential aspect of the role of the registered nurse (AACN, 2014). Nurses educated at the ADN level may not have had formal education on the concept of leadership. However, there is no doubt ADNs have experience with the concept in everyday practice. Nurses are called to be leaders because part of their daily work, while delivering patient care and when working with colleagues to address concerns, influences the practice of nursing. Studying leadership will help you to be well prepared to meet the demands of nursing today. It will provide you with the knowledge and skills to be a leader at the bedside across a variety of settings. Although you might not be entertaining the idea now, it will also assist you should you be interested in a formal leadership position in the future. For example, our nation's Magnet® hospitals are requiring all nurse managers/leaders to have a baccalaureate or graduate degree in nursing (ANCC, 2014).

LEADERSHIP EXPECTATIONS OF THE PROFESSIONAL NURSE

The AACN has established *The Essentials of Baccalaureate Education for Professional Nursing Practice* (2008). This document outlines what is expected of a BSN graduate and takes into account the recommendations of National Academy of Medicine (formerly the Institute of Medicine) regarding the core knowledge necessary for healthcare professionals. The AACN *Essentials of Baccalaureate Education for Professional Nursing Practice* clearly notes that leadership is an essential expectation of the professional nurse. In particular, the document notes professional nurses should acquire leadership skills that involve making ethical decisions, establishing and maintaining collegial relationships, using civil collaboration and communication in interprofessional teams, coordinating care, delegating, and demonstrating effective conflict-resolution techniques. Professional nurses need to understand complex systems as well as the influence of power, policy, politics, and regulatory standards on these systems.

According to AACN (2008), some of the leadership expectations of the professional nurse are as follows:

- Apply leadership concepts, skills, and decision-making in provision of high-quality nursing care, healthcare team coordination, and the oversight and accountability for care delivery in a variety of settings.
- Demonstrate leadership and communication skills to effectively implement patient safety and quality improvement initiatives within the context of the interprofessional team.
- Demonstrate an awareness of complex organizational systems.

- Demonstrate a basic understanding of organizational structure, mission, vision, philosophy, and values.
- Participate in quality and patient safety initiatives, recognizing that these are complex system issues, which involve individuals, families, groups, communities, populations, and other members of the healthcare team. (p.14)

The competencies, skills, and decision-making that are discussed throughout this book will help you to develop the capacity to be an effective leader. The process requires self-assessment, reflection, and much time and effort. To get started, refer to Box 1.2 to assess your

BOX 1.2 SELF-ASSESSMENT

Self-assessment: Are you a leader?

This is not a scientific self-assessment but rather is intended to foster reflection. Please answer "yes" or "no" to the following questions:

- Do colleagues ask you for your clinical opinion/expertise regarding patient care?
- Do colleagues ask your opinion regarding ethical issues in your practice area?
- Do people ask you to help resolve conflicts?
- Do people confide in you?
- Do people turn to you for guidance in unclear situations?
- Do people find what you have to say as important even though they might disagree?
- Do people consider you a role model?
- Do you solve problems in your work environment?
- Do you develop solutions to workplace issues?
- Do you have a vision for how things should be done?
- Do you bring out the best in people?
- Do you encourage the growth and development of your colleagues?
- Are you currently driven by a set of career goals?
- When you recognize a negative issue in your healthcare setting, are you comfortable with developing an argument for change?
- Are you persuasive?
- Are you approachable?
- Is your communication style clear and direct?

If you answered "yes" to most of these questions, you are most likely already a leader in your area. Do not worry if you did not answer "yes" to many of these questions. Sometimes it is easier to learn evidence-based skills the first time rather than having to relearn skills that might not be backed by any evidence. Remember, leadership is a learned skill you can hone through education and practice. This book provides you with information to develop your leadership competencies, skills, and decision-making.

leadership. Although completing a self-assessment is a good start to becoming an effective leader, you should also engage in reflective practice to increase your self-awareness coupled with education, training, and experience.

QUALITY AND SAFETY EDUCATION for NURSES (QSEN) CONSIDERATIONS

As you read the following QSEN competencies (Box 1.3) related to leadership, ask yourself:

- Which of these competencies do I meet and which competencies do I need to develop more fully?
- What plan of action can I take to enhance those competencies in which I am weak and to develop those which I lack at this time?

BOX 1.3 LEADERSHIP: SELECT RELEVANT QSEN COMPETENCIES

- Describe own strengths, limitations, and values in functioning as a member of a team
- Initiate plan for self-development as a team member
- Act with integrity, consistency and respect for differing views
- Appreciate importance of intra- and inter-professional collaboration
- Recognize contributions of other individuals and groups in helping patient/family achieve health goals
- Assume role of team member or leader based on the situation
- Value the perspectives and expertise of all health team members
- Respect the unique attributes that members bring to a team, including variations in professional orientations and accountabilities
- Describe impact of own communication style on others
- Discuss effective strategies for communicating and resolving conflict
- Demonstrate a commitment to team goals
- Solicit input from other team members to improve individual, as well as team, performance
- Value teamwork and the relationship upon which it is based
- Participate in designing systems that support effective teamwork

Source: Quality and Safety Education for Nurses Institute. (2014). QSEN competencies. Retrieved from http://qsen.org/competencies/pre-licensure-ksas

HOW DO LEADERSHIP SKILLS DIFFER FROM MANAGEMENT SKILLS?

In this book, we not only address leadership skills but also consider management skills. As we have discussed, leadership skills involve the development of a vision, setting goals effectively, and motivating others to reach those goals. Leadership requires the ability to influence to achieve desired outcomes. Management skills, on the contrary, involve overseeing operations and processes. Management skills involve how you handle the day-to-day operations of the unit and help people to work together efficiently and harmoniously. It helps to understand those with whom you work and what motivates them so you can identify the right approach. Chapter 3 will further help you distinguish between leadership and management behaviors.

CONCLUSIONS

Leaders are needed at the bedside to help inspire others to achieve patient outcomes. Leadership is not just about the position you hold but about self-awareness, knowledge of processes, and relationships with others. In addition to improving patient care, your leadership abilities can potentially benefit you with personal as well as professional satisfaction. Learning about leadership will build upon the knowledge you have from your ADN education and prepare you for the essential expectations of the baccalaureate-prepared professional nurse. Throughout this book, we focus on leadership and management competencies, skills, and decision-making necessary for the professional nurse. This information coupled with self-reflection and practice/experience will help you become the effective leader that healthcare needs you to be.

CRITICAL THINKING QUESTIONS AND ACTIVITIES

- Develop your own definition of leadership in one or two sentences.
- Interview two nurses who you feel are leaders. Ask them for their definition of leadership. How does their definition compare to what you learned in this chapter and compare to your personal definition of leadership? What are the qualities that led you to see them as leaders? How do these leaders influence your leadership style at this time?
- Do you feel it is important for nurses to support and value leadership at all levels of an organization? Explain.

REFERENCES

American Association of Colleges of Nursing. (2008). *Essentials of baccalaureate education for professional nursing practice.* Washington, DC: Author.

American Association of Colleges of Nursing. (2014). *Fact sheet: The impact of education on nursing practice.* Washington, DC: Author.

American Nurses Credentialing Center. (2014). *2014 Magnet application manual.* Silver Spring, MD: Author.

Downey, M., Parslow, S., & Smart, M. (2011). The hidden treasure in nursing leadership: Informal leaders. *Journal of Nursing Management, 19*(4), 517–521. doi:10.1111/j.1365-2834.2011.01253.x

Duffy, N., & Smith, S. B. (2013). Leading at the bedside and beyond. *American Nurse Today, 8*(12). Retrieved from https://www.americannursetoday.com/leading-at-the-bedside-and-beyond

Feldman, H. R. (Ed.). (2012). *Nursing leadership: A concise encyclopedia* (2nd ed.). New York, NY: Springer Publishing.

George, V., Burke, L., Rodgers, B., Duthie, N., Hoffmann, M. L., Koceja, V., ... Gehring, L. L. (2002). Developing staff nurse shared leadership behavior in professional nursing practice. *Nursing Administration Quarterly, 26*(3), 44–59. doi:10.1097/00006216-200204000-00008

Glazer, G., & Fitzpatrick, J. J. (Eds.). (2013). *Nursing leadership from the outside in.* New York, NY: Springer Publishing.

Grindel, C. G. (2016). Clinical leadership: A call to action. *Medsurg Nursing, 25*(1), 9–16. Retrived from https://www.amsn.org/sites/default/files/documents/practice-resources/clinical-leadership-development-program/CeceGrindelArticleMSNJ.pdf

Huber, D. L. (2014). *Leadership and nursing care management.* Maryland Heights, MO: Elsevier Saunders.

Lauren1021. (2006, December 23). ADN v. BSN education (Blog). Retrieved from http://nursingleadershipandeducation.blogspot.com

Mahaffey, E. H. (2002). The relevance of associate degree nursing education: Past, present, future. *Online Journal of Issues in Nursing, 7*(2). Retrieved from http://ojin.nursingworld.org/MainMenuCategories/ANAMarketplace/ANAPeriodicals/OJIN/TableofContents/Volume72002/No2May2002/RelevanceofAssociateDegree.html

Mannix, J., Wilkes, L., & Daly, J. (2013). Attributes of clinical leadership in contemporary nursing: An integrated review. *Contemporary Nurse, 45*(1), 10–21. doi:10.5172/conu.2013.45.1.10

Morton, J. L., & Hyrkas, K. (2012). Management and leadership at the bedside. *Journal of Nursing Management, 20*(5), 579–581. doi:10.1111/j.1365-2834.2012.01476.x

Quality and Safety Education for Nurses Institute. (2014). QSEN competencies. Retrieved from http://qsen.org/competencies/pre-licensure-ksas

Taylor, R., & Martindale, S. (2013). Clinical leadership in primary care. *Primary Health Care, 23*(5), 32–38. doi:10.7748/phc2013.06.23.5.32.e795

2

LEADERSHIP ATTRIBUTES

AUDREY MARIE BEAUVAIS

LEARNING OBJECTIVES

After completion of this chapter, the reader will be able to

- Describe personal attributes of effective leaders.
- Discuss a variety of leadership styles.
- Explain the significance of self-awareness in leading others.
- Describe a variety of methods to increase one's level of self-awareness.
- Explain how to overcome barriers that obstruct one's level of self-awareness.
- Discuss the concept and benefits of emotional intelligence.
- Apply the concept of emotional intelligence to a leadership case scenario.

As you develop further into your leadership roles, you will need to develop certain personal attributes and skills to enhance your success. In this chapter, we review personal attributes of effective leaders and discuss ways to promote your level of self-awareness. The topic of emotional intelligence (EI) is explored as an ability that can enhance your leadership effectiveness.

PERSONAL ATTRIBUTES OF EFFECTIVE LEADERS

Leadership attributes are the personal qualities and characteristics that describe how an individual conducts himself or herself. These qualities and characteristics include the person's character, motives, behaviors, and skills. Personal attributes not only describe the leader's personal character but also help establish direction and mobilize the commitment of others.

Think of a leader you admire. What personal attributes come to mind? Now think about your own personal attributes. How would your friends and coworkers describe you? A sample of personal attributes of effective leaders is given in Table 2.1. Highlight each word that you think applies to you.

As an associate's degree nurse, you already possess many personal attributes that will promote your success as a leader. However, there may be other attributes that you can further cultivate. As you can see from the list in Table 2.1, there are numerous leadership attributes—and those are only a sample of them! However, there are some essential qualities we should highlight for you. An essential personal attribute for an effective nurse leader includes a strong ethical core in which human dignity and caring are at the center of decisions and actions. Effective leaders act with integrity and honesty to keep and carry through with their promises. At certain times in your role as a leader, you will need to enlist the help of your coworkers. To encourage coworkers' assistance, you should be likable and authentic, which in turn will help you develop genuine relationships. Leaders often have to address problems calmly, giving people the benefit of doubt and being careful not to humiliate others. Such attributes highlight the essential characteristics that will promote your success as a leader.

Another leadership attribute gaining attention in the literature is "grit." Angela Duckworth, an associate professor of psychology at the University of Pennsylvania, has spent time examining this concept. Duckworth has

TABLE 2.1 SAMPLE PERSONAL ATTRIBUTES OF EFFECTIVE LEADERS

accountable	decisive	optimistic
authentic	dedicated	passionate
calm	energetic	patient
candid	engaging	politically sensitive
caring	enthusiastic	positive
clinical expert	ethical	proactive
collaborative	fair	reliable
committed	good communicator	respected
compassionate	honest	self-aware
competent	inspirational	self-directed
confident	integrity	self-reliant
consistent	moral	transparent
courageous	nondefensive	trustworthy
creative	nonreactive	understanding
critical thinker	open-minded	visionary

BOX 2.1 EXERCISE

Access Duckworth's website www.angeladuckworth.com and listen to the TEDtalk on grit in which she discusses the power of passion and perseverance. In addition, access the Grit Scale, a 10-question quiz, which will help you assess how "gritty" you are.

defined "grit" as perseverance and passion for long-term goals. She believes that to be successful it is not just about your talent and intelligence but about your tenacity. Grit encompasses several characteristics such as courage (ability to manage your fear of failure), achievement orientation (work tirelessly to complete a task), endurance, resilience, optimism, confidence, creativity, and a desire for excellence (Perlis, 2013). Box 2.1 provides you with additional resources and an exercise on grit.

Most likely you possess some of the qualities noted in the self-assessment of great leaders listed in Box 2.2. Perhaps you developed those qualities or maybe you were born with them. However, there may be other qualities that you are lacking. The good news is that you can set out to gain those skills you do not currently possess. As a leader, you need to look to improve yourself. Tracy (2014) mentions four steps to improve your leadership attributes:

1. Do more: Spend more time on the activities that are of greater value to you and on the activities that are important in achieving your leadership goals.
2. Do less: Likewise, decrease the amount of time you spend on the activities that will not help you achieve your leadership goals or will hinder your accomplishments as a leader.
3. Do things you should be doing: Identify the skills, knowledge, and competencies that are needed to be a successful leader. Once those qualities are identified, learn and/or acquire them.
4. Stop doing other things: Reflect on all your activities with the perspective of what you want to achieve as a leader. Perhaps what you are spending your time on is no longer pertinent to your leadership goals. You may realize that the activities that were once valuable are no longer valuable and are taking up precious time.

QUESTIONS TO ASK BEFORE READING ON

How do you typically conduct yourself?
If you are given a task, how do you go about getting it done?
If a crisis comes up, how do you handle it?
When you need help from others, how do you go about garnering support and mobilizing people to help you?

BOX 2.2 SELF-ASSESSMENT

The following qualities have been identified by Bornstein and Bornstein (2016) as contributing to making "great leaders." How many of these qualities of "great leaders" do you possess?

- Focus: Are you distracted by minor issues or are you able to focus on major concerns?
- Confidence: Do you instill confidence in others? Do you have a clear vision? Do you show empathy? Do you like to coach others?
- Transparency: Are you authentic? Do you engender the trust of others?
- Integrity: Do you need to be right or do you do what is right? Are your words and actions consistent?
- Inspiration: Are you driven? Are you powered by your values and beliefs? Do you have an internal drive? Are you able to motivate others?
- Passion: Do you love your job? Are you obsessed with your career? Are you never satisfied and strive for something better? Do you lead by example?
- Innovation: Are you creative? Do you like to solve challenging issues? Do you like to think outside the box to address issues and concerns?
- Patience: Are you able to stay the course when you have a vision or a cause? Do you know when to abandon the cause?
- Stoicism: Are you able to anticipate the worst-case scenario? In difficult situations, are you able to regulate your emotional reaction?
- Authenticity: Have you learned from other great leaders but retained your own character and voice?
- Open-mindedness: Do you keep an open mind? Are you flexible and able to adjust if necessary?
- Decisiveness: Are you wishy-washy when making decisions? Do you second guess your decisions? Or do you make decisions with conviction and do not look back?
- Personableness: Are you able to make genuine connections with people? Do you look for ways to help others (as opposed to look for ways they can help you)?
- Empowerment: Do you appropriately delegate responsibility? Or do you feel it is easier to do it yourself?
- Positivity: Are you able to create optimism? Are you able to make the impossible seem possible?
- Generosity: Are you able to build up others? Do you help others to grow as individuals?
- Persistence: Do you feel that great accomplishments can take time? Do you have the tenacity needed to accomplish your goals?
- Insightfulness: Do you have the wisdom to know what is important and what is not?
- Communication: Are you a good communicator? Are you able to express your expectations? Do you treat your job as a collaboration?
- Accountability: Do you take responsibility for your behavior? When you make a mistake, do you take steps to make it right?
- Restlessness: Do you think that you and your team have all the answers? Are you willing to look outside your group to find information and answers?

LEADERSHIP STYLE PREFERENCE

In your role as an associate's degree nurse, you have developed a leadership style but perhaps have not given it much thought. As you develop in your BSN role, it is helpful to contemplate your leadership style and decide how you would like to develop it further. There are different leadership styles based on different assumptions and leadership theories. The first major study about leadership was conducted by Lewin, Lippit, and White (1939), which outlined several major leadership styles. Table 2.2 highlights several leadership styles.

Additional leadership theories such as transformational leadership, servant leadership, situational leadership, and authentic leadership are presented in Chapter 3.

Your leadership style will be based on your values, beliefs, and preferences as well as your organization's culture and norms. Your leadership attributes are combined to create your overall leadership style. Understanding your baseline leadership style preference will help you to further develop your leadership awareness and skills. Box 2.3 will help you assess your leadership style.

Chances are that as an associate's degree nurse, you have been using a number of different styles at different times. Your style may involve expecting excellence and often exemplifying it yourself. If someone in your team is not performing well, perhaps you demand more of them and maybe even step in to help them. At other times, maybe you are all about keeping the peace. At those times, harmony and working in a collaborative manner that focuses on emotional needs over work issues might take precedence. Emergency medical conditions with your patient might require you to take quick decisive action. However, if you are working on a policy change, you might choose to gather key stakeholders to get their input and foster their commitment while making a group decision about policy revision. No matter what your leadership style is, you should make sure it is aligned with the mission, vision, and philosophy of your organization. Think about what kind of a leader you want to be. Also, consider how your leadership style can assist you in becoming a successful leader. Refer to Box 2.4 for a critical thinking exercise that will help you apply leadership styles to practice.

SELF-AWARENESS

Self-awareness is an important leadership attribute and crucial to effective leadership. Self-awareness requires an honest self-appraisal of your motives, mental state, emotions, attitudes, personality, abilities, beliefs, and values (McKenna, 2017; Showry & Manasa, 2014).

If you answered the previous questions with a concrete response such as "I am a nurse and a mother," then we ask you to reflect a little deeper.

TABLE 2.2 LEADERSHIP STYLES

Leadership Style	Definition	Decision Maker	Disadvantages	Example of When It Is Used
Authoritarian	The leader tells staff what to do and does not solicit their input	Leader	Doesn't allow for others' opinions Can result in strikes and disputes, can produce frustration Impedes development of employees May lead by fear and force Leader takes responsibility for decisions	Used to facilitate quick decisions, prompt action, and unity of direction Used with a new employee who is learning the role Used in an emergency situation when time is of the essence
Paternalistic or maternalistic	Like the authoritarian leader, this leadership style involves a dominant authority figure; however, the paternalistic/maternalistic leader treats staff like members of a family; the leader expects the staff to be loyal and obedient	Leader	Leader functions like a father/mother Leader guides and protects staff (like family members) When staff are treated like children, then they act like children Staff may not think for themselves Staff wait to be told what to do Staff don't want to be held accountable	Used commonly in small family-run businesses
Democratic	The power is vested in the staff and executed by their leader. The leader leads by persuasion. The leader and staff share responsibility.	Group	Collaboration can take time especially if people aren't in agreement Difficult to make fast decisions Can be dangerous to depend on consensus of people who may be misinformed or lack accurate information	Used to solve safety issues

Participative	Leader includes staff in the decision-making process but often makes the final decision	Leader with group input	Must set priorities and delegate certain tasks Can blame others when things go wrong Can backfire if people feel their input is ignored	Used with employees who know their role Used if the leader is aware there is a problem but doesn't have all the information Used when creating new policies and procedures
Laissez-faire	Allows staff to make decisions but the leader is responsible for the decisions that are made	Group	Leader avoids power and responsibility Responsibility passed to subordinates Leader takes minimum initiative with administration Leader gives no direction Group establishes own goals Group works out own problems Organization is likely to struggle	Used when employees are experienced, skilled, and self-starters

BOX 2.3 LEADERSHIP STYLE SELF-ASSESSMENT

To help you to understand your leadership style, consider taking the following online leadership style surveys: www.nwlink.com/~donclark/leader/survstyl.html and www.yourleadershiplegacy.com/assessment/assessment.php

BOX 2.4 CRITICAL THINKING EXERCISE

Let us put some of these styles into practice by reviewing some scenarios in which different leadership styles (such as authoritarian, paternalistic, democratic, participative, and laissez-faire) are used. Describe the style being used. Would you use the same style or would you handle it differently? Although there is no right or wrong ways to handle each situation, there may be more effective ways to get the results you want. As you work through each scenario, try to cultivate your ability to act like a leader in each scenario.

1. The nursing manager at a long-term care facility wants to order new bed alarms for her unit. She has different vendors come in to show the staff their products. Although the team discusses the pros and cons of each product, the nurse manager will make the final decision.
2. The nurse manager at the rehabilitation facility is told she needs to reduce the fall rate. She immediately starts telling the staff what changes will be implemented. When staff offer their thoughts, she tells them she will be making the decision and does not need their input.
3. The outpatient clinic has no nursing supervisor. The staff are expected to function on their own to find staffing and to provide safe patient care.
4. The charge nurse has to clear all decisions regarding staffing and patient assignments with her nurse manager before taking action.
5. The physician's office in which you work performs similar functions each day. The office manager needs to get information to the staff. She chooses to send an email to convey this information rather than calling a meeting or talking to people face-to-face.

QUESTIONS TO ASK BEFORE READING ON

Who are you?
What kind of impression do you make?
What do you want to achieve?
What do you believe in?

However, if you answered the previous questions with well-articulated values such as "I am caring, honest, and competent," then you are more apt to respond to challenges with integrity and consistency (Flanagan, 2013). Cultivating self-awareness will help to free you of dysfunctional habits and self-defeating behaviors, which in turn can lead to personal transformation (Flanagan, 2013). Knowing your strengths and weaknesses, looking for feedback from others, and obtaining insight from mistakes can allow you to expand your self-awareness and thus improve your leadership skills (Glazer & Fitzpatrick, 2013, p. 249).

An effective leader is willing to obtain self-awareness from a number of sources. Two such sources are introspection and social comparison (Showry & Manasa, 2014). "Introspection" is an internal process of examining who you are (your thoughts, feelings, character, traits, etc.). Effective leaders can also see how other people view them ("social comparison") and understand the impact of their actions (Showry & Manasa, 2014). If you can be honest about your strengths and weaknesses, then you will have an opportunity to change your weaknesses into strengths by developing yourself (Showry & Manasa, 2014). Self-awareness can help change how you think and what you think, and thus provide the opportunity to transform your behavior (Flanagan, 2013).

Showry and Manasa (2014) note the following obstacles to gaining self-awareness:

- Incompetence: You need to be competent to engage in self-assessment. If you are not competent to assess yourself free from biases and prejudices, then you will not obtain an accurate self-reflection.
- Motives: There may be conflict between your need to be accurate in your self-perception and your desire to feel good about yourself. Hence, if your motive is to feel good about yourself, then it can prevent you from getting objective feedback.
- Self-presentation: Self-presentation is your ability to persuade public perceptions. You are what you are able to lead others to believe you are. However, deliberately creating a false impression is destructive and will create a fake identity, which will lead to a high degree of distortion.
- Core self-evaluation: Core self-evaluation is the bottom line assessment you make about your self-worth. It is made up of self-esteem, self-efficacy, and self-confidence. Having low self-esteem, self-efficacy, and self-confidence can hinder your ability to see what others see in you, which can lead to a distorted self-assessment.
- High self-monitors: High self-monitors refer to those individuals who present an impressive representation of themselves versus low self-monitors who tend to present their true selves. High self-monitors also have the ability to present different impressions depending on what the situation requires. This can present a problem when they change their core values to suit a specific situation.

BOX 2.5 SELF-REFLECTION EXERCISE

Consider keeping a daily journal to reflect on the events of your day. Which events went well? What could you have done to make the day go better? What sources of feedback did you use to help make judgments about the day?

- Self-deception: Self-deception may protect you from the truth that could potentially cause pain and anxiety. Self-deception happens when you lack openness and objective self-evaluation.
- Defense mechanisms: Defense mechanisms like denial, displacement, and isolation can promote feedback-avoiding behavior. This can influence the way you gather information and derive conclusions about yourself.
- Distorted feedback: People's misconceptions about you can affect your self-awareness. The more power you have, the less candid feedback you tend to receive because of people's fear of the repercussions. As a result, it is vital to assess the feedback for its honesty and disregard the feedback if it is detrimental to you.
- Narcissism: Narcissism refers to people who are obsessively interested in themselves and tend to be emotional authoritarian decision makers. Their self-absorption is done at the expense of others via displays of egotism, dominance, and aggression. They tend to have a distorted self-concept, which makes them blind to their weaknesses.

Being aware of these obstacles will help you avoid the pitfalls to self-awareness. Leaders who succeed are aware of who they are and what they want to achieve. Rather than not acknowledging their weaknesses, successful leaders embrace this information and make needed changes. How might you foster your self-awareness? For starters, you need to be open to feedback. Participate in self-reflection activities that can help you analyze, understand, and gain meaning from the feedback you are given. See Box 2.5 for a self-reflection exercise.

EMOTIONAL INTELLIGENCE

Emotional intelligence (EI) has been identified as an important leadership attribute for nurses (Doe, Ndinguri, & Phipps, 2015; Sadri, 2012). But what exactly is EI? EI is often defined by either an ability-based model or by an expansive model. For the purposes of this chapter, we focus on the ability-based model by Mayer, Salovey, and Caruso (2004) who define EI as the ability to reason with emotions to enhance thinking. In this model, EI encompasses four abilities: to accurately perceive emotions, to use emotion to facilitate thoughts, to understand emotions, and to manage emotions. This model is measured by the Mayer–Salovey–Caruso Emotional Intelligence Test (MSCEIT). Box 2.6 will help us put this into practice with questions to consider and a case scenario.

BOX 2.6 CASE SCENARIO

Keep the following questions in mind as you read the following case scenario. The first part of this case scenario focuses on the EI ability to perceive emotions.

Perceiving emotions:

- What are Nancy's feelings?
- What might the nurse manager be feeling?

A year ago, the nurse manager who was feeling stretched by her numerous responsibilities decided to delegate the task of developing the staffing schedule to a trusted certified nursing assistant who had been working with the organization for over 30 years. Although this arrangement worked well for the first 6 months, the staff are now starting to feel that the system is unfair and that the certified nursing assistant is playing favorites and not taking their requests into account. Nancy, a staff nurse and leader on the unit, has spoken with her colleagues who have also expressed concerns. Nancy worked with her peers to develop a viable alternative solution to developing the staffing schedule. The scheduling issue has become personal for Nancy because she requested a day off to go to her grandmother's surprise 85th birthday party but was denied this request. Frustrated by the situation, Nancy is anxious to present the problem and the potential solution to the nurse manager. On Friday afternoon, Nancy goes to find the nurse manger to discuss this but she is not in her office. The unit secretary shares that the nurse manger was called to an emergency budget meeting with the chief financial officer and the senior vice president/chief nursing officer. The unit secretary also shares that the nurse manager was hoping to leave early given her plans to get away for the weekend to celebrate her wedding anniversary.

How do you think Nancy was feeling? It is safe to say that Nancy is feeling frustrated perhaps even downright angry that she was not allowed to go to her grandmother's surprise 85th birthday party, especially when the nurse manager will be leaving early for her own personal reason (wedding anniversary). Nancy is also anxious to speak to the nurse manger to express her feelings and get this resolved.

How might the nurse manager be feeling? Although there are no emotions listed in the above-mentioned scenario, one can deduce that the nurse manager might have a host of feelings related to the emergency budget meeting that was called. Chances are the emergency meeting did not deliver happy news such as the institution has a surplus of money they need her to spend. Chances are that there is a crisis that needs to be managed. Hence, most likely the manager may feel anxious, upset, or even angry. In addition to this emergency budget meeting on a Friday, remember the nurse manager wanted to leave early to celebrate her anniversary. Hence, she might have additional feelings about this meeting imposing on her time when she wanted to leave and celebrate. Let us continue this case scenario and focus on the EI ability of using emotion to facilitate thought.

BOX 2.6 CASE SCENARIO *(continued)*

As you continue with this case scenario, consider the following questions that will focus on the EI ability of using emotion to facilitate thought.

Using emotion to facilitate thought:

- What is the impact of Nancy's feelings on the situation?
- What might the impact of the nurse manager's feelings be on the situation?
- How can Nancy use her feelings to help her make decisions that are healthy for her and others involved?
- Should Nancy redirect and prioritize her thinking on the basis of the associated feelings to focus on the goal at hand?

Nancy decides to wait for the nurse manager to discuss the perceived staff scheduling problem and to present her solution. Nancy has been upset about the situation and is anxious to get this off her chest. The nurse manager returns to the unit and is visibly preoccupied and troubled from her previous emergency budget meeting. Despite this, Nancy heads to the nurse manager and asks to speak with her. The nurse manager explains that she does not have much time as she needs to leave work early. Nancy insists they speak and says it will not take much of the nurse manager's time. The nurse manager does not appear pleased but agrees to hear what she has to say if she can make it quick.

The impact of Nancy feeling anxious and frustrated about the scheduling situation was that she insisted on speaking with the nurse manager that day. Nancy seems to have not noticed (or perhaps ignored) that the nurse manager was upset on returning from her emergency budget meeting. The impact of the nurse manager's feeling on this situation is that she may not be open to hear about Nancy's problem because she has other pressing issues at hand. Using the information that the nurse manger is upset could help Nancy to redirect and prioritize her thinking to achieve her goal of changing how the schedule is created.

As you continue with this case scenario, consider the following questions that will focus on the EI ability of understanding emotions and managing emotions.

Understanding emotions:

- What were the goals of the interaction for Nancy?
- What were the goals of the interaction for the nurse manager?
- Can you understand the reasons for Nancy's emotions?
- Can you understand the reasons for the nurse manager's emotions?
- What is the purpose of the emotions that each person felt?
- How have these emotions impacted the outcomes?
- Does Nancy understand why the nurse manager has reacted this way?

Managing emotions:

- How could Nancy have channeled her emotions in a positive fashion? Do you think Nancy can identify the negative emotions expressed and channel them in a positive fashion?

(continued)

BOX 2.6 CASE SCENARIO *(continued)*

- How could Nancy work through the situation in a constructive manner? How can Nancy use emotional data and cues to achieve a positive outcome?

Nancy sits down in the manager's office and begins to recount how she and her fellow colleagues feel the current system of determining the staffing schedule is "unfair." As Nancy talks, the nurse manager appears uncomfortable and is fidgeting in her chair. Nancy cannot tell if the nurse manager is upset or angry or feeling some other emotion. Nancy continues on with discussing the problem and the potential solutions. Once Nancy finishes talking, the nurse manager takes a deep breath and says, "As I shared with you, I don't have much time. I can't believe it has been a year and this is the first I am hearing about this. I can't make a decision about this right now. In fact, I have a lot going on and frankly have bigger and more immediate problems to deal with. I am going to think about this and get back to you." Nancy leaves the meeting feeling hurt, misunderstood, and defeated. The nurse manager feels blindsided and frustrated to have yet another problem to deal with. Although the nurse manager did not share with Nancy, she had just been told at her budget meeting that she has to eliminate two positions.

Nancy's goal for the interaction was to feel heard and understood. She wanted to present the problem and a potential solution to how the schedule is created. The nurse manager in this case has a very different goal. Her goal most likely is around leaving early to celebrate with her husband. These competing goals lead each individual to have unique feelings. These feelings then impact outcomes. Seeing that the manager was just delivered difficult news about the budget and wants to leave early, she is not receptive to what Nancy has to say. If Nancy was able to identify and understand the nurse manager's feelings, the outcome may have been different. If Nancy was able to perceive that the nurse manager was upset and anxious, she could have used the information to help make decisions. She could have attempted to manage her own emotions and realize that the timing was not right to have such a conversation with her manager. Perhaps she could have asked to set up a meeting for next week to discuss the problem when hopefully they would both be in a better place emotionally.

The case above provides one example of how EI might influence nursing leaders. There are many other reasons that EI is needed in nursing leadership. For example, EI is helpful in fostering mutual respect with colleagues, superiors, and subordinates (Băeşu & Bejinaru, 2015). EI can be helpful in times of stress/crisis, because those abilities will help you to acknowledge the thoughts and feelings of others and to anticipate their reaction and decide the best option (Băeșu & Bejinaru, 2015). EI can be useful as you manage projects, build effective teams, and create educational programs (Powell, Mabry, & Mixer, 2015).

EI is believed to develop with age much like your intelligence quotient (IQ). What happens if you do not have the level of EI you want? Does that mean it is a lost cause? No, the good news is that it is believed that EI skills can be enhanced with educational strategies. This is promising as many of us can benefit from enhancing these skills!

BOX 2.7 WHAT IS YOUR LEVEL OF EMOTIONAL INTELLIGENCE?

This is not a scientific self-assessment but rather is intended to foster reflection. Please answer "yes" or "no" to the following questions.

Identify emotions:

I am aware of my emotions.
I am able to accurately identify how other people are feeling.
I am able to express my emotions.
I am able to express my needs related to my emotions.
I do not read too much into people.

Use emotions:

I redirect my thinking based on how I am feeling.
I am able to use my emotions to facilitate problem-solving ability and creativity.
I am able to use my feelings to help me make healthy decisions.

Understand emotions:

I am able to determine the cause of emotions.
I am able to determine the consequences of emotions.
I can understand complex feelings.
I can understand transitions among emotions.
I often know the right thing to say.
I make good predictions about what people may feel.

Manage emotions:

I am open to feelings (pleasant and unpleasant).
I reflect on my emotions.
I can manage my own emotions.
I can manage the emotions of others.
I am able to turn unpleasant emotions into positive learning opportunities.

If you answered "yes" to the majority of these questions, then you most likely have high emotional intelligence. If you have answered "no" to some or many of these questions, you have an opportunity to hone your emotional intelligence skills.

Research supports that higher levels of EI can help improve patient outcomes, enhance nurse–patient relationships, and lead to organizational improvement (Doe et al., 2015; Powell et al., 2015). EI abilities such as managing emotions can lead to higher levels of overall well-being, reduced occurrences of burnout, and generation of improved patient outcomes (Powell et al., 2015).

Despite all the above-mentioned positives, it should be noted that the concept/measurement of EI has faced criticism. The criticism is mainly because of inconsistent theoretical and operational definitions as well as inconsistent measurements of EI. Such inconsistencies make it challenging to synthesize the literature and translate it into practice. Regardless of these issues, EI continues to be of interest as evidenced by the numerous articles found in the literature. EI continues to be a promising concept but will require further research to determine the utility of EI in nursing.

QUALITY and SAFETY EDUCATION for NURSES (QSEN) CONSIDERATIONS

As you read the following QSEN competencies related to leadership attributes, ask yourself:

- Which of these competencies do I meet and which competencies do I need to develop more fully?
- What plan of action can I take to enhance those competencies in which I am weak and to develop those which I lack at this time?

BOX 2.8 LEADERSHIP ATTRIBUTES: SELECT RELEVANT QSEN COMPETENCIES

- Demonstrate awareness of own strengths and limitations as a team member
- Act with integrity, consistency and respect for differing views
- Function competently within own scope of practice as a member of the healthcare team
- Communicate with team members, adapting own style of communicating to needs of the team and situation

Source: Quality and Safety Education for Nurses Institute. (2014). QSEN competencies. Retrieved from http://qsen.org/competencies/pre-licensure-ksas

CONCLUSIONS

In this chapter, we discussed how your personal attributes can contribute to your effectiveness as a leader. Your leadership attributes help to create your overall leadership style. You may use different leadership styles depending on the situation to achieve maximum results. Keep in mind that your leadership style needs to be congruent with the mission and vision of your organization. An essential personal attribute that is critical to effective leadership is self-awareness. We discussed sources of information to promote self-awareness as well as obstacles to gaining self-awareness. Finally, we examined the concept of EI as it relates to effective leadership.

CRITICAL THINKING QUESTIONS AND ACTIVITIES

- Personal attributes of effective leaders: Name three personal attributes of an effective leader that you possess. Name three personal attributes you would like to develop.
- Leadership style: Give an example when you (or another leader) used the leadership styles discussed in this chapter: authoritarian, paternalistic/maternalistic, democratic, participative, and laissez-faire. What style do you prefer to use? What style do you see used most often at your place of employment?
- Self-awareness exercise: What do you want people to think about you as a leader? What do you not want people to think about you? Is it more important that people like you or that you do your job well? Explain.
- EI: Think of a "put down" (critical remark) someone in nursing leadership has said to you or a coworker. How did it make you feel when you heard that remark? How do you think the leader felt after making such a comment? Why do you think your leader made that comment? What was the purpose of such a statement? What negative words/phrases affect you the most? How often do you hear them at work? If no one at work ridiculed others, what would happen? Would you or your coworkers lose anything? What are the benefits of not using critical remarks?

REFERENCES

Băeșu, C., & Bejinaru, R. (2015). Innovative leadership styles and the influence of emotional intelligence. *USV Annals of Economics and Public Administration, 15*(Special issue), 136–145. Retrieved from http://www.seap.usv.ro/annals/ojs/index.php/annals/article/viewFile/814/733

Bornstein, A., & Bornstein, J. (2016). What makes a great leader? *Entrepreneur, 3*(16), 36–44.

Doe, R., Ndinguri, E., & Phipps, S. T. (2015). Emotional intelligence: The link to success and failure of leadership. *Academy of Educational Leadership Journal, 19*(3), 105–114.

Flanagan, J. (2013, August). Self-awareness. *Training Journal*, pp. 45–49.

Glazer, G., & Fitzpatrick, J. J. (2013). *Nursing leadership from the outside in*. New York, NY: Springer Publishing.

Lewin, K., Lippit, R., & White, R. K. (1939). Patterns of aggressive behavior in experimentally created social climates. *Journal of Social Psychology, 10*, 271–301. doi:10.1080/00224545.1939.9713366

Mayer, J. D., Salovey, P., & Caruso, D. (2004). Emotional intelligence: Theory, findings and implications. *Psychological Inquiry, 15*(3), 197–215. doi:10.1207/s15327965pli1503_02

McKenna, P. J. (2017). Analyzing a leadership candidate's strengths. *Of Counsel, 36*(1), 5–8.

Perlis, M. M. (2013). 5 characteristics of grit: How many do you have? *Forbes*. Retrieved from https://www.forbes.com/sites/margaretperlis/2013/10/29/5-characteristics-of-grit-what-it-is-why-you-need-it-and-do-you-have-it/#6c2467c44f7b

Powell, K. R., Mabry, J. L., & Mixer, S. J. (2015). Emotional intelligence: A critical evaluation of the literature with implications for mental health nursing leadership. *Issue in Mental Health Nursing, 36*, 346–356. doi:10.3109/01612840.2014.994079

Quality and Safety Education for Nurses Institute. (2014). QSEN competencies. Retrieved from http://qsen.org/competencies/pre-licensure-ksas

Sadri, G. (2012). Emotional intelligence and leadership development. *Public Personnel Management, 41*(3), 535–548. doi:10.1177/009102601204100308

Showry, M., & Manasa, K. V. (2014). Self-awareness—Key to effective leadership. *IUP Journal of Soft Skills, 8*(1), 15–26.

Tracy, B. (2014). *Leadership*. New York, NY: American Management Association.

3

LEADERSHIP AND MANAGEMENT ROLES IN PROFESSIONAL NURSING

JAMES CYRUS

LEARNING OBJECTIVES

After completion of this chapter, readers will be able to

- Define and describe leadership.
- Distinguish between leadership and management behaviors.
- Discuss key leadership theories.
- Apply leadership theories to nursing practice and clinical situations.
- Identify essential components of effective followership.
- Evaluate one's own leadership potential.

The climate of healthcare is dynamic, often changing in response to varying economic situations, the availability of resources, advancements in technology, numerous regulatory requirements, and the rising costs of providing services. The impact of these factors may be seen through the restructuring or merging of healthcare institutions, reductions in workforce, elimination of employee benefits, or the overall expectation to do more with less. This can translate to workplace stress or turmoil throughout an organization, from executive offices to the clinical care areas. To address the turbulence or excel in spite of it, strong leadership is required. Nurses can adapt to new and different circumstances by practicing and developing specific leadership knowledge, skills, and attitudes (Table 3.1). Nurse leaders can influence positive change and help mold environments that are supportive, inclusive, and engaging instead of chaotic.

Leadership is a fundamental component and core competency of nursing practice. As a registered nurse, you have likely been expected to assume leadership responsibilities that require delegation or the supervision and direction of others. This may have been as a charge nurse or team leader or in everyday practice working with clients to achieve goals of care. Because these circumstances involve human interaction and an implication of authority, they can sometimes be challenging to navigate. Understanding the principles of leadership theory can strengthen your aptitude as a leader and effectively prepare you to face diverse clinical situations or interpersonal encounters.

In every practice setting and in all positions, regardless of official title or designated role, nurses must exhibit effective leadership, management, and followership skills to remain successful. The development of such skills should be viewed as a lifelong journey of personal and professional growth. Just as you have advanced your clinical knowledge and honed nursing techniques over time, through training, commitment, and experience, you can likewise cultivate proficiency in the areas of leadership, management, and followership. These competencies can build upon your nursing skills, bolster your clinical performance, and strengthen your professional judgment. This chapter describes four key leadership theories, encourages you to reflect on your personal experiences, and helps you identity concepts that resonate for you and which you can apply to your individual practice as you continue to grow in your role as a registered nurse.

Review Table 3.1 and consider how well you meet each of the Quality and Safety Education for Nurses (QSEN) competencies. In which competencies are you particularly strong? In what areas can you improve?

TABLE 3.1 DEVELOPING LEADERSHIP SKILLS: RELEVANT QSEN COMPETENCIES
• Describe own strengths, limitations, and values in functioning as a member of a team (teamwork and collaboration: knowledge) • Assume role of team member or leader based on the situation (teamwork and collaboration: skills) • Describe impact of own communication style on others (teamwork and collaboration: knowledge) • Communicate respect for team member competence in communication (teamwork and collaboration: skills) • Act with integrity, consistency, and respect for different views (teamwork and collaboration: skills) • Value the perspectives and expertise of all health team members (teamwork and collaboration: attitudes) • Respect the unique attributes that members bring to a team, including variations in professional orientations and accountabilities (teamwork and collaboration: attitudes) • Initiate actions to resolve conflict (teamwork and collaboration: skills) • Value teamwork and the relationships upon which it is based (teamwork and collaboration: attitudes) • Practice aligning the aims, measures and changes involved in improving care (quality improvement: skills) • Appreciate the value of what individuals and teams can to do to improve care (quality improvement: attitudes)

Source: Quality and Safety Education for Nurses Institute. (2014). QSEN competencies. Retrieved from http://qsen.org/competencies/pre-licensure-ksas

QUESTIONS TO CONSIDER BEFORE READING ON

Reflect on your experience as a registered nurse and identify a major change that occurred in your workplace. What specific behaviors were helpful during this time of transition? Are they leadership or management behaviors?

Think about the skills which you possess at this point in your nursing career. Do you currently have more leadership or more management traits?

LEADERSHIP AND MANAGEMENT

The words "leadership" and "management" are sometimes used interchangeably. Although they are closely linked and at times their functions overlap, there are important distinctions in behaviors and characteristics that separate leaders from managers (Table 3.2). Recognizing these differences can assist you in selecting an approach that is best suited to each situation.

LEADERSHIP

Leadership is the process of influencing and inspiring others to accomplish important tasks or achieve specific objectives. Leaders are individuals who motivate others to willingly change their behavior and empower others to act in ways that lead to goal attainment. In all organizations, there are formal and informal leaders. Formal leaders are those who are appointed to a position that carries with it overt, legitimate authority. Examples of formal leaders in nursing include nurse managers, nursing directors, or chief nursing officers. Although formal leaders have an official title and a designated position within an organization's hierarchy, they derive true power and effectiveness by knowing their employees and developing rapport with those whom they lead. Informal leaders are individuals whom a group chooses to follow, despite the fact that they do not have official authority to direct others. In nursing, informal leaders are often staff nurses who have seniority, expert clinical skills, or a charismatic personality. They may frequently assume the roles of a charge nurse, a preceptor, or an educator. Informal leaders derive power through influence and persuasion. Ideally, formal and informal leaders share common goals and figure out ways to work together to contribute to the success of their team.

Leaders have a long-range, future-focused perspective, which can also be called a "vision." Barker, Sullivan, and Emery (2006) describe a vision as an image of a possible and desirable future state that can serve as a guiding light to illuminate a desired pathway. Leaders are those who create or embrace a vision, internalize it, frequently communicate it to others, and allow the vision to guide their attitudes and approaches in decision-making.

Truly effective leaders can articulate a vision in ways that stimulate thought and motivate action of their followers. Visions help develop a sense of mutual purpose or shared meaning by linking efforts to successful outcomes (Taylor, Cornelius, & Colvin, 2014).

Leadership, like nursing, is an activity that is profoundly personal, in the sense that it is essentially a matter of human interaction and social exchange. Effective leaders view interpersonal relationships as important instruments in reaching group goals. They see the potential and bring out the best in their followers by engaging their hearts and minds. Leaders not only build employee performance through intellectual stimulation but also inspire passion and commitment by embracing emotions and crafting connectedness (Colan, 2009). Bennis (1994) asserts that to leaders, "relationships have to do with outstanding people working in harmony and openness, where everyone feels empowered, where all members feel included and at the center of things, where they feel competent and significant" (p. xiv).

MANAGEMENT

Management is the process of planning, organizing, directing, and controlling the use of resources to accomplish performance objectives. In contrast to leaders being formal or informal, managers always have an official position within an organization through which they derive power and exert influence. The official status of managers serves as a basis for their relationship with subordinates (McEwen & Wills, 2007). Generally, in healthcare institutions, managers are charged with the responsibility of overseeing the use of organizational assets and maintaining a balance of operations. This involves coordinating the time and efforts of staff and managing the use of money, supplies, and space to meet organizational goals.

Managers have a short-range, current-focused perspective, and are concerned with day-to-day operations. Where leadership centers on relationships and influencing people, the primary focus of management is on organizational systems and processes (Bennis, 1994). The management process can be categorized into the following five core functions (Fayol, 1949):

1. *Planning*—having forethought, determining goals, and developing courses of action for achievement; deciding in advance what is to be done
2. *Organizing*—forming lines of responsibility and authority and building structure to activities by configuring material and human resources
3. *Commanding*—communicating goals and expectations, giving orders and clear instructions, in addition to supervising subordinates in their daily work

4. *Coordinating*—synchronizing elements and orchestrating efforts, as well as motivating and influencing others to follow a specific direction
5. *Controlling*—ensuring conformity to established standards; checking that proper procedures are followed and outcomes are as desired and making adjustments when needed to make sure the process remains within control

Both leadership and management are concerned with achieving goals, and, although divergent in application, the processes are highly interconnected. Leadership and management are both equally vital to the success of a team or an organization. The need for each varies according to the specific circumstances of a situation. To maximize achievement and obtain optimal results, a balance of leadership and management is necessary. Nurses at all levels are required to use both leadership and management skills. As a registered nurse, while providing care, you are expected to empower, motivate, persuade, and influence others just as leaders do; and as a manager of care, you are also expected to assess situations, plan actions, coordinate resources, and facilitate interdisciplinary collaborations. Understanding the functions, behaviors, and characteristics of leadership and management and recognizing when to apply each can enhance your nursing practice and increase your effectiveness as a caregiver. Table 3.2 identifies 20 differences in leadership and management. To help you apply the above information to clinical practice, complete the case scenario in Box 3.1.

TABLE 3.2 TWENTY DIFFERENCES IN LEADERSHIP AND MANAGEMENT

Leadership	Management
1. Has a vision and sets the course to fulfill it	1. Has an objective and makes a plan to achieve it
2. Sells	2. Tells
3. Provides guidance and inspiration	3. Provides direction and instruction
4. Goal-oriented	4. Task-oriented
5. Enables flexibility	5. Ensures stability
6. Future focus, long-range thinking	6. Current focus, short-range thinking
7. Encourages participation	7. Assigns duties
8. Empowers	8. Approves
9. Mentoring	9. Monitoring
10. Strategic	10. Tactical
11. Participative	11. Directive
12. Cultivates	12. Constructs
13. Focuses on people	13. Focuses on systems
14. Motivates	14. Coordinates
15. Fosters transformation	15. Oversees change
16. Permits creativity	16. Expects consistency
17. Relationship based on rapport	17. Relationship based on position
18. "Coach," "mentor," "servant"	18. "Boss," "supervisor," "director"
19. Innovators	19. Administrators
20. Does the right thing	20. Does things right

BOX 3.1 CASE SCENARIO

As you read this case scenario, consider the following questions:

- What information presented in the case scenario relates to Rachel's leadership role?
- What information relates to her management role?

Rachel has been the nurse manager of a 20-bed medical intensive care unit (MICU) for 5 years. During this time, she has dedicated herself to creating a workplace culture built on trust, respect, and fairness. Recently, the hospital for which she works was acquired by a large healthcare organization, which has resulted in a reorganization of leadership and the addition of new roles and responsibilities. Rachel will soon be required to assume management of an adjacent 12-bed observation unit, in addition to the MICU. Some of the MICU staff have expressed worry about the uncertainty of the future, whereas others seem to be upset or angry about the upcoming changes. Rachel realizes that any change, especially as significant as this, can disrupt the workplace atmosphere. Accordingly, she schedules a staff meeting to develop a vision for the future and to develop plans for the transition.

Before the staff meeting, Rachel prepares by speaking with her supervisor to make specific plans for when she will assume leadership of the other unit. They discuss potential challenges and develop strategies for managing the increased workload. One particular challenge that is discussed is that the observation unit currently has several RN vacancies resulting in deficient staffing levels. Conversely, the MICU has good staffing. To reduce overtime costs, Rachel recognizes an opportunity for the MICU staff to assist with covering the observation unit, but she also knows that this will most likely not be a popular idea.

During the staff meeting, Rachel first asks the MICU staff about their feelings and concerns for the transition. She displays empathy by listening to various perspectives and allowing the staff to share their opinions. Then, Rachel clearly communicates her goals and details her plan for coverage of the two units. To ensure transparency, she also shares the probable need for MICU staff to periodically work in the observation unit.

LEADERSHIP THEORIES

Theory is a group of specific concepts, definitions, and propositions of relationships used to describe events or explain phenomena. Theory provides structure to ideas and organization to knowledge and offers a systematic means of collecting data to explain, predict, and guide practice (McEwen & Wills, 2007). Theory provides a framework for understanding the relationships among a set of facts or principles. As a registered nurse, exploring and comprehending leadership theory can broaden your perspectives and help you develop a personal approach to leadership that can be used in daily practice.

BOX 3.2 SELF-ASSESSMENT OF LEADERSHIP AND MANAGEMENT SKILLS

Instructions: Give yourself 1 point for each statement that is true for you. Add up the number of points in each column.

Results: Column A corresponds to management behaviors. Column B corresponds to leadership behaviors. A higher number in column A reflects that you have a tendency to manage. A higher number in column B reflects that you have a tendency to lead. Equal numbers in each column indicate that you use a combination of management and leadership skills.

TABLE 3.3 MANAGEMENT AND LEADERSHIP SELF-ASSESSMENT

Column A	Column B
I like to maintain the day-to-day functioning. Yes (1 point) _____ No (0 points) _____	I like to develop things. Yes (1 point) _____ No (0 points) _____
I like to focus on systems and structure. Yes (1 point) _____ No (0 points)_____	I like to focus on people. Yes (1 point) _____ No (0 points) _____
I like to control things. Yes (1 point) _____ No (0 points) _____	I like to inspire trust. Yes (1 point) _____ No (0 points) _____
I tend to have a short-range view. Yes (1 point) _____ No (0 points) _____	I tend to have a long-range view. Yes (1 point) _____ No (0 points) _____
I tend to ask the questions "how" and "when." Yes (1 point) _____ No (0 points) _____	I tend to ask the questions "what" and "why." Yes (1 point) _____ No (0 points) _____
I tend to have my eye on the bottom line. Yes (1 point) _____ No (0 points) _____	I tend to have my eye on the horizon. Yes (1 point) _____ No (0 points) _____
I tend to accept the status quo. Yes (1 point) _____ No (0 points) _____	I tend to challenge the status quo. Yes (1 point) _____ No (0 points) _____
I do things right. Yes (1 point) _____ No (0 points) _____	I do the right thing. Yes (1 point) _____ No (0 points) _____
Total number of points in Column A: _____	Total number of points in Column B: _____

Literature from within the discipline of nursing, and from without, describes many diverse leadership theories from which to draw conclusions and develop understanding. This chapter describes four key leadership theories (Table 3.4) that are particularly applicable to nursing, meaningful in today's organizational environments, and can remain relevant throughout the constantly evolving landscape of healthcare.

TRANSFORMATIONAL LEADERSHIP

Transformational leadership was first described by Burns (1978) as two or more persons engaging with each other in such a way that leaders and followers raise one another to higher levels of motivation and morality. Barker et al. (2006) assert that transformational leadership is a philosophical point of view about the leader–follower relationship rather than a prescriptive set of rules. Transformational leadership focuses on producing revolutionary change through a commitment to the organization's vision (Sullivan & Decker, 2005). In transformational leadership, the leader and the follower mutually support a common purpose. Transformational leadership is a relationship in which "both the leader and follower find meaning and purpose in their work, and grow and develop as a result of the relationship" (Barker et al., 2006, p. 16). Transformational leadership is a moral leadership versus a technical leadership. It is an inspirational leadership that raises aspirations and gets people to accomplish more in achieving high performance (Schermerhorn, 2004).

Transformational leadership can be further described as containing the following four components (Bass, 1998; Bass & Avolio, 1990):

1. Inspiration
2. Charisma
3. Intellectual stimulation
4. Individualized consideration

"Inspiration" refers to motivation or a leader's ability to produce enthusiasm within his or her followers. Chief components of inspiration are communicating a sense of direction or a vision and setting clear expectations. Transformational leaders are effective in developing interest in shared goals and excitement about accomplishing tasks.

"Charisma" can also be called "idealized influence." It refers to leaders influencing others by acting as role models and using the power of personal reference. In doing so, transformational leaders gain respect, loyalty, and trust and create passion and pride within their followers. Followers will identify with leaders, adopt their ideals, and want to emulate them.

"Intellectual stimulation" occurs when leaders solicit the input of followers. Transformational leaders are not satisfied with the status quo but rather seek for new approaches and encourage followers to explore new ways of doing things. They stimulate thought, creativity, and imagination among followers by creating awareness of problems, gathering opinions and ideas, and jointly formulating solutions.

"Individualized consideration" implies a respect for the uniqueness of each follower and the honoring of individual differences. Transformational leaders create workplace climates that celebrate diversity. Transformational leaders display empathy and support by listening to the concerns and remaining attentive to the needs of each individual. They recognize the potential in each follower and provide personalized coaching and mentoring.

While exploring transformational leadership, it is also important to review the contrasting concept of "transactional" leadership. Burns (1978) defines transactional leadership as one person taking the initiative to make contact with others for the purpose of an exchange of something valued. In transactional leadership, there is no concern for a common vision or unified direction; it is merely a function of exchanging one thing for another. It is, in a sense, the trading of commodities, a give-and-take for reciprocal benefits. Transactional leaders give followers something they want in return for something the leaders want (Kuhnert & Lewis, 1987), for example, exchanging salary for hours worked. Transactional leaders identify the needs of followers and provide rewards in exchange for performance. Transactional leaders focus on the maintenance and management of day-to-day operations (Huber, 2006). Transactional leadership also includes management by exception, which involves identifying and addressing only areas that deviate from the norm. In this model, if followers are performing as expected, the leaders will not take action.

Although transactional leadership may be effective in producing effort and obtaining performance as expected, the concept of transformational leadership is more useful and applicable to nursing (Huber, 2006). In fact, the American Nurses Association (ANA) includes transformational leadership as an expected professional competency for registered nurses (ANA, 2013). The nursing profession is characterized by progress and change. Transformational leadership is especially relevant under these circumstances (Bass & Avolio, 1990).

SERVANT LEADERSHIP

Servant leadership was originally conceptualized by Robert Greenleaf in 1970 and holds to the idea that leaders are initially driven from a desire within themselves to serve others, and then they make a conscious choice to aspire to leadership to accomplish this goal (Greenleaf, 2002). Servant leaders are servants above all else. They put serving others, including employees, customers, and community, as the number one priority. Servant leadership is, in essence, a way of being and a long-term approach to life and work (Spears & Lawrence, 2004). Spears expounded on these concepts and identified the following 10 characteristics as central to the development of servant leadership:

1. *Listening*—being mindfully present during conversations; listening actively, receptively, and intently; allowing others to voice their concerns and express their needs; asking clarifying questions to develop deep understanding; reflecting on what was discussed
2. *Empathy*—considering followers not only as employees but also as people; striving to understand, relate to, and accept others; assuming that others have positive intentions, regardless of their behavior or performance; appreciating diversity and recognizing the uniqueness of individuals
3. *Healing*—approaching situations with the intention of promoting wholeness for others as well as oneself; viewing interactions as opportunities to help make whole those with whom one comes in contact; solving problems and resolving conflicts
4. *Awareness*—recognizing one's own strengths, weaknesses, and values; maintaining a sense of what is happening around and within oneself; honoring the styles, preferences, values, and needs of others
5. *Persuasion*—using inspiration, rather than official position, to influence individuals and groups to make decisions for the benefit of the whole; convincing versus coercing; building consensus within groups
6. *Conceptualization*—looking beyond the details of day-to-day realities; practicing broad-based thinking; seeing the "big picture"; focusing on long-term goals
7. *Foresight*—having the ability to anticipate the likely outcome of a situation; integrating lessons learned from past experiences, understanding the realities of the present, and anticipating the future implications of decisions or actions; having intuition
8. *Stewardship*—caring for resources responsibly, to include human, environmental, financial, physical, material, and organizational resources; being committed to serving the needs of others; holding one's institutions in trust for the greater good of society
9. *Commitment to the growth of others*—investing in the development of others; nurturing the personal and professional growth of employees; believing in the intrinsic value of people beyond their tangible contributions as workers; helping people become independent servant leaders themselves
10. *Building community*—creating spaces and environments that foster teamwork and collaboration; promoting group identity and shared purpose; building relationships and strengthening bonds; facilitating interactions and intentionally getting to know others

The theory of servant leadership aligns closely with the work and purpose of nursing, considering that nursing is a profession that is dedicated to the service of others. Like nursing, servant leadership emphasizes a holistic manner of relating to people. It is strongly based in ethical and caring behavior and focuses on enhancing the well-being of others (Spears & Lawrence, 2004).

SITUATIONAL LEADERSHIP

Hersey, Blanchard, and Johnson (2001) describe a situational leadership model, which recommends leaders adjust their style of leadership depending on the readiness of followers to perform in a given situation. Situational leadership theory examines the interplay of three specific dimensions: task behavior, relationship behavior, and the readiness of the follower.

"Task behavior" is the amount of guidance required by the leader to ensure that the task is accomplished. Task behavior is the extent to which the leader engages in one-way communication by explaining what is to be done by each follower and where, when, and how it is to be completed. Task behavior involves defining roles, setting goals, organizing, setting timelines, directing, and controlling.

"Relationship behavior" is the amount of socioemotional support the leader provides to followers. This is the extent to which the leader engages in two-way communication and maintains personal relationships with followers. Relationship behavior involves encouraging, listening, facilitating actions, and providing feedback to followers.

"Readiness" is the extent to which the follower demonstrates the ability and willingness to accomplish a particular task. Ability refers to the follower's actual knowledge, experience, and skill; willingness refers to the follower's confidence, commitment, and motivation. Readiness has to do with the preparedness of the follower in specific situations. It is not the evaluation of personal character traits, nor does it refer to the follower's overall aptitude or attitude. Situational leaders must diagnose the readiness of followers in each situation and tailor their leadership approach accordingly.

Hersey et al. (2001) define the following four leadership styles within the model of situational leadership:

1. *Delegating*—allowing followers to make decisions and take responsibility for task completion; leader is involved through observing, monitoring, and evaluating; a low-task, low-relationship style
2. *Participating*—allowing for follower input and practicing participative decision-making; leader is involved through encouraging and collaborating; a low-task, high-relationship style
3. *Selling*—explaining task directions; leader is involved through clarifying and persuading; a high-task, high-relationship style
4. *Telling*—giving specific instructions; leader is involved through guiding and directing; a high-task, low-relationship style

Situational leadership is not as much about leadership as it is about recognizing and meeting the needs of followers. In this model, no one style of leadership is considered optimal. To be effective, leaders must remain flexible and adapt their approach according to each situation. Situational leadership is applicable to nursing, considering that the nursing workforce is particularly diverse. A nursing unit or workgroup often includes individuals at different points in their careers and with varying levels of experience, training, and expertise. Situational leadership encourages leaders to practice assessment and critical thinking by weighing the variables of group dynamics together with the context of situations to choose the leadership style that best fits their goals, circumstances, and staff (Hersey et al., 2001).

AUTHENTIC LEADERSHIP

Authentic leadership refers to developing a personal leadership style that is consistent with one's own personality and character. Simply stated, it means being your own person as a leader. This requires leaders to be true to themselves, accepting their faults, and capitalizing on their strengths (George, 2003). Avolio and colleagues define authentic leaders as "those individuals who are deeply aware of how they think and behave and are perceived by others as being aware of their own and others' values/moral perspective, knowledge, and strengths, aware of the context in which they operate, and who are confident, hopeful, optimistic, resilient, and high on moral character" (as cited in Avolio, Gardner, Walumbwa, Luthans, & May, 2004, p. 804). Authentic leaders can be described as individuals who are self-aware, transparent, ethical, and balanced in the way they gather information to make their decisions (Riggio, Chaleff, & Lipman-Blumen, 2008). Authentic leadership consists of the following five dimensions:

1. *Purpose*—having a passion and a genuine desire to serve others through leadership; seeking to empower people instead of striving for power, prestige, or financial reward
2. *Values*—following a moral compass; differentiating right from wrong and choosing to do the right thing; ensuring that one's behavior is based on integrity; remaining ethical and transparent
3. *Heart*—having sincere empathy for people; being compassionate to others and also engaging in self-compassion
4. *Relationships*—creating connectedness; nurturing close and enduring relationships with others
5. *Self-discipline*—practicing consistency; remaining dependable, reliable, fair, and balanced (George, 2003)

An important concept of authentic leadership is the view of leadership as a journey, rather than a destination. Authentic leaders realize that becoming an effective leader involves a lifetime of personal development and that all of one's life experiences, especially the challenges and setbacks, contribute to overall success. Developing authenticity through a foundation of self-awareness and self-acceptance can lead to self-actualization and allow leaders to maximize their potential (George, 2015).

Authentic leaders are credible and believable and consequently gain legitimacy and garner trust. By practicing authenticity, leaders can construct healthy workplace settings that encourage self-determination and facilitate employee engagement. Authentic leadership is guided as much by the qualities of the heart, as by the qualities of the mind (George, 2003). This resembles the concept of caring, which is an essential component of nursing practice. The caring process promotes self-knowledge, self-control, and self-healing, which helps to build trusting, caring, self-aware relationships (Watson, 2005). Nurses can implement authentic leadership by forming high-quality relationships and genuinely connecting with others in meaningful and purposeful ways.

TABLE 3.4 SUMMARY OF LEADERSHIP THEORIES

Leadership Theory	Framework
Transformational leadership	• Charisma • Inspiration (vision) • Intellectual stimulation • Individualized consideration
Servant leadership	• Listening • Empathy • Healing • Awareness • Persuasion • Conceptualization • Foresight • Stewardship • Commitment to the growth of others • Building community
Situational leadership	• Task behavior • Relationship behavior • Readiness • Delegating • Participating • Selling • Telling
Authentic leadership	• Purpose (passion) • Values (integrity) • Heart (compassion) • Relationships (connectedness) • Self-discipline (consistency)

BOX 3.3 THE CASE SCENARIO CONTINUES TO UNFOLD

As you read this case scenario, try to determine the leadership styles used by Rachel as well as by Kevin. Offer evidence to support your answer.

Regarding the plan to float staff to the observation unit, some of the MICU nurses are against it; and they openly voice their dissatisfaction. In contrast, Kevin, a seasoned MICU nurse, shows support for Rachel and commitment to the organization by volunteering to work in the observation unit whenever needed. Kevin also offers to collaborate with the charge nurse of the observation unit to develop a competency checklist that will ensure that the MICU nurses are properly prepared when working in the different area. Rachel is grateful for Kevin's help, trusts his judgment, and facilitates his participation by allowing protected time for him to work on the competency checklist project.

When the merger of the hospitals concluded, Rachel assumed full leadership accountability for both the MICU and the observation unit. Although her responsibilities grew significantly, the change was made less challenging due to the supportive attitudes and actions of Kevin and other staff. At first, Rachel was consumed with the increased workload and spent very little time interacting directly with the staff. However, she soon realized this and made necessary adjustments. Rachel then made a concerted effort to be present in both units, to take time out to listen to concerns, and to make herself available for any staff in need.

QUESTIONS TO CONSIDER BEFORE READING ON

- Consider the leadership style of your current supervisor. Does he or she display transformational, transactional, servant, situational, or authentic leadership? Does your supervisor vary styles on the basis of differing situations?
- Consider where you may be on your own journey as a leader. What type of leader do you aspire to be?

FOLLOWERSHIP

Without followers, there can be no leaders. Furthermore, the success of any group depends on the actions of both leaders and followers. The relationship between leaders and followers is reciprocal and characterized by interdependence. Leaders and followers both rely on each other to create conditions under which mutual influence is possible (Reicher, Haslam, & Hopkins, 2005). "Followership" is the concept of an individual actively following a leader. Kelley (1988) describes followership as an interactive process of participation in which followers exercise self-reliance, intelligence, and enthusiasm in the pursuit of organizational objectives. Followership can have varying degrees of effectiveness and engagement. Kelley (1988) defines five categories of followers in terms of their capacity for independent, critical thinking, as well as their degree of active versus passive engagement. These categories include the following:

1. *"Sheep"*—passive employees who rely on the leader to do the thinking for them and to provide them with motivation. These individuals lack commitment and initiative. They require close supervision and instruction from the leader.
2. *"Yes-people"*—positive employees who are always supportive of the leader. They do not question the decisions or actions of the leader. They look to the leader for the thinking and the vision, but they will do what is asked of them and will energetically follow direction.
3. *"Pragmatics"*—employees who preserve the status quo. They avoid risks and see which way the wind blows. They are not trendsetters or early adopters, but, rather, will go along with the group, once they see where things are headed.
4. *"Alienated" followers*—skeptical, cynical employees who have negative energy. They are often unsupportive and critical of the leader or fellow group members. These individuals think for themselves, but may hamper progress by questioning the decisions or actions of the leader.
5. *"Star" followers*—exemplary employees who participate and have a positive energy. They will not accept the decisions or actions of the leader without their own, comprehensive evaluation. They take initiative and actively contribute to the success of the group. (Riggio et al., 2008)

Kelley (1988) further explains that effective followers manage themselves well, are able to think independently, and can work without close supervision. They demonstrate commitment to a cause, an idea, or the organization; that is to say, their hearts are in their work. Effective followers also display competence and focus. They are committed to professional development and continuing education; they master skills that prepare them to perform successfully and meet personal and organizational goals. In addition, they are critical thinkers whose knowledge and judgment can be trusted; and they stand up for what they believe in. Effective followers are honest, credible, and courageous (Kelley, 1988).

Chaleff (2009) reinforces the notion of courage as an essential component of effective followership. He explains that courageous followership involves the courage to support the leader and contribute to the leader's success; the courage to assume responsibility for a common purpose and act with or without direct orders from the leader; the courage to constructively challenge the behaviors of the leader or the group and to question policies if these threaten the common purpose; the courage to participate in any transformation needed to improve the leader–follower relationship or enhance the group's performance; and the courage to take a moral stand, if necessary, to prevent ethical abuses or to refuse to participate in them (Riggio et al., 2008).

The word "followership" should not be viewed as a pejorative term. On the contrary, followership is an honorable and legitimate role that is essential to the success of any group. In achieving organizational objectives, followership is equally as important as leadership. Indeed, the majority of work in organizations is done by followers (Riggio et al., 2008). Although followers lack formal authority, they do not lack power or influence. Engaged followers are actually effective agents of change; their behaviors and attitudes impact the outcomes of their teams.

In the nursing profession, there are many different specialty areas and the work of a nurse can be highly variable. A nurse can be a caregiver, a teacher, an advocate, a team leader, a researcher, a counselor, a supervisor, a coordinator, or a manager of care. Depending on the context of each situation, nurses are called to be both followers and leaders, or perhaps even both simultaneously. By recognizing and using the practices of effective followership, you can help create workplace environments that are conducive to increased safety, improved quality, and high performance. Table 3.5 offers a list of actions that will support your personal development and professional growth in the areas of leadership and followership.

QUESTIONS TO CONSIDER BEFORE READING ON

- Review Kelley's followership information. Currently, what type of follower are you?
- Consider the qualities of effective leadership and effective followership. What are the similarities? What are the differences?

CONCLUSIONS

Leadership is inextricably tied to nursing; it is woven into the fabric of the nursing profession. There is a need and an expectation that all registered nurses maintain and develop leadership knowledge, skills, and attitudes (Table 3.1). Nurses can demonstrate leadership at any level of experience and in any stage of their careers. Leadership has little to do with an organizational chart and more to do with how one relates to others. A leader's true power is not in position, but rather in his or her ability to inspire and influence others to accomplish goals.

TABLE 3.5 PRACTICAL IDEAS FOR PERSONAL DEVELOPMENT AND PROFESSIONAL GROWTH

Leadership
• Share power and collaborate with others • Encourage diversity of ideas and consider the opinions of others • Remain humble and admit your mistakes • Maintain ethical and moral bearings • Stay in touch with reality • Fulfill responsibilities • Do not make commitments you cannot keep • Know your limits and seek support when necessary • Surround yourself with experts in your areas of weakness • Constantly seek to improve and gain knowledge • Remember the mission and vision • Stay balanced, fair, and impartial • Be actively self-aware through introspection and reflective practice • Work towards an acceptable work–life balance • Develop a personal support system, network with others, and build coalitions • Strive for stakeholder balance by connecting with all followers, not just a select few • Practice self-discipline and develop good habits
Followership
• Be an engaged, active participant • Think independently and share ideas eagerly • Be prepared to question and challenge others and be questioned and challenged yourself • Do what you know is right • Speak up when something seems wrong • Find allies and take collective action • Demonstrate teamwork and offer assistance • Verify that information is correct and complete • Do not spread rumors or gossip • Hold leaders accountable • Willingly fulfill your responsibilities • Maintain awareness of goals and pay attention to detail • Take breaks and practice self-care • Maintain optimism and positivity • Arrive on time • Put group goals before personal goals

Source: Candy, W. (2008). Bad leadership. In J. L. Pierce & J. W. Newstrom (Eds.), *The manager's bookshelf: A mosaic of contemporary views* (8th ed., pp. 206–210). Upper Saddle River, NJ: Pearson; Kellerman, B. (2004). *Bad leadership: What it is, how it happens, why it matters.* Boston, MA: Harvard Business School Press; Kellerman, B. (2007). What every leader needs to know about followers. *Harvard Business Review, 85*(12), 84–91; Whitlock, J. (2013). The value of active followership. *Nursing Management, 20*(2), 20–23. doi:10.7748/nm2013.05.20.2.20.e677; Willson, A. (2012). *Attaining peak performance.* Cardiff, UK: 1000 Lives Plus. Retrieved from http://www.1000livesplus.wales.nhs.uk/sitesplus/documents/1011/Attaining%20Peak%20Performance.pdf

Mintzberg (1998) describes three separate levels at which leadership can be exercised: individual, group, and organizational. At the individual level, leaders mentor, coach, and motivate. At the group level, leaders build teams and resolve conflicts. At the organizational level, leaders build culture.

This chapter presented a leadership self-assessment tool which can be used to identify leadership strengths in addition to areas with room for growth. Leadership and management were differentiated. Explanations of four key leadership theories were provided: transformational leadership, servant leadership, situational leadership, and authentic leadership. The concept of followership was described and practical suggestions were offered to assist with personal development and professional growth.

CRITICAL THINKING QUESTIONS AND EXERCISES

- Review Tables 3.2 and 3.5 and consider how to apply the information personally. What deliberate actions will you take as an RN to enhance your leadership, management, or followership skills?
- Think of supervisors you know or with whom you have worked who can be categorized into each type of leadership style (transformational, servant, situational, or authentic). As an employee, which style do you prefer? As a leader, which style do you favor?
- Reflect on your experiences as a follower. What specific situations have called for courageous followership?

REFERENCES

American Nurses Association. (2013). ANA Leadership Institute: Competency model. Retrieved from https://www.nursingworld.org/~4a0a2e/globalassets/docs/ce/177626-ana-leadership-booklet-new-final.pdf

Avolio, B. J., Gardner, W. L., Walumbwa, F. O., Luthans, F., & May, D. R. (2004). Unlocking the mask: A look at the process by which authentic leaders impact follower attitudes and behaviors. *Leadership Quarterly, 15*(6), 801–823. doi:10.1016/j.leaqua.2004.09.003

Barker, A. M., Sullivan, D. T., & Emery, M. J. (2006). *Leadership competencies for clinical managers: The renaissance of transformational leadership*. Sudbury, MA: Jones & Bartlett.

Bass, B. M. (1998). *Transformational leadership: Industry, military, and educational impact*. Mahwah, NJ: Lawrence Erlbaum Associates.

Bass, B. M., & Avolio, B. J. (1990). *Transformational leadership development: Manual for the multifactor leadership questionnaire*. Palo Alto, CA: Consulting Psychologists Press.

Bennis, W. (1994). *On becoming a leader*. Cambridge, MA: Perseus.

Burns, J. M. (1978). *Leadership*. New York, NY: Harper & Row.

Candy, W. (2008). Bad leadership. In J. L. Pierce & J. W. Newstrom (Eds.), *The manager's bookshelf: A mosaic of contemporary views* (8th ed., pp. 206–210). Upper Saddle River, NJ: Pearson.

Chaleff, I. (2009). *The courageous follower: Standing up to and for our leaders* (3rd ed.). San Francisco, CA: Berrett-Koehler.

Colan, L. J. (2009). *Engaging the hearts and minds of all your employees: How to ignite passionate performance for better business results*. New York, NY: McGraw-Hill.

Fayol, H. (1949). *General and industrial management*. London, UK: Pitman & Sons.

George, B. (2003). *Authentic leadership: Rediscovering the secrets to creating lasting value*. San Francisco, CA: Jossey-Bass.

George, B. (2015). *Discover your true north*. Hoboken, NJ: Wiley.

Greenleaf, R. K. (2002). *Servant leadership: A journey into the nature of legitimate power and greatness*. New York, NY: Paulist Press.

Hersey, P., Blanchard, K. H., & Johnson, D. E. (2001). *Management of organizational behavior: Utilizing human resources* (8th ed.). Upper Saddle River, NJ: Prentice Hall.

Huber, D. L. (2006). *Leadership and nursing care management* (3rd ed.). Philadelphia, PA: Elsevier.

Kellerman, B. (2004). *Bad leadership: What it is, how it happens, why it matters*. Boston, MA: Harvard Business School Press.

Kellerman, B. (2007). What every leader needs to know about followers. *Harvard Business Review, 85*(12), 84-91.

Kelley, R. (1988). In praise of followers. *Harvard Business Review, 66*(6), 142–148. Retrieved from https://hbr.org/1988/11/in-praise-of-followers

Kuhnert, K. W., & Lewis, P. (1987). Transactional and transformational leadership: A constructive/developmental analysis. *Academy of Management Review, 12*(4), 648–657. doi:10.2307/258070

McEwen, M., & Wills, E. M. (2007). *Theoretical basis for nursing* (2nd ed.). Philadelphia, PA: Lippincott Williams & Wilkins.

Mintzberg, H. (1998). Covert leadership: Notes on managing professionals. Knowledge workers respond to inspiration, not supervision. *Harvard Business Review, 76*(6), 140–147. Retrieved from https://hbr.org/1998/11/covert-leadership-notes-on-managing-professionals

Quality and Safety Education for Nurses Institute. (2014). QSEN competencies. Retrieved from http://qsen.org/competencies/pre-licensure-ksas

Reicher, S., Haslam, S. A., & Hopkins, N. (2005). Social identity and the dynamics of leadership: Leaders and followers as collaborative agents in the transformation of social reality. *Leadership Quarterly, 16*, 547–568. doi:10.1016/j.leaqua.2005.06.007

Riggio, R. E, Chaleff, I., & Lipman-Blumen, J. (Eds.). (2008). *The art of followership: How great followers create great leaders and organizations*. San Francisco, CA: Jossey-Bass.

Schermerhorn, J. R. (2004). *Core concepts of management*. Hoboken, NJ: Wiley.

Spears, L. C., & Lawrence, M. (Eds.). (2004). *Practicing servant-leadership: Succeeding through trust, bravery, and forgiveness*. San Francisco, CA: Jossey-Bass.

Sullivan, E. J., & Decker, P. J. (2005). *Effective leadership and management in nursing* (6th ed.). Upper Saddle River, NJ: Pearson/Prentice Hall.

Taylor, C. M., Cornelius, C. J., & Colvin, K. (2014). Visionary leadership and its relationship to organizational effectiveness. *Leadership & Organization Development Journal, 35*(6), 566–583. doi:10.1108/LODJ-10-2012-0130

Watson, J. (2005). *Caring science as sacred science*. Philadelphia, PA: F. A. Davis.

Whitlock, J. (2013). The value of active followership. *Nursing Management, 20*(2), 20–23. doi:10.7748/nm2013.05.20.2.20.e677

Willson, A. (2012). *Attaining peak performance*. Cardiff, UK: 1000 Lives Plus. Retrieved from http://www.1000livesplus.wales.nhs.uk/sitesplus/documents/1011/Attaining%20Peak%20Performance.pdf

4

FOUNDATIONAL ASPECTS OF EFFECTIVE LEADERSHIP

MARY E. QUINN ● MARY T. QUINN GRIFFIN

LEARNING OBJECTIVES

After completion of this chapter, the reader will be able to

- Describe the characteristics of effective leadership.
- Define the meaning of ethical leadership as it relates to various healthcare settings.
- Identify situations where ethical leadership can be strengthened on important issues in the work setting.
- Explain key strategies to address ethical issues and challenges.
- Describe legal implications for nurse leaders.
- Define spiritual leadership.
- Identify positive outcomes of workplace spirituality.
- Identify strategies to promote workplace spirituality.
- Describe the four-tier model of professional nursing practice.

Being a leader doesn't require a title; having a title doesn't make you one.

—Author Unknown

Nurse leaders are not defined by an administrative title. Each professional nurse is a leader and has responsibilities inherent in the role that encompasses leadership skills and behaviors. A nurse leads his or her patients, families, and communities to wellness and a healthier state; a nurse leads by acting as an advocate for each patient and intervening as needed; a nurse leads through his or her contribution and collaboration to improve the work environment; a nurse leads through application of evidence-based practice to improve the quality of care and outcomes; a nurse leads by understanding the healthcare and political environment and actively engaging in organizational forums to protect and advance the profession of nursing; and a nurse leads through continuous learning. Nurses use basic leadership skills in their day-to-day practice, in varying practice environments, as advocates for their patients to make sure their patients get the resources needed or escalate their concerns when issues arise so that care is not compromised.

Google the term "effective leadership" and a myriad of terms and definitions can be found with common themes highlighted. Effective leadership includes strong character, in which the leader exhibits honesty, integrity, trustworthiness, and ethics. Leaders act in line with how they speak. Think about the sayings over the years, such as "actions speak louder than words" and more recently "walk it like you talk it." These describe effective leadership traits. An effective leader demonstrates clear communication skills. Effective leaders inspire loyalty and goodwill in others because they themselves act with integrity and trust. They are capable of bold and courageous moves and adapt as each situation arises.

As an associate's degree nurse (ADN), you have foundational leadership skills that you use in the prioritization and delivery of nursing care to include critical thinking, problem-solving, judgment, and reasoning in processing information in the formulation of a plan of care. In addition, the ADN must possess essential emotional and coping skills in managing the day-to-day potential stressors in the delivery of care as determined by professional standards of practice such as conflicts with end-of-life decisions and goals of care discussions. The ADN exercises good judgment, establishes empathic and therapeutic relationships with patients, families, and others from diverse populations, age groups, races, socioeconomic and ethnic backgrounds. This includes patients with varying mental, physical, and substance use diseases and disorders.

In this chapter, a review of the foundations of effective leadership is presented—ethical, spiritual, legal, and professional advocacy. Case studies and reflective questions are used to provoke self-assessment and awareness of your professional practice with regards to ethical dilemmas that you may have encountered or experienced in your work environment. The goal of these reflective exercises is to stimulate a greater understanding of your role as a nurse leader and as an advocate for both patients and nurses. Take a moment now to reflect and consider how you think about, evaluate, and act to ensure that nursing professional standards of practice are promoted and followed regardless of the clinical setting. Remember, you do not need a title to be an effective nurse leader.

QUESTIONS TO CONSIDER BEFORE READING ON

- What ethical concepts did you learn in your basic nursing program and/or continuing education?
- How do you see the concepts you learned applied in your agency by nurses?

continued

QUESTIONS TO CONSIDER BEFORE READING ON *(continued)*

- Does your organization have policies regarding ethical behavior?
  - If yes, have you ever reviewed them and understand how they pertain to your role as a professional nurse and leader?
  - If not, take a moment to review and describe what they are.
- Consider and reflect on your experiences in which you felt your ethics as a professional nurse were supported and/or challenged.
- Is there an anonymous process available for nurses to use in reporting breaches of ethics?
- What are the top ethical issues at your organization?

ETHICAL ASPECTS OF EFFECTIVE LEADERSHIP

It is not fair to ask of others what you are not willing to do yourself.

—Eleanor Roosevelt

Ethics involves the moral obligation of determining what is good and what is bad. According to the Gallup 2016 survey of Americans' rating of "Honesty and Ethical Standards in Professions," nurses continue to be ranked highest with 84% of the public rating nurses' standards and ethics as "high" or "very high" (Norman, 2016). A core component of professional nursing practice is an understanding of one's values and behaviors (American Association of Colleges of Nursing [AACN], 2008). Kubsch, Hansen, and Huyser-Eatwell (2008) conducted a study comparing the professional values of 198 nurses according to their level of nursing education and other factors. The highest level of perceived professional values was found among RN-BSN students (Kubsch et al., 2008). Professional nurses need to be aware of their values and beliefs and how they influence their behavior and interactions with patients, families, and colleagues.

QUESTIONS TO CONSIDER BEFORE READING ON

- Building upon what you have learned in your basic and continuing education programs, describe ethical behaviors and values required of a nurse leader.
- Do you consider yourself a nurse leader?
- Describe the nursing professional values; review the following five professional values; perform your own self-assessment in how you apply these values to your nursing practice.

As a nurse leader, it is important to understand the underpinnings of nursing professional values and ethics. The AACN (2008) outlines core foundational requirements of baccalaureate education for professional nursing practice known as the *Essentials.* Essential VIII, Professionalism and Professional Values, defines five professional values in which nurses demonstrate ethical behavior in the interactions with colleagues and in the care of their patients (pp. 27–28):

1. **Altruism** is a concern for the welfare and well-being of others. In professional practice, altruism is reflected by the nurse's concern and advocacy for the welfare of the patient, other nurses, and other healthcare providers.
2. **Autonomy** is the right to self-determination. Professional practice reflects autonomy when the nurse respects patients' rights to make decisions about their healthcare.
3. **Human dignity** is respect for the inherent work and uniqueness of individuals and populations. In professional practice, concern for human dignity is reflected when the nurse values and respects all patients and colleagues.
4. **Integrity** is acting in accordance with an appropriate code of ethics and accepted standards of practice. Integrity is reflected in professional practice when the nurse is honest and provides care based on an ethical framework that is accepted within the profession.
5. **Social justice** is acting in accordance with fair treatment regardless of economic status, race, ethnicity, age, citizenship, disability, or sexual orientation.

The American Nurses Association (ANA) *Code of Ethics* (2015) outlines key guiding principles within nine provisions and provides a framework related to professional nursing practice (Table 4.1). As a nursing leader, you incorporate this *Code of Ethics* into your daily practice.

Nurses have an ethical obligation to address the care of the patients. However, as a professional nurse and leader, your ethical responsibilities are even broader. You will have an obligation to also address any overall organizational system or process concerns that may influence patient care (Grande, 2015). Ethical nurse leaders have humility, integrity, and knowledge regarding the role of the leader. As a baccalaureate-prepared nurse leader, you are required to serve as a role model who helps create an ethical environment that is just and fair, establishes standards of conduct and a culture of integrity. Gilbert (2007) focused on the relationship between ethics and organizational performance. Gilbert surmised that the ethical culture of an organization is more than a compilation of credos and value statements; it relies on ethical wisdom. "Ethical wisdom" is defined as the individual and collective knowledge, experience, and good sense to make sound ethical decisions and judgments everywhere and every day (Gilbert, 2007). Nurse leaders are critical to establishing and maintaining an ethical

TABLE 4.1 AMERICAN NURSES ASSOCIATION CODE OF ETHICS FOR NURSES	
Provision 1	The nurse practices with compassion and respect for the inherent dignity, work, and unique attributes of every person.
Provision 2	The nurse's primary commitment is to the patient, whether an individual, family, group, community, or population.
Provision 3	The nurse promotes, advocates for, and protects the rights, health, and safety of the patient.
Provision 4	The nurse has authority, accountability, and responsibility for nursing practice; makes decisions; and takes action consistent with the obligation to provide optimal patient care.
Provision 5	The nurse owes the same duties to self as to others, including the responsibility to promote health and safety, preserve wholeness of character and integrity, maintain competence, and continue personal and professional growth.
Provision 6	The nurse, through individual and collective effort, establishes, maintains, and improves the ethical environment of the work setting and conditions of employment that are conducive to safe, quality health care.
Provision 7	The nurse, in all roles and settings, advances the profession through research and scholarly inquiry, professional standards development, and the generation of both nursing and health policy.
Provision 8	The nurse collaborates with other health professionals and the public to protect human rights, promote health diplomacy, and reduce health disparities.
Provision 9	The profession of nursing, collectively through its professional organizations, must articulate nursing values, maintain the integrity of the profession, and integrate principles of social justice into nursing and health policy.

Source: American Nurses Association. (2015). *Code of ethics for nurses with interpretive statements.* Silver Spring, MD: Author. Retrieved from http://nursingworld.org/DocumentVault/Ethics-1/Code-of-Ethics-for-Nurses.html

culture within their work environment. To establish an ethical culture, Gilbert outlined a framework that includes the following five disciplines:

1. *Mindfulness*: Being aware of your practice and work environment.
2. *Voice*: Staff's ability to speak up without fear of retribution, especially when raising concerns and challenging common work practices.
3. *Respect*: A critical building block in building team cohesiveness and trust so that critical conversations or concerns may be voiced.

4. *Tenacity*: Looking to what is best for patients, staff, and community.
5. *Legacy*: Taking action on the basis of decisions that are aligned with overall organizational mission and vision.

QUESTIONS TO CONSIDER BEFORE READING ON

On the basis of your review of the five disciplines just discussed, reflect on:

- Your practice and rate yourself as to how you currently incorporate these disciplines in your day-to-day practice as you work with your colleagues and patients/clients
- Your work environment and how these disciplines are within the culture of your work environment
- Whether there are opportunities for improvement within your practice and work environment. If yes, as a nurse leader, what strategies could you use for improvement?

ETHICAL ISSUES AND CHALLENGES

The concept of ethics is not new to professional nursing practice. It is a critical component of daily nursing practice (Rushton & Broome, 2015). Ethical conflicts are encountered by nurses in all clinical settings and go beyond end-of-life care and treatment issues. Foundational to the development of ethical skills and behaviors in nurses is a self-awareness and understanding of the motivations in addressing ethical issues (Robichaux, 2017). Robichaux (2017) emphasizes the importance of nurses being actively engaged in continuous learning to advance their knowledge and skills to effectively address ethical issues and challenges. The case scenario in Box 4.1 describes the conflict that nurses have experienced at some point in their career—taking risk with process workarounds versus following prescribed steps for performing a task.

BOX 4.1 CASE SCENARIO

As you read this case scenario, consider the AACN's five professional values and the ANA *Code of Ethics*, and reflect on how you would handle such a situation.

Nurse Mary is a new hire within the unit. She is an RN with several years of experience and is now working on obtaining a BSN degree. She has a defined professional development plan to continue education and enhance her learning and leadership skills through participation in various organizational committees and projects. She speaks with her manager about her desire to lead unit-based projects and other committees. Her nurse manager commends her plan and states she will "look out for something."

(*continued*)

BOX 4.1 CASE SCENARIO *(continued)*

Later on, a family member openly raises concerns to the nurses that some nurses check the ID bands before giving medications, whereas others do not and feels that family members have to be at the bedside all the time to make sure the right medications are given to their loved ones. When the nurse manager spoke with the family member who observed this, the family member indicated "not wanting to get anyone in trouble" and declined to give any specific information. Nurse Mary begins to observe some practice workarounds related to patient verification and wonders why practice varies and sees this as a potential performance improvement project for her unit. As she begins to talk with her colleagues, she is dismayed to hear that they did not think it was important because "nothing bad" has happened in the past so "why bother." Nurse Mary continues to feel this variation in practice is unsafe but feels uncomfortable in approaching any of her colleagues with her observations and is uncertain of how to proceed.

Nurse Mary deliberates on the situation and wonders how other nurses have dealt with this in the past. She conducts a review of the literature using key phrases such as "medication safety events" and "patient verification" and finds a wealth of articles that cite the risks and the steps nurses can take to minimize the risks of error. She also goes to the State Board of Nursing (BON) website to see if there are any violations or enforcement actions taken against nurses related to patient verification issues and is alarmed to find how many nurses were suspended and/or fined related to lack of following standards of care and professional practice related to patient verification errors. She presents her information to her nurse manager and proposes a project to improve patient verification processes through a full process review and use of barcode scanning compliance data for medication administration. Nurse Mary also shares the information she found with her colleagues and gains support that there are issues with overall medication management and that a "fresh" look and approach may enhance the system. The nurse manager has a staff meeting and gets consensus for a unit-based project with Nurse Mary leading it and a number of other nurses volunteering to participate. An interdisciplinary team was formed with several system and process issues identified with use of barcode scanning technology. Actions were taken locally on that unit with positive outcomes. Nurse Mary proudly presented the results of her unit's project work and outcomes to other nurses with the spread of those improvement strategies throughout the organization.

The case scenario highlights the leadership taken by Nurse Mary in not letting go of a potentially unsafe practice with variation in how patient verification was performed. Nurse Mary's actions are in accordance with the professional values of altruism and integrity. Nurse Mary demonstrated the leadership behavior and disciplines needed in ethical practice through mindfulness (being aware of the work environment practices), a voice (speaking with her colleagues), and respect (speaking with colleagues in a nonconfrontational manner). She also demonstrated tenacity (not settling for status quo but using the evidence on the risks to patient safety to get stakeholder support to make change) and legacy (through promotion of professional nursing practice and role in patient safety). She did not need to be the nurse manager to make changes happen; she gathered supporting evidence and discussed her findings with her manager and colleagues and highlighted the current risk in their practice environment that was in their control to address and upon which to improve.

QUESTIONS TO CONSIDER BEFORE READING ON

- Have you been faced with an ethical dilemma involving care of vulnerable populations as noted earlier? How have you responded in the past?
- Are you aware of any bias you may have or have observed when caring for vulnerable populations? How would you handle any conflict that may arise within your practice?

As you read the case scenario in Box 4.2, reflect on your own attitudes and beliefs and how they may have influenced your interactions with patients and colleagues and decisions related to your practice. Have you experienced or observed situations in which the professional value of social justice (acting in accordance with fair treatment regardless of economic status, race, ethnicity, age, citizenship, disability, or sexual orientation) has been lacking? If yes, reflect on those situations: How did you address the situation when confronted? What did you do when observing situations where nursing professional values were not upheld?

BOX 4.2 CASE SCENARIO

Nurse Patricia, a new employee, works in a school-based clinic where a 15-year-old patient comes in and asks for contraception information and supplies. Nurse Patricia is surprised to hear this request and begins to counsel the patient on the importance of abstinence and the risks of premarital sex. The patient persists in asking for information to avoid pregnancy. Nurse Patricia continues to instruct the patient on the high incidence of teenage pregnancy, asks the patient about her religious upbringing, speaks about the immoral behavior of sex before marriage, and again mentions abstinence from any sexual encounters. Nurse Debbie overhears the conversation and observes the patient crying and fears that the nurse will call her mother.

As you read the continuation of the case scenario, consider the following questions:

- What would be the best way for Nurse Debbie to handle this situation?
- Should the nurse manager intervene? If so, what strategies can she or he take?

BOX 4.2 CASE SCENARIO *(continued)*

Nurse Debbie enters the room and apologizes for the interruption and asks Nurse Patricia to step outside for a moment to assist her and says that they would be a few minutes and return. They proceed to the workroom where Nurse Debbie advises Nurse Patricia that she overheard the patient crying and asked how she could help. She asked Nurse Patricia why she is taking that approach with the patient. Nurse Patricia admitted she had a similar experience with her family member getting pregnant as a teenager that "ruined" her family member's life and wants to prevent it from happening to other teenagers. Nurse Debbie verbalized she understood and sympathized with her experience but pointed out the patient's right to get the information and resources needed to prevent pregnancy and to provide a safe environment for the patient to ask questions and come back with any concerns in the future. Nurse Patricia then realized her own personal influence on the way she interacted with the patient. Nurse Patricia returned to the patient and apologized for her abruptness, provided her with the necessary information and referral appointment, and advised the patient that the information would be confidential and not shared with her mother.

Nurse Debbie's actions highlight her leadership skills and all five of the professional values—altruism (concern for the welfare of the patient), autonomy (the right of the patient to get contraceptive information and resources), human dignity (respect for the patient and colleague in understanding the situation first before taking action), integrity (making sure appropriate care is given), and social justice (fair treatment given to the teenager regardless of personal opinions).

APPLICATION TO PRACTICE—SELF-AWARENESS AND ADVOCACY

Essential VIII—Professionalism and Professional Values (AACN, 2008) for the baccalaureate-prepared nurse highlights that one behavior of a professional nurse is the awareness and responsibility to understand the impact of their attitudes, values, and expectations when caring for others, especially those vulnerable populations, such as the economically disadvantaged, racial and ethnic minorities, the uninsured, low-income children, the elderly, the homeless, those with human immunodeficiency virus (HIV), those with severe mental illness, and even those who chose an alternative lifestyle (e.g., same-sex partners). In the case scenario presented in Box 4.2, Nurse Debbie exemplifies this professional behavior in that she took the leadership role in assisting her colleague in understanding how her personal experience was influencing her care of her patient and how she needed to acknowledge her bias but still render the care needed.

The case scenario in Box 4.3 describes how nurses advocate for their patients. Think of an example where you had to advocate for your patient, where you felt you were "heard," and had respectful collaboration to assist you in dealing with the situation at hand. Have you experienced moral distress and powerlessness where you felt your voice was not heard or disregarded? How did you handle that situation?

BOX 4.3 CASE SCENARIO

Nurse Jose is caring for his patient Paul in the medical ICU, a 42-year-old male with end-stage liver disease. Upon admission, Paul is alert and oriented; he has full knowledge and understanding of his disease and prognosis. In speaking with Paul, Nurse Jose gains an understanding of his patient's wishes with regards to end-of-life care; he knows his patient is "at peace" and although he does not wish to die, he does not want futile attempts and prolonged use of artificial means to support his life. Nurse Jose asks Paul if he has an advance directive but Paul was advised he did not need one—because his family "knows his wishes and what to do." Paul's clinical condition deteriorates and he loses the capacity for decision-making; his family indicates that "all measures" should be taken to "keep him alive." Nurse Jose attempts to share his understanding of the patient's wishes with the team, but the team indicates "not your decision." Aggressive measures are implemented; 2 weeks pass with no improvement with full life-sustaining treatment maintained. Nurse Jose asks for help in addressing his concerns, but was surprised that his colleagues reported it was up to the medical team to get an ethics consult and shared their frustrations with "the system." Nurse Jose persists and contacts the ethics consult and gets assistance in coordinating a meeting with the medical team, nursing, and patient's family to discuss goals of care. Not satisfied with the current system to address ethical concerns, Nurse Jose works with his colleagues to develop a proposal for a nurse-driven ethics consult and educational program in collaboration with the ethics department in the hospital. The proposal was accepted and the program implemented.

APPLICATION TO PRACTICE—ROLE-MODELING

In the case scenario discussed in Box 4.3, Nurse Jose demonstrated a core skill of a baccalaureate nurse in not settling when he saw a need to advocate for his patient in accessing the resources needed to resolve the ethical dilemma he identified in the conflict with the patient's known wishes and the plan of care. He demonstrated his leadership in communicating and raising the system issue that did not permit nurse autonomy to call for an ethics consultation when needed, lack of adequate educational programs to enhance nurses' skills in managing difficult ethical situations, and a structured forum in which nurses had an opportunity to debrief with peers. Nurse

Jose established a team of nurses and other key stakeholders to develop and implement systematic changes not only for his unit but also throughout the organization.

In this case scenario, the safety and quality of care to leadership. Sorrell (2012) highlights the role impact of the 2010 Institute of Medicine (IOM) report, the *Future of Nursing: Leading Change, Advancing Health,* in ensuring that nurses practice to the fullest extent of their education and training. For the promotion of patient safety and care, it is essential for nurses to be accountable and responsible for the delivery of safe and quality patient care.

As you read this case scenario in Box 4.4, think about your role and work environment. What ethical challenges have you encountered? How have you handled situations where you have observed lapses in nursing professional practice and care? How would you approach ethical situations now as a baccalaureate nurse and leader? What makes the difference?

BOX 4.4 CASE SCENARIO

Annie, a nurse, was at the bedside of her father in the cardiac ICU. During the course of his hospitalization, Annie was surprised at the variation of competence and care among the nurses assigned to her father. She was dismayed to see the lack of critical thinking and initiative by the nurses and residents in addressing some of her concerns related to her father's plan of care. Annie struggled with escalation of what she considered inadequate care and the possible "reaction" from the staff, but also weighed her duty as a professional nurse for ensuring that quality and safe care is provided. As a result, she had to escalate her concerns to the nurse manager and medical team for resolution.

STRATEGIES TO ADDRESS ETHICAL ISSUES AND CHALLENGES

Rushton and Broome (2015) highlighted the collaborative work of the Johns Hopkins University School of Nursing and Berman Institute of Bioethics in the creation of "A Blueprint for 21st Century Nursing Ethics" as a resource for organizations and nurses to use to support ethical nursing practice and culture. The blueprint highlights the need for a system that integrates ethics within clinical practice, nursing education, research, and nursing policy. It also stresses the importance of establishing an inventory of available resources (standards, guidelines, and best practices), clear policies, and metrics to assess outcomes related to ethics to sustain an ethical culture (www.bioethicsinstitute.org/nursing-ethics-summit-report). Other strategies found in the literature that nurses can take the lead and implement within their work environment include (Raines, 2000):

- *Provide Nursing Ethics Resources*: Organize resources (articles, policies and other resources) related to ethics and ethical leadership into a central repository for easy staff access.
- *Sponsor and Engage in Activities*: Colleagues should gather to form a nursing ethics committee; to form an ethics journal club; to establish nursing grand rounds focusing on ethical leadership.
- *Standardize and Incorporate Discussion of Ethics and Ethical Leadership*: Ethics should be included as a standing staff meeting agenda item for nurses to openly raise ethical dilemmas encountered and strategies from peers on best practices to handle them.
- *Participate*: Nurses should have representation on the organization/agency's ethics committee.

Other actions that each nurse leader may use to enhance his or her ethical leadership include:

- *Knowledge/Competency*: Know the rules (laws, standards of practice, organizational policies and procedures) under which you work. Engage in continuous learning to maintain skills and competency related to your work environment and nursing role.
- *Communicate*: Your beliefs, concerns with colleagues—ask yourself: "What is the goal; what am I trying to achieve?"; ask for help if needed when faced with a difficult ethical decision.
- *Scrupulous*: Be rigorous in difficult challenging situations. Think twice before taking shortcuts—stop when thinking: "It should be okay—just this once." Think instead of: "Is this really okay to proceed in this manner?" and "Is it ethical?"
- *Stop and Think*: Before any action, make sure you have the facts, take out any emotional bias, pause, and test your decision; ask questions such as: "Can I discuss my decision with people whom I respect and trust openly?" Consider the consequences of your decision before taking action—ask yourself, "Who could be negatively impacted by my decision?"
- *Storytelling*: Share experiences related to ethical dilemmas and discuss how they were addressed or not. What were the consequences or "lessons learned"—either positive or negative—from that decision or actions taken. Storytelling can be a great motivator for making ethical choices.
- *Celebrate*: Praise sound ethical decisions during staff meetings, educational programs, and encourage staff to share their examples. Ethical exemplars should be the "norm" and not the singled out "heroic" measures.
- *Encourage*: Open discussions on ethical challenges experienced by staff; make it a safe haven to candidly discuss different viewpoints; as a team discuss strategies on how to handle resources that are available when confronted with these challenges.

- *Formalize*: Establish an ethics program—at unit and/or department level.
- *Lead by Example*: Remember: you do not need a title to be a nurse leader. Lead by example and behave ethically in all you do. Avoid complacency when confronted with colleagues' comments and attitudes that "it has always been done this way." Assist your colleagues when you observe them struggling with a situation or an unsafe practice that needs to be addressed.

There are several tools to assess ethical leadership. Thornton (2013), an educator in ethical leadership, developed questions that leaders may use to perform an annual self-assessment of their ethical leadership behaviors. Thorton posed 10 questions for business leaders, which were modified for nurse leaders (Box 4.5).

BOX 4.5 SELF-ASSESSMENT ON ETHICAL LEADERSHIP

Use this Ethical Leadership checklist to perform a self-assessment of your ethical leadership. When you have responded to the questions, develop a plan to improve those areas where you perceive improvement is needed. Within your improvement plan prioritize actions with a defined timeline for completion because you cannot work on all areas at once. Reassess your ethical leadership behaviors at least annually.

As a nurse leader:

1. How do I define "ethical leadership"?
2. How do my professional values influence my ethical behavior?
3. As a nurse leader, would others recognize that I am an ethical leader? Describe your behaviors that demonstrate ethical leadership.
4. Do I create an ethical environment that is just and fair for my colleagues and patients?
5. How consistently do I show respect when my views do not align with someone else's views?
6. How do I meet my ethical obligation to address the care of patients?
7. How well do I meet my ethical responsibility to address the organizational system or process concerns that may influence patient care?
8. Are there opportunities to be more proactive and intentional about ethics—my behavior and culture of ethics within my work setting?
9. How well do I mange ethical conflicts encountered in the clinical setting?
10. How much importance do I put on engaging in continuous education to enhance my knowledge and skills to be an effective ethical leader, especially when addressing ethical issues?

Resources: Tools related to self-assessment of ethical leadership may be found at:

- https://leadingincontext.com/2013/12/18/10-ethical-leadership-questions-for-the-new-year
- https://ache.org/newclub/career/ethself.cfm

SPIRITUAL ASPECTS OF EFFECTIVE LEADERSHIP

What defines a spiritual leader? Strack and Fottler (2002) posed an interesting question in their review of the literature on spirituality and effective leadership as follows, "Does the level of a leader's spirituality affect his or her effectiveness as a leader?" (p. 3). Reave (2005) also explored the relationship between spirituality and leadership effectiveness. Although years apart in their studies of spirituality and effective leadership, similar themes emerged. Reave (2005) highlighted that spiritual leadership is the embodiment of spiritual values such as integrity ("walking the talk") and behaviors such as the expressing of caring and concern. It is the demonstration of actions in the consistent application of ethics in practice, respect, and concern shown to others. As a nurse leader, you will have an opportunity to promote an environment that enhances not only the quality care but also the growth of employees. Being a nurse requires a commitment to our patients' well-being, but being a nursing leader requires that you also care for the nursing team (Caldeira & Hall, 2012). One way to promote both is to foster spiritual leadership that leads to the provision of spiritual care for patients and spiritual growth for employees (Burkhart, Solari-Twadell, & Haas, 2008). Spirituality is an important dimension of nursing care but it is also a factor in the workplace because it helps us have meaning and fulfillment in our profession. Workplace spirituality has to do with the meaning and purpose of our work and that our roles as nurses make a difference. Nurses work in healthcare settings that can be challenging and may leave nurses questioning the meaning of life and reflecting on their own life journeys. For example, a nurse working in a neonatology unit, an oncology unit, or an intensive care unit may be faced with suffering, which can leave one contemplating the purpose of life. Given how demanding the work of a nurse can be, it is imperative that nurses feel they are cared about by nurse leaders. A spiritual leader cares about the team's well-being as well as each member individually. A nurse leader can inspire nurses to find meaning in their nursing profession.

Workplace spirituality has many positive outcomes (International Institute for Spiritual Leadership, n.d.):

- Increased job satisfaction
- Increased commitment
- Improved productivity, creativity, and flexibility
- Reduced absenteeism
- Reduced turnover
- Less fearful employees
- More ethical employees
- More committed employees

It is important to note that workplace spirituality is not about a specific religion or a specific belief system. Workplace spirituality is about leaders and workers who have a sense of calling that provides meaning and purpose for their lives. In addition, it involves an environment where employees feel a sense of belonging as well as connectedness to each other and their patients.

As a nurse leader, what can you do to promote workplace spirituality? You can accomplish this by giving yourself and your colleagues an opportunity to reflect on your work experiences (Burkhart et al., 2008). The reflective process can be transformative. Some institutions may choose to do this through brown-bag lunch sessions and staff meetings whereas others may choose to have retreats. Facilitators can help guide the discussion with many institutions tapping into resources available through pastoral care services. A critical aspect of the reflection process is storytelling, which reflects on the meaning of those experiences. McCann (2012) outlines other strategies to promote spiritual leadership, such as:

- *Mindfulness*: Approach life and work in a calm manner and an awareness of the work environment. Acknowledge one size does not fit all and that you may not have the answers, but are willing to learn.
- *Mission*: Understand your organization's culture and mission with an ability to promote change as needed.
- *Engagement*: Work with teams in a collaborative manner where everyone, at all levels, is encouraged to participate and offer an opinion on how to address the situation at hand.
- *Balance*: Promote work–life balance for health and well-being in self and others. It is the ability to recognize when you need to step out of the moment and not react to the initial emotions that arise with "heart versus head" and understand how your reactions and actions may influence others both positively and negatively.

LEGAL ASPECTS OF EFFECTIVE LEADERSHIP

As a nurse leader, you need to be familiar with the legal aspects of your role. For starters, it helps to be familiar with key terms. The term "law" often refers to a system of rules of conduct are binding and may be enforced. Sources of law include the U.S. Constitution (Bill of Rights), legislation (statutes such as Nurse Practice Acts), administration (government agencies, state boards), and common law (judicial decisions that are not codified in statutes or laws but used as precedent for future cases). Nursing practice is governed by established regulations and laws that serve as professional guidelines to ensure quality of care and to protect the public. Standards are used as the foundation in determining what is the "reasonable" care that a patient/client should receive and how nurses should act given the same situation. Standards and regulations are derived from various sources such as internal organization/agency (policies and procedures), professional organizations (guidelines, community standards, and evidence-based practices), state (Department of Health Regulations, Nurse Practice Acts), and national (Patient's Bill of Rights, The Joint Commission Accreditation Standards, and Centers for Medicare and Medicaid Services Conditions of Participation Regulations).

Styles, Schumann, Bickford, and White (2008) established the Model of Professional Nursing Practice Regulation, which illustrates the foundation of regulation (specific laws and guidelines) of nursing practice as a four-level tier that supports the provision of outcomes of safe, quality, evidence-based nursing practice (Figure 4.1). The first level is Nursing Professional Scope of Practice, Standards of Practice, Code of Ethics, and Specialty Certification. The second level is Nurse Practice Acts and Rules and Regulations. The third level comprises Institutional Policies and Procedures. At the top of the pyramid is Self-Determination. The baccalaureate nurse leader has the professional responsibility and accountability to know these laws and guidelines and to apply these rules in determining his or her own practice. When confronted with ethical dilemmas or scope of practice problems, the nurse leader could seek clarification from the organization's policies and procedures, progress to the applicable state nurse practice act (NPA) as needed, and access other resources within the code of ethics to determine what is needed in the provision of safe, quality care that is evidence based.

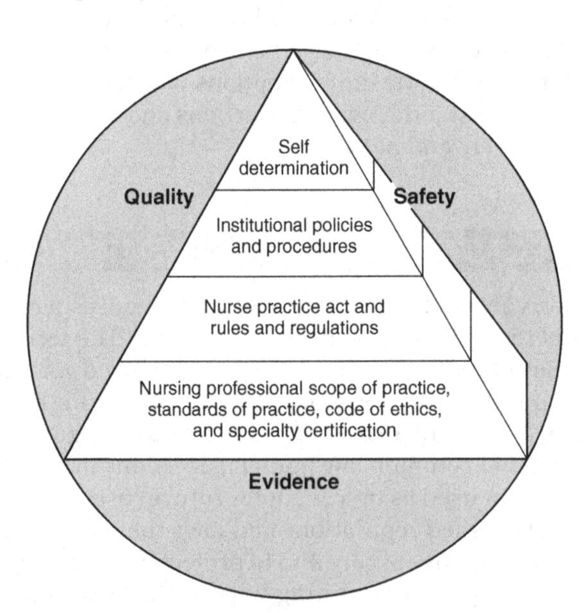

FIGURE 4.1 Model of Professional Nursing Practice Regulation.

Styles, M. M., Schumann, M. J., Bickford, C. J., & White, K. (Eds.). (2008). *Specializing and credentialing in nursing revisited: Understanding the issues, advancing the profession*. Silver Spring, MD: American Nurses Association.

NURSE PRACTICE ACT

Each state and territory within the United States has enacted an NPA (National Council of State Boards of Nursing [NCSBN], 2017), which defines the laws for the professional practice of nursing. Each state and territory has an established state Board of Nursing (BON) to further define the rules and regulations related to the NPA. As a general rule, all NPAs include language governing (NCSBN, 2017):

- Authority, power, and composition of a BON
- Educational program standards
- Standards and scope of nursing practice
- Types of titles and licenses
- Requirements for licensure
- Grounds for disciplinary action, enforcement action, and reinstatement rules

The case scenarios in Boxes 4.6 and 4.7 describe practice situations faced by nurses. It is critical for nurses to fully understand their state's Nurse Practice Act (NPA). As you read these case scenarios think about the following:

- How it would play out in your state?
- What do you know about your own NPA which governs your practice as a registered professional nurse? If you are not familiar with your state's NPA to to its website and review the scope of nursing practice.

BOX 4.6 CASE SCENARIO

Nurse Rachel, a travel nurse, was working in the triage area in the emergency department (ED), where a patient presented with chest pain. Nurse Rachel went to immediately initiate an ECG, conduct lab tests, initiate oxygen supply, administer aspirin and an IV on the patient. Nurse Amy, who was team leader in the ED, stopped her from taking actions and immediately notified the ED physician of the patient's status. Orders were written and Nurse Rachel implemented those orders. Afterwards, Nurse Rachel questioned why she could not act independently given the emergency situation and her assessment of the patient and reported that in her prior assignment in another state she was permitted to do so. Nurse Amy explained that in this state, it was outside the scope of nursing practice to implement this type of nonpatient–specific standing order and a patient-specific order from the provider was needed. When she questioned the accuracy of her statement, Nurse Amy showed her the hospital's policy related to orders and the state's BON webpage, which outlined the scope of practice for nursing for that state.

BOX 4.7 CASE SCENARIO

As you read this case scenario, consider as a nurse leader how you would have responded in the following situation. Are you aware of the policies and procedures within your work environment related to the scope of nursing practice?

Nurse Mary observes an unsafe practice by Nurse Joyce, a nurse with seniority, in administering medications without completing the five rights check and use of a secondary source (medication orders or medication administration record) as required by hospital policy. Nurse Mary tried to raise the issue with Nurse Joyce about her safety concern when Nurse Joyce stated: "I know the rules—but I know what to do and know my patients...I have never made any medication errors... worry about your own practice." Nurse Mary feels she attempted to raise this safety issue with her peer to no avail. She believes that the nurse manager is aware of this unsafe practice and allows it to continue. Nurse Mary feels she is not the "leader" of the unit and therefore it is not her responsibility to intervene further.

PATIENT BILL OF RIGHTS

Nurse leaders should be familiar with the Patient's Bill of Rights. A Patient's Bill of Rights was first established by the American Hospital Association (AHA) in 1973, to promote and standardize care practices related to the rights of hospitalized patients (Pecorino, 2002). In 1992, the AHA modified the document to include additional rights and clarifying language to better define a patient's rights. The last modification occurred in 2001 with repacking of the information by changing "A Patient's Bill of Rights" to "The Patient Care Partnership: Understanding Expectations, Rights, and Responsibilities" (AHA, 2003). Patients' rights remain the same and are organized into six sections:

1. High-quality hospital care
2. A clean and safe environment
3. Patient involvement in care
4. Protection of your privacy
5. Preparing you and your family for when you leave the hospital
6. Help with your bill and filing insurance claims

In addition, the Joint Commission's accreditation standards "Rights and Responsibilities of the Individual" outlines requirements organizations must successfully demonstrate related to their commitment to a patient's rights through the ways that staff and caregivers interact with the patient and involve him or her in care, treatment, and services (The Joint Commission, 2017). The Patient's Bill of Rights is mandated for provision of healthcare services and is adapted on the basis of the clinical healthcare setting (hospital, nursing home residential facilities, clinics, etc.).

QUESTIONS TO CONSIDER BEFORE READING ON

Have you ever read the Patient's Bill of Rights? Do you provide this to your patients/clients upon orientation to the unit/facility?

The case scenario in Box 4.8 describes the application of the bill of rights in your day to day practice as a nurse in caring for your patients. As you read this case scenario, consider the following questions:

- Do you know the mandatory reporting requirements by RNs for the state in which you practice?
- Think about how you would deal with the conflicting advice Nurse Patty received from her colleague on how to deal with her concerns for her patient's safety. How would you respond when you get feedback to just "let it go"?

BOX 4.8 CASE SCENARIO

Nurse Patty has been caring for a patient Jane who is an 80-year-old female admitted for failure to thrive and dementia. The patient has capacity which waxes and wanes at times. Her husband is deceased and her son, also on staff with the organization and who lives with her, visits frequently. The staff has had to intervene with the son who was observed to be yelling at the patient and slapping her arm on several occasions. The son appeared contrite, apologized indicating he was having a "bad day." Nurse Patty told the son she understood because she had a parent she cared for who had similar issues. The patient frequently asked for her son. After the son left the unit, Nurse Patty asked the patient about her home life and if she was treated well at home. Jane looked away and indicated she was "fine." When assisting the patient out of bed, Nurse Patty noted slight bruising on the patient, which may have been attributed to her history of falls, but Nurse Patty was unsettled about the patient's assessment and asked the patient about how she got the bruise. Jane was noncommittal and just indicated "I want to go home." Nurse Patty thought about her own mother who bruised easily and debated escalating to her manager because the patient's son was on staff and did not want to cause "trouble" for him. She spoke with her colleague on the unit who advised her not to make waves and let the social worker deal with it. Despite this advice, Nurse Patty thought about her role to keep the patient safe and went to her manager and social worker. A case was opened with Adult Protective Services to investigate the home environment and support needed for a safe discharge.

PROFESSIONAL ADVOCACY

Professional advocacy is part of the nurse leader's role. Consider the term "advocacy" and how it is defined. Grace (2001) and Mahlin (2010) highlight the lack of a clear definition of advocacy. Most nurses would consider advocacy in relation to their role in the provision of care to patients. The ANA *Code of Ethics* (2015) specifically highlights advocacy in Provision 3, which defines one standard of practice of professional nursing in the promotion and advocacy for the rights, health, and safety of patients. But advocacy goes beyond the role of patient advocate by the nurse and work environment. Other provisions of the ANA *Code of Ethics* (2015) indeed highlight the critical role of nurses as advocates for their own health, their professional development, the overall promotion and advancement of the profession of nursing, development of professional standards, as well as nursing and health policy. Foundational to ethical leadership is the promotion of professional advocacy. Grace (2001) argues that a broader view of professional advocacy is needed that encompasses the nurse leader's role in advocating and furthering health to both individuals and society. A nurse's advocacy responsibilities are viewed as central to ethical leadership and can extend beyond taking actions on behalf of patients to investigation and improvement of organizational systems and processes, and even collaborative political action at the professional organizational, local, and/or national levels (Grace, 2001; Mahlin, 2010).

QUALITY AND SAFETY EDUCATION for NURSES (QSEN) CONSIDERATIONS

Reflect on QSEN knowledge, skills, attitudes (KSA) competencies related to ethical skills development (AACN, 2012; Cronenwett et al., 2007). Conduct a self-assessment of your skills in day-to-day practice related to the following competencies presented in Table 4.2 QSEN competencies.

- Describe how you incorporate these skills into your practice.
- Describe one or two actions you can take to enhance your skills/ practice.

TABLE 4.2 QSEN COMPETENCIES

QSEN Graduate-Level Competencies (Knowledge, Skills, Attitudes): ● Patient-Centered Care ● Quality Improvement ● Safety	Describe how you incorporate this skill in your practice today—what is your attitude regarding this value?	Describe additional steps you could take to enhance your skills.
Patient-Centered Care: Recognize the patient or designee as the source of control and full partner in providing compassionate and coordinated care based on respect for patient's preferences, values, and needs.		
Knowledge: Analyze multiple dimensions of patient-centered care, including patient/family/community preferences and values, as well as social, cultural, psychological, and spiritual contexts.		
Skill: On the basis of active listening to patients, elicit patient values, preferences, and expressed needs as part of clinical interview, diagnosis, implementation of care plan, as well as coordination and evaluation of care.		
Knowledge: Analyze ethical and legal implications of patient-centered care.		
Skill: Work to address ethical and legal issues related to patients' rights to determine their care.		
Knowledge: Describe the limits and boundaries of patient-centered care.		
Skill: Support patients in their decisions even when a decision conflicts with personal values.		
Knowledge: Analyze concepts related to conflictual decision-making by patients.		
Skill: Assess level of patient's decisional conflict and provide appropriate support, education, and resources.		
Knowledge: Analyze personal attitudes, values, and beliefs related to patient-centered care.		

(continued)

TABLE 4.2 QSEN COMPETENCIES *(continued)*

QSEN Graduate-Level Competencies (Knowledge, Skills, Attitudes): • **Patient-Centered Care** • **Quality Improvement** • **Safety**	**Describe how you incorporate this skill in your practice today—what is your attitude regarding this value?**	**Describe additional steps you could take to enhance your skills.**
Skill: Continuously assess and monitor own efforts to be patient centered.		
Quality Improvement: Use data to monitor the outcomes of care processes and use improvement methods to design and test changes to continuously improve the quality and safety of healthcare systems.		
Knowledge: Analyze ethical issues associated with continuous quality improvement.		
Skill: Participate in the design and monitoring of ethical oversight of continuous quality improvement projects; maintain confidentiality of any patient information.		
Safety: Minimize risk of harm to patients and providers through both system effectiveness and individual performance.		
Knowledge: Identify best practices that promote patient, community, and provider safety in the practice setting.		
Skill: Integrate strategies and safety practices to reduce risk of harm to patients, self, and others.		
Knowledge: Analyze human factors safety design principles as well as commonly used unsafe practices (e.g., work-arounds, risky behavior, and hazardous abbreviations).		
Skill: Demonstrate leadership skills in creating a culture where safe design principles are developed and implemented. Skill: Engage in systems focus when errors or near misses occur. Skill: Promote systems that reduce reliance on memory.		

(continued)

TABLE 4.2 QSEN COMPETENCIES *(continued)*

QSEN Graduate-Level Competencies (Knowledge, Skills, Attitudes): • Patient-Centered Care • Quality Improvement • Safety	Describe how you incorporate this skill in your practice today—what is your attitude regarding this value?	Describe additional steps you could take to enhance your skills.
Knowledge: Summarize methods to identify and prevent verbal, physical, and psychological harm to patients and staff.		
Skill: Encourage a positive practice environment of high trust and high respect. Skill: Develop culture where a hostile work environment is not tolerated. Skill: Use best practices and legal requirements to report and prevent harm.		

As you read the case scenario in Box 4.9, consider how the nurse leader is demonstrating professional advocacy.

- What does professional advocacy mean to you as a nurse leader?
- What behaviors exemplify professional advocacy?

BOX 4.9 CASE SCENARIO

During a staff meeting, the director of nursing reviewed clinical data on implementation of orders; gaps in practice were highlighted related to nurses applying oxygen and other interventions without orders. Clinical nurses expressed their frustration at not being able to independently act using approved protocols as other nurses do in other states and were reminded it was out of scope of practice within their state and subject to disciplinary action. Clinical nurses sought guidance from their chief nurse officer (CNO) as to how to change the rule to permit them autonomy in implementing an approved protocol and interventions on the basis of their nursing assessment and plan of care. The CNO provided several strategies they could do at the "grassroots" level, including reaching out to the local professional nursing organizations for additional information. The CNO offered to be an advisor for the project and encouraged the staff to get involved. Subsequently, the nurses joined their local organization task force to address nonpatient-specific standing orders.

CONCLUSIONS

Let us never consider ourselves finished nurses ... we must be learning all of our lives.

—Florence Nightingale

In summary, this chapter provided a review of the foundations for effective leadership. Knowledge and behaviors related to ethical practice, spiritual awareness, legal requirements, and professional advocacy are core dimensions of an effective nurse leader. Attention to ethical leadership in nursing has diminished over the years (Makaroff, Storch, Pauly, & Newton, 2014). Ethical nurse leaders are responsible with regard to their practice to be aware of the organizational work environment, to establish systems to enhance nurse's knowledge of ethics within their practice, and to facilitate discussion of ethics in the day-to-day practice environment.

Ethical behavior is knowing and doing what is right. Defining what is "right" is the dilemma often faced by nurses and in many instances there is no "right" answer that will apply to all circumstances. As discussed in this chapter, within the nursing profession there are several resources available to nurses to inform and guide nurse leaders as to the behaviors expected. Nurses, in every clinical setting, spend the majority of the time with patients and their families and as a result are in a unique position to understand and identify the core principles, values, and beliefs of their patients/families and how they impact their healing and well-being. This information should be integrated within the patients' goals and plans of care and communicated to other members of the healthcare team. Nurses' ability to appropriately identify, discuss, and address ethical issues is contingent upon their own skill level as well as the organizational system in which they work. Strategies to enhance ethical skill development have been provided—it starts with each nurse performing his or her own self-assessment, a review of the organizational support to provide educational programs on ethics topics (both clinical and professional behavioral focus), and unit-level support to provide a "safe haven" to share ethical concerns with peers and other team members.

A nurse leader is the person who influences and guides direction, opinion, and actions to achieve goals. People know effective leadership when they see it. An effective leader has intrinsic qualities of integrity, spirituality, courage, initiative, and resilience. An effective leader consistently demonstrates critical thinking in provision of care and development of solutions to address system or process problems to improve the quality of care. An effective leader is self-aware and strives for excellence through engaging with others in obtaining feedback and providing feedback as needed. An effective nurse leader takes the time to understand and listen to others and incorporates purposeful mindfulness in all interactions with patients, families, colleagues, and others to promote collaboration and teamwork to achieve desired outcomes and goals. An effective nurse leader does not settle for the status quo, but takes an active role in self-assessment and continuous learning, and advocates for patients and the advancement of the profession of nursing. Think about your own professional practice: Do you consider yourself an effective leader? If not, why? If not, what are you going to do today and tomorrow to become an effective leader? What is your path to effective leadership: What changes can you make now?

> *Leading with positive ethical values builds trust and brings out the best in people, which brings out the best in the organization, which leads to great results....*
>
> —Author Unknown

CRITICAL THINKING QUESTIONS AND ACTIVITIES

- The establishment of effective and ethical nursing leadership was highlighted in the directives written by Florence Nightingale (2009, p. 767)

> The person in charge of everyone must see to be just and candid, looking at both sides, not moved by entreaties, or by likes and dislikes, but only by justice; and always reasonable, remembering and not forgetting the wants of those of whom she is in charge. She must have a keen though generous insight into the characters of those she has to control. They must know that she cares for them even when she is checking them; or rather that she checks them because she cares for them.
>
> [L]et whoever is in charge keep this simple question in her head (*not*, how can I always do the right thing myself, but) how can I provide for this right thing to be always done?

These directives are further illustrated in the ANA *Code of Ethics*. Carefully re-read and consider these directives as written by Florence Nightingale; review the ANA *Code of Ethics*. Then, perform your own self-assessment:

- How have you incorporated these principles within your daily practice as a baccalaureate nurse?
- What changes can you make now to improve your practice as a nurse leader?
- Perform an assessment of your organization's approach to effective leadership. Do you see evidence of effective, ethical, and spiritual leadership? Provide some examples of each. How have nursing leaders in your organization demonstrated professional advocacy? Provide examples of the legal aspects of leadership within your organization.

(*continued*)

CRITICAL THINKING QUESTIONS AND ACTIVITIES *(continued)*

- How does your organization support nurses' knowledge of ethics? What changes can you propose to enhance nurses' knowledge of ethics as it applies to their practice?
- Shared Learning: Within your work environment, identify one or two ethical situations that you felt were challenging. Openly raise these issues with your peers and lead a team discussion on how to address these issues; use resources within your organization, such as the ethics consult, to partner with you in this discussion.
- Identify ethics resources within your organization and assess your peer's knowledge of these resources and how to access resources.
  - On the basis of the results, explore opportunities to establish a standing forum to discuss ethical issues experienced by nurses in your clinical setting, and explore other educational programs to foster an awareness of ethical leadership among nurses.
  - Present at least one or two opportunities to your local nurse leader and/or chief nursing officer. On the basis of feedback, be part of the team to develop and implement a program(s) to increase knowledge of ethics for nurses in your organization.
- Locate your organization's policy and procedures related to nursing scope of practice and your state board of nursing (BON). Locate your state BON website; resource to access specific state BON information is the National (www.ncsbn.org). On the state BON page, find the Nursing Practice Act and Enforcement sections; review the content and become familiar with definitions for enforcement actions, and if available, recent actions taken.
  - Identify one or two things that you were not previously aware of related to the practice of nursing within your state.
  - As a nurse leader, consider sharing this information with your colleagues.

REFERENCES

American Association of Colleges of Nursing. (2008, September). *The essentials of baccalaureate education for professional nursing practice.* Retrieved from http://www.aacnnursing.org/Portals/42/Publications/BaccEssentials08.pdf

American Association of Colleges of Nursing QSEN Education Consortium. (2012, September 24). Graduate-level QSEN competencies: Knowledge, skills and attitudes. Retrieved from http://www.aacnnursing.org/Portals/42/AcademicNursing/CurriculumGuidelines/Graduate-QSEN-Competencies.pdf?ver=2017-07-15-135425-900

American Hospital Association. (2003). The patient care partnership. Retrieved from https://www.aha.org/system/files/2018-01/aha-patient-care-partnership.pdf

American Nurses Association. (2015). *Code of ethics for nurses with interpretive statements.* Silver Spring, MD: Author. Retrieved from http://nursingworld.org/DocumentVault/Ethics-1/Code-of-Ethics-for-Nurses.html

Burkhart, L., Solari-Twadell, P. A., & Haas, S. (2008). Addressing spiritual leadership: An organizational model. *Journal of Nursing Administration, 38*(1), 33–39. doi:10.1097/01.NNA.0000295629.95592.78

Caldeira, S., & Hall, J. (2012). Spiritual leadership and spiritual care in neonatalogy. *Journal of Nursing Management, 20*(8), 1069–1075. doi:10.1111/jonm.1234

Cronenwett, L., Sherwood, G., Barnsteiner, J., Disch, J., Johnson, J., Mitchell, P., ... Warren, J. (2007). Quality and safety education for nurses. *Nursing Outlook, 55*(3), 122–131. doi:10.1016/j.outlook.2007.02.006

Gilbert, J. A. (2007). *Strengthening ethical wisdom: Tools for transforming your health care organization.* Washington, DC: Health Forum.

Grace, P. J. (2001). Professional advocacy: Widening the scope of accountability. *Nursing Philosophy, 2,* 151–162. doi:10.1046/j.1466-769X.2001.00048.x

Grande, D. (2015). Ethical leadership. *American Nurse.* Retrieved from http://www.theamericannurse.org/2015/05/01/ethical-leadership/

International Institute for Spiritual Leadership. (n.d.). What is spiritual leadership? Retrieved from http://iispiritualleadership.com/spiritual-leadership

The Joint Commission. (2017, January 9). *Comprehensive accreditation and certification manual for hospitals: The official handbook.* Oak Brook, IL: Author.

Kubsch, S., Hansen, G., & Huyser-Eatwell, V. (2008). Professional values: The case for RN-BSN completion education. *Journal of Continuing Education in Nursing, 39*(8), 375–384. doi:10.3928/00220124-20080801-05

Mahlin, M. (2010). Individual patient advocacy, collective responsibility and activism within professional nursing associations. *Nursing Ethics, 17*(2), 247–254. doi:10.1177/0969733009351949

Makaroff, K. S., Storch, J., Pauly, B., & Newton, L. (2014). Searching for ethical leadership in nursing. *Nursing Ethics, 21*(6), 642–658. doi:10.1177/0969733013513213

McCann, M. (2012, July 2). Spiritual leadership for management and activities. Retrieved from https://www.mcknights.com/news/spiritual-leadership-for-management-and-activities/article/248550

National Council of State Boards of Nursing. (2017). What are U.S. Boards of Nursing? Retrieved from https://www.ncsbn.org/about-boards-of-nursing.htm

Nightingale, F. (2009). Florence Nightingale's addresses to nurses. In L. McDonald (Ed.), *The Nightingale school: Collected works of Florence Nightingale* (Vol. 12). Waterloo, ON, Canada: Wilfrid Laurier University Press.

Norman, J. (2016, December 19). Americans rate healthcare providers high on honesty, ethics. *Gallup.* Retrieved from http://www.gallup.com/poll/200057/americans-rate-healthcare-providers-high-honesty-ethics.aspx

Pecorino, P. A. (2002). Bill of rights. In *Medical ethics: Rights, truth and consents.* Retrieved from http://www.qcc.cuny.edu/SocialSciences/ppecorino/MEDICAL_ETHICS_TEXT/Chapter_6_Patient_Rights/Readings_The%20Patient_Bill_of_Rights.htm

Raines, M. L. (2000). Ethical decision making in nurses: Relationships among moral reasoning, coping style, and ethics stress. *JONA'S Healthcare Law, Ethics and Regulation, 2*(1), 29–41. doi:10.1097/00128488-200002010-00006

Reave, L. (2005). Spiritual values and practices related to leadership effectiveness. *Leadership Quarterly, 16,* 655–687.

Robichaux, C. (2017). Developing ethical skills: A framework. In C. Robichaux (Ed.), *Ethical competence in nursing practice: Competencies, skills, decision-making* (pp. 23–46). New York, NY: Springer Publishing.

Rushton, C. H., & Broome, M. E. (2015). Safeguarding the public's health: Ethical nursing. *Hastings Center Report, 45*(1), insidebackcover. doi:10.1002/hast.410

Sorrell, J. (2012, July 3). Ethics: Creating a culture of ethical watchfulness. *Online Journal of Issues in Nursing, 17*(3), 9. Retrieved from http://ojin.nursingworld.org/MainMenuCategories/ANAMarketplace/ANAPeriodicals/OJIN/Columns/Ethics/Ethics-Culture-of-Ethical-Watchfulnes.html

Strack, G., & Fottler, M. D. (2002). Spirituality and effective leadership in healthcare: Is there a connection? *Frontiers of Health Services Management, 18*(4), 3–18. doi:10.1097/01974520-200204000-00002

Styles, M. M, Schumann, M. J, Bickford, C. J., & White, K. (Eds.). (2008). *Specializing and credentialing in nursing revisited: Understanding the issues, advancing the profession.* Silver Spring, MD: American Nurses Association.

Thornton, L. F. (2013). *7 Lenses: Learning the principles and practices of ethical leadership.* Richmond, VA: Leading in Context.

II

LEADERSHIP SKILLS ESSENTIAL TO THE PRACTICE OF NURSING

5

HANDLING STRESS IN THE WORKPLACE

SUSAN DENISCO

LEARNING OBJECTIVES

After completion of this chapter, the reader will be able to

- Explore the numerous factors that increase stress in the healthcare workplace.
- Discuss the effects of pathological stress on healthcare workers.
- Describe how workplace stress can negatively affect individuals and organizations.
- Identify stress management techniques.
- Develop an individual resilience self-care plan.

Stress is a common phenomenon in today's rapidly changing world. Healthcare workers are under enormous pressure to do more with less resources. As nurses, you should already be familiar with the physiology of stress and stress-related diseases. Stress management is an important life skill that will ensure success in your professional and personal life. Undoubtedly, you most likely use a variety of techniques outside of the workplace to control stress. As the worldwide nursing shortage continues, the aged population with chronic illnesses becomes larger, and technology continues to advance, nurses continually will be faced with numerous workplace stressors. As the largest group of healthcare professionals, it is imperative that nurses understand the physiology of stress, sources of stress, symptoms of stress, and strategies to prevent and alleviate stress and burnout. Adjustment to typical life cycle changes such as marriage, pregnancy, divorce, death, and retirement will also produce individual stress reactions and different coping responses for the same situation.

The ways in which individuals are affected depends on a number of factors such as level of confidence, adaptability, and resources available. In the workplace, nurses witness misfortune, suffering, and human distress on a routine basis. These stressors, which are associated with helping patients and families to overcome adversity, call upon the nurse's individual resilience. "Resilience" is the ability of an individual to positively adjust to adversity, and can be applied to building personal strength and capacity in nurses through the development of a self-reflective resilience action plan (Tusaie & Dyer, 2004). Building resilience and achieving positive levels of stress control have the potential to decrease fatigue, injury, and thus increase job satisfaction. It is well known that nurses working long hours under duress are more prone to making mistakes and medical errors where patient safety may suffer (Gulavani & Shinde, 2014).

"Self-care" refers to activities and practices that the nurse can engage in on a regular basis to reduce stress and both enhance and maintain health and well-being. Self-care is necessary for being effective in meeting professional nursing goals and honoring personal commitments. The nurse who practices self-care will become skilled at identifying and managing general challenges and stressors, will increase recognition of personal vulnerabilities, and will achieve a higher degree of balance in the different life domains.

This chapter provides a framework for the professional nurse to understand the causes and consequences of stress and develop an affinity for stress management strategies to bridge the gap between home and workplace. The benefits of strengthening personal resilience include lowering vulnerability to adversity, improving well-being, and achieving better care outcomes and a safer work environment.

HEALTHCARE SAFETY, BACCALAUREATE ESSENTIALS, AND QUALITY AND SAFETY EDUCATION for NURSES (QSEN)

HEALTHCARE SAFETY

In 2011, U.S. healthcare personnel experienced seven times the national rate of musculoskeletal disorders compared with all other private sector workers. To reduce the number of preventable injuries among healthcare personnel, the Centers for Disease Control and Prevention (CDC) collaborated with the National Institute for Occupational Safety and Health (NIOSH) to create the Occupational Health Safety Network (OHSN) to collect detailed injury data to help target prevention efforts (CDC, 2017). At 114 U.S. healthcare facilities surveyed, 10,680 OSHA-recordable injuries were reported: patient handling and movement injuries (4,674); slips, trips, and falls (3,972); and workplace violence injuries (2,034) occurring from January 1, 2012 to September 30, 2014 (Gomaa et al., 2015). Nursing personnel has the highest injury rates of all occupations examined (Figure 5.1). Focused interventions such as stress reduction strategies, practice of self-awareness, reciprocal trust, and enhanced communications can mitigate some of these injuries.

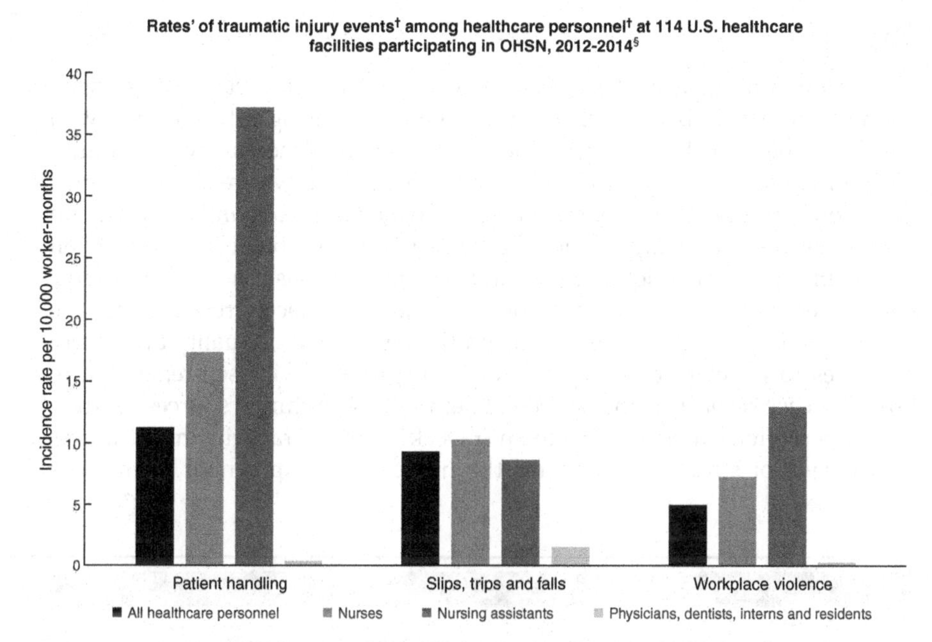

FIGURE 5.1 Rates of traumatic injury events among healthcare personnel at 114 U.S. healthcare facilities participating in OHSN, 2012–2014.

OHSN, Occupational Health Safety Network.

Source: Centers for Disease Control and Prevention. (2017). Data and injury trends among OHSN-participating facilities. Retrieved from https://www.cdc.gov/niosh/topics/ohsn/newinjury.html

BACCALAUREATE ESSENTIALS

When the American Association of Colleges of Nursing (AACN) endorsed the revision of the essentials for baccalaureate education (AACN, 2008), a seismic shift was occurring in the healthcare industry to include competencies that would support safe, quality, and cost-effective patient-centered care. Organizational and systems leadership, quality improvement, and safety are critical to promoting high-quality patient care. It became apparent that additional nursing skills were needed emphasizing ethical decision-making, maintaining mutually respectful communication, and successful collaboration within intra- and interprofessional teams. Baccalaureate education includes the essential development of professional values and value-based behavior. Understanding the values that patients and other health professionals bring to the therapeutic relationship is critically important in providing quality patient care. As healthcare systems become more complex and work demand increases, it is imperative that the baccalaureate-prepared nurse develop conflict resolution and stress management strategies including critical reflection, self-analysis, and valuing diversity in patients and colleagues.

QUALITY AND SAFETY EDUCATION IN NURSING

The overarching goal of the QSEN Institute and the Robert Wood Johnson Foundation (RWJF) is to meet the challenge of preparing future nurses who will have the knowledge, skills, and attitudes (KSAs) necessary to continuously improve the quality and safety of the healthcare systems within which they work (AACN, 2012; Cronenwett et al., 2007). Teamwork and collaboration are among the core competencies that nurses must be able to practice. When the healthcare team is not cohesive and communications cease to be productive, patient safety may be compromised and workplace stress become the norm. Nursing education must focus on the integration of quality and safety measures to develop a healthy workforce beginning with self-reflection. In Box 5.1, a case scenario is introduced to demonstrate common sources of stress that nurses often experience (Sullivan & Decker, 2005). Practicing mindfulness as a means of stress reduction for the nurse has the potential to increase

BOX 5.1 CASE SCENARIO

As you read this case scenario, reflect on the following questions:

- What are the sources of stress for Allison?
- What symptoms of stress are Allison and her family experiencing?

Allison is a registered nurse with 7 years of experience in general medical–surgical nursing in a mid-sized community teaching hospital. She is a single parent of two school-aged children who attend a before and after school program while she is at work. Allison was recently promoted to be a nurse manager over 32-bed medical–surgical unit. In this role, she has 24-hour responsibility for staffing and problems that arise on the evening and night shifts. She finds herself returning to the unit on weekends or after hours once or twice a week, which necessitates her finding a babysitter for her young family. With a 20% nurse vacancy rate on her units, she finds herself constantly scrambling for nursing coverage. She has had to resort to mandating nurses to work double shifts, which has caused low morale and conflict among her staff. The hospital recently announced that it is being acquired by a large corporation effective in 3 months and layoffs are being planned. Allison has been assigned to four departmental committees and was asked to lead the implementation of a nurse residency program for new graduate students. Allison feels burdened with all her responsibilities and finds herself taking work home to complete tasks such as performance reviews and quality improvement reports. Recently, Allison's 6-year-old daughter has started wetting the bed and she has been called to school to discuss her 8-year-old son's disruptive behavior in the classroom. Allison finds herself not being able to sleep, having overeating tendencies, and having frequent headaches. Despite what should be a positive experience of "the promotion," Allison and her family are experiencing physical and emotional signs of stress.

caregiver presence, build personal resilience, and stimulate empathy thereby contributing to positive patient outcomes (Antanaitis, 2015).

PHYSIOLOGY OF STRESS AND RELATION TO PATHOLOGY

"Stress" can be defined as the nonspecific reaction of the body to a perceived threat or demand. The purpose of stress is to prepare the body for physical action and can be both positive and negative. Eustress is a positive force that adds excitement and challenge to life, which can be motivating and a constructive mechanism to help us achieve our goals. Conversely, distress is a negative force where perceived demands or pressures exceed current resources resulting in unhealthy, negative, and destructive responses (Borkowski, 2011). The way an individual responds to a stressor is dependent on a variety of factors including the person's perception of the stress, physical and mental well-being, and involvement in meaningful relationships.

When the sympathetic nervous system becomes activated by a perceived threat, the chemicals epinephrine (adrenaline) and norepinephrine (noradrenaline) are released by the adrenal medulla and cortisol by the nervous system (McCance & Huethe, 2014). Table 5.1 outlines the physiological responses to stress.

TABLE 5.1 PHYSIOLOGICAL RESPONSES TO STRESS

Physiological Activation	Physical Reactions
Nervous system (NS) • Sympathetic NS—hormone release • Parasympathetic NS—resting state	Dry mouth Heart palpitations Elevated blood pressure Blood pressure rises Sweating Fatigue Loose stools
Stress hormones • Adrenaline • Noradrenaline • Cortisol	
Cortisol • Corticotropin releasing hormone (CRH) • Adrenal stimulation • Production of extra glucose and fatty acids	Immune suppression Heart disease Cancer Osteoporosis Aging

TABLE 5.2 GENERAL ADAPTATION SYSTEM STRESS RESPONSES
Alarm reaction phase: Mobilization of resources ready for either fight or flight
Resistance phase: Use of resources to fight the stressor; flight response disappears
Exhaustion phase: The depletion of individual's energy reserve

These fight and flight hormones are released in response to imminent danger. The heart rate increases, and blood flow increases to core organs and muscles, and decreases to peripheral or nonessential areas, for example, the gut. This results in increased blood pressure, sweating, rapid and shallow breathing, and tension in the muscles (Selye, 1950). These physiological responses result in the development of the general adaptation system (GAS). The GAS describes the three sequential phases of responses to a stress event as the alarm phase, the resistance phase, and the exhaustion phase (Selye, 1950; Table 5.2).

QUESTIONS TO CONSIDER BEFORE MOVING ON

Reflect on the case scenario presented earlier and consider the following questions:

- What organizational factors are contributing to Allison's stress?
- What internal factors are contributing to Allison's stress?
- Is Allison experiencing any consequences related to her work environment?

WORK-RELATED STRESS

Nurses experience workplace stress from a variety of external and internal factors (Table 5.3). These stressors can be described as either acute or chronic in nature. External stressors encompass both organizational and interpersonal factors related to environmental conditions in the workplace, demands of the role, and relationships with colleagues (Wright, 2014). These stressors can result from intense skill set acquisition requirements, ethical dilemmas, caring for those who are suffering or dying, working with limited resources, challenging interpersonal relationships, and patient safety concerns.

"Patient safety" as defined by the QSEN is minimizing risk of harm to patients and providers through both system effectiveness and individual performance (AACN, 2008). With the stakes higher than ever for nurses to attain patient safety goals when a serious safety event does occur, nurses are often unrecognized "second victims." When nurses are involved in an unanticipated adverse patient event, in a medical error, and/or a patient-related injury, they often become traumatized by the event (Scott, Hwang, & Rogers, 2006). Commonly, these individuals feel personally responsible for the adverse outcome and begin to doubt their clinical decision-making skills and competence. They may experience emotional abuse, bullying, intimidation, humiliation, and neglect from coworkers (Lee et al., 2015).

TABLE 5.3 WORKPLACE STRESSORS: EXTERNAL AND INTERNAL

External Stressors	Internal Stressors
Organizational factors: • Environmental—lack of equipment, poor lighting, extreme temperatures, noise, alarms, tight workspace, violence • Managerial style—authoritarian, laissez-faire, or crisis-centered • Tasks and work load demands • Norms and expectations • Organizational integration **Interpersonal factors:** • Communication issues • Interdisciplinary conflict • Discrimination • Peer pressure • Personality conflict: passive, rude, domineering, aggressive	**Life cycle factors:** • Marriage, pregnancy, birth, moving, changing jobs, home purchase, death • Excess calories, excess caffeine, tobacco use, alcohol misuse, drugs, lack of sleep, lack of exercise **Mental health factors:** • Pessimistic, deficiency focusing, self-effacing, inflexible, unrealistic expectations, learned helplessness, lack of confidence in skills, level of resilience **Personality traits:** • Perfectionist, workaholic, types A and B personalities, perception of control

Internal stressors have to do with the individual nurse's physiological well-being, psychological tendencies, life cycle factors, and personality traits. Disproportional physical workplace stress exists including back injuries, chemical spills, and exposure to blood-borne pathogens resulting in both physical pain and consequent psychological stress. These stressors may lead to negative sequelae including physical symptoms, impaired mental health, compassion fatigue, resignation, job turnover, and burnout (Lachman, 2016).

CONSEQUENCES OF STRESS ON THE INDIVIDUAL AND THE ORGANIZATION

Stress has consequences for the individual nurse, the patient, the interdisciplinary healthcare team, and the organization at large. Workplace stress can be described as the physical and emotional effects that occur when there is disparity between the demands of the job and the ability of control the nurse has in meeting those demands. Whenever stress occurs, it is an indication that the demands placed upon the person have exceeded the person's personal resources, whether these resources are physical, emotional, economic, social, or spiritual (Lambert & Lambert, 2008). Thus, workplace stress occurs when the challenges and demands of work become excessive, the pressures of the workplace exceed the worker's ability to handle them, and job satisfaction turns to frustration and exhaustion.

QUESTIONS TO CONSIDER BEFORE MOVING ON

What physiological red flags should the nurse be aware of if he or she or a coworker is experiencing stress?

CONSEQUENCE OF INDIVIDUAL STRESSES

According to Lambert and Lambert (2008), consequences of stress in an individual can be categorized as cognitive, physical, emotional, and behavioral. Cognitive symptoms can include, but are not limited to, memory impairment, indecisiveness, poor concentration, lack of insight, seeing only the negative side of an issue, rumination, constant worrying, and fearful expectancy that something bad will happen. Physical symptoms may manifest as headache, myalgia, gastrointestinal issues, dizziness, insomnia, chest pain, palpitations, weight gain or loss, hives, loss of libido, and frequent upper respiratory infections. Emotionality may become apparent in moodiness, irritability, restlessness, short temper, impatience, inability to relax, and feeling "keyed up." Often individuals feel overwhelmed, which may lead to loneliness or isolation, and finally depression. Finally, behavioral symptoms can include disruption in eating patterns; insomnia or hypersomnia; social isolation; procrastination; neglecting responsibilities; self-medicating with alcohol, cigarettes, or drugs; nail biting; pacing; teeth grinding; jaw clenching; overreacting to unexpected problems; and picking fights with others (Khamisa, Oldenburg, Peltzer, & Ilic, 2015; Lambert, Lambert, & Yamase, 2003).

There are certain red flags that indicate that the individual is not coping well and may need a formal intervention or enrollment in a comprehensive health promotion program (Table 5.4). It is imperative that the individual brings his or her stress level under control in an effort to prevent long-term

TABLE 5.4 FOUR RED FLAGS

Psychological Red Flags	Physical Red Flags
• Prolonged anxiety, phobias, persistent fear • Depression that causes isolation from family and friends • Feeling worthless, helpless, not enjoying normal activities • Erratic behavior and mood swings that can cause self-harm or harm to others • Excessive use of alcohol or mood-altering substances • Perfectionism • Workaholic	• Excessive weight gain • Excessive weight loss • Colitis • Gastric ulcer • Heart palpitations • Chest pain • Chronic daily headaches • Hypertension

effects that can result in disruption of physical and psychological homeostasis. These include persistent anxiety and depression that is noted by others, erratic behavior and mood swings that may cause the nurse to self-medicate, and physical illnesses. It should be noted that any of these symptoms may also be the result of other comorbid psychological or physical conditions warranting a complete evaluation by a primary care provider.

ORGANIZATIONAL CONSEQUENCES

In the past, the term "healthy organizations" almost always implied that an organization was fiscally strong. Recent studies indicate that healthcare institutions that have policies and programs that benefit employees' health also benefit the organizations' bottom line (Borkowski, 2011). Today "healthy organizations" connotes not only financial soundness but also a culture that supports the physical and mental well-being of the employees. When nurses and other healthcare professionals experience stress, the healthcare organization will suffer repercussions if not managed properly. This may take the form of loss of work days because of physical complaints, reduced performance, poor judgment, lack of appropriate documentation, and not addressing patients' best interests (Jenkins & Warren, 2012). Decreased productivity, decreased efficiency, increased patient error, and decreased quality of care are hallmarks. Stressed employees will experience job dissatisfaction and a lower professional quality of life, which may lead to individuals leaving the nursing profession altogether. Avoidance or dread of working with certain patients or coworkers as well as workplace rage has become too common (Boyle, 2015; Harris & Griffin, 2015).

"Coping with stress at work" can be defined as an effort by a person or an organization to manage and overcome demands and critical events that pose a challenge, threat, harm, or loss to the person's functioning or to the organization as a whole. "Stress management" can be referred to as a narrow set of individual-level interventions such as meditation, biofeedback, and relaxation techniques or can have a broader meaning such as the implementation of stress management interventions where the organization targets individual employee characteristics, job demands, and the organizational culture as a whole. Organizational prevention is designed to enhance an employee's health and performance at work by anticipating and eliminating the stressors. These methods include modifying work demands and improving relationships in the workplace (Pipe et al., 2010; Sergeant & Laws-Chapman, 2012).

QUESTIONS TO CONSIDER BEFORE MOVING ON

- What individual strategies can the nurse use to manage stress in the workplace?
- What constitutes self-care practices?
- Is resilience a personal trait or a quality that can be developed?

MANAGING STRESS, SELF-CARE, AND RESILIENCE

We all have events in our lives that create stress and most of them cannot be eliminated. A certain degree of stress can be positive and constructive, acting as a catalyst to move us forward to achieve our goals and optimize our performance at work and home. Learning to manage stress in a healthy manner is an important skill to master to enhance our productivity rather than allowing stress to deplete our energy. Physical and psychological symptoms of stress can be experienced when demands exceed our internal and external resources. Developing healthy mental habits by centering one's self brings the body back into a state of equilibrium and balance. Building personal resilience by identifying and strengthening innate protective traits and internal resources is another approach to managing stress (Pines et al., 2011).

WORKPLACE STRATEGIES

One of the first steps in managing stress is to recognize stressors in one's environment and control them. Nurses by their nature tend to be self-sacrificing, so it is important to improve one's self-awareness regarding stressors and triggers. Self-care in the context of eating well, exercising regularly, getting enough sleep, taking time out for oneself, and developing a habit of positive self-talk are important strategies for coping with stress. Developing interpersonal skills and nurturing supportive relationships can also facilitate stress management. Altering, avoidance, and acceptance techniques are sets of strategies to deal with stress in the workplace (Barker, Taylor-Sullivan, & Emery, 2006). Using these techniques requires that the source of workplace stress has been identified by the individual. As previously mentioned, stress may be experienced for a variety of reasons including, but not limited to, feeling underappreciated, unrealistic role expectations, having no voice, or being a victim of harassment or discrimination. Other occupational stressors include fear of organizational mergers, having difficulty keeping up with technology, and inadequate training. Using a mix of the behavioral techniques listed in Table 5.5 will require self-reflection, change in communication patterns, and tempering reactions to stress.

SELF-CARE

Self-care is not simply about limiting or addressing professional stressors. It is also about enhancing one's overall well-being and is often considered to be an important aspect of resiliency. Those who are able to adequately meet their needs are often able to better cope with everyday stressors. Self-care efforts are aimed at regulating psychosocial and physical health, fostering and sustaining relationships, and achieving a work–life balance. Centering one's self brings the mind and body back into balance. Nurses are most likely

TABLE 5.5 STRESS MANAGEMENT TECHNIQUES IN THE WORKPLACE

Altering Techniques	Avoidance Techniques	Acceptance Techniques
• Problem-solving • Communication • Gathering information • Time management • Priority setting • Planning ahead • Delegating tasks • Conflict management	• Practice assertiveness • Say no • Let go • Avoid toxic people • Awareness of personal limitations • Compartmentalize negative thoughts	• Practice optimism • Minimize negativity • Practice forgiveness • Look at the big picture • Adjust standards • See humor in the moment

familiar with self-care strategies such as diaphragmatic breathing, meditation, yoga, music, massage, progressive relaxation, nutrition, and exercise. Engaging in creative activities, hobbies, humor, or prayer are other possibilities to build resilience and minimize stress reactions (Dellve & Wikström, 2009).

An abbreviated list of self-care practices can be found in Table 5.6, which will help you set personal goals by making healthy lifestyle choices in the form of rest, relaxation, and self-nurturance.

RESILIENCE

"Resilience" is generally defined as a phenomenon of positive adjustment or adaptation in the face of adversity. Working in the healthcare environment is fast paced and challenging requiring nurses to respond quickly and recover rapidly. Nurses are constantly pressured to make high-stake decisions

TABLE 5.6 SELF-CARE PRACTICES

Physical Self-Care	Psychological Self-Care	Spiritual Self-Care
• Eat healthy foods regularly • Avoid overeating • Exercise regularly • Avoid self-medicating • Get regular medical care • Take time off when sick • Engage in fun physical activities • Get enough sleep • Take vacations • Make time away from technology	• Make time for self-reflection • Write in a journal • Read literature that is unrelated to work • Do something at which you are not expert or in charge • Spend time with others whose company you enjoy • Stay in contact with important people in your life • Give yourself affirmations	• Make time for reflection • Spend time with nature • Find a spiritual connection • Be open to inspiration, cherish your optimism and hope • Be open to not knowing • Identify what is meaningful to you and notice its place in your life • Meditate • Read motivational literature

requiring both teamwork and accurate communications. The innate challenges to this work can be both rewarding and exciting; however, over time the constant pressures and stressors can take a toll on the individual quickly deteriorating into poor job performance and a decline in health.

Healthcare providers should be aware that resilience is a personality trait that can moderate the negative effects of stress and promote adaption. Resilience is dynamic and by the development of action-based interventions can help individuals strengthen dispositional traits, personal resources, capacity, and assets, which will moderate stressors in the workplace. Personal assets include physical, intellectual, social, and psychological elements. Correlates of resilience include protective factors such as optimism, meaning, purpose, social, and emotional support (Wagnild & Young, 1990). Psychological research methodologies indicate that people with traits of resilience are optimistic, zestful, curious, open to new life experiences, and have high positive emotionality (Jackson, Firtko, & Edenborough, 2007).

Personal and perceived competence, good intellectual functioning, positive self-worth, and the ability to self-regulate are other traits. Relational attributes of resilience are characterized by the ability to seek out and relate to positive role models and have positive social interactions and support (Hunter & Warren, 2014; Jacelon, 1997; Polk, 1997). Perseverance or exercising grit and persistence in the face of adversity or discouragement can be learned. Self-reliance, or the belief in one's self and one's capabilities, can be strengthened by identifying the inner resources and confidence to manage one's life despite adversity. Finding meaningfulness is the realization that one's life has purpose and value and that stressors can be opportunities for personal growth and satisfaction (Tugade & Fredrickson, 2004; Wagnild & Young, 1990). Self-acceptance by having the ability to feel joy, gratitude, and comfort in one's aloneness can be another source of strength to moderate stress. Having a positive attitude toward life and the ability to see that good times lie ahead are paramount. Positive emotions such as a sense of humor, the ability to use relaxation techniques, and positive thinking have emerged as important elements of resilience (Jones, 2012; Pipe et al., 2010).

Adopting effective personal stress management techniques to build resilience can translate into better awareness of self and others and more effective communication and, therefore, into a safer patient care environment. Taking time to reflect on both personal and professional goals as well as identifying barriers to goal achievement will assist the nurse in increasing resilience (Table 5.7). Box 5.2 provides a resource that may be useful as you conduct your own self-assessment of your stress threshold and personal strength.

MINDFULNESS

The literature is full of evidence of disappointment, discouragement, and exhaustion that arises from nursing practice as the stresses of increased patient acuity, changing models of care, and expectations to meeting the

TABLE 5.7 GOAL SETTING TO BUILD PERSONAL RESILIENCE				
Read the personal domains in the left-hand column. Check yes or no and write a goal that comes to mind. Consider perceived barriers to your goals and how you plan to overcome them.				
	Yes	**No**	**Goal**	**Perceived Barriers**
SLEEP Do I usually get sufficient sleep—enough that I feel refreshed (average is 8 hours)?				
FOCUS Do I spend sufficient time to feel focused in the activities I am doing—where I feel I am "in the zone"?				
EXERCISE Do I get enough physical exercise?				
ALONE TIME Do I spend time in solitude and self-reflection—with no goal or agenda?				
RELAXING Do I spend enough time just relaxing—nothing else to do?				
RELATING Do I spend enough time with those closest to me?				
RELATING Am I satisfied with how much time I spend with friends, socializing, in community activities, or making new acquaintances?				
PLAY Do I spend time doing things I enjoy, that are new, or just for "fun" (gardening, reading, playing with children, playing with pets)?				
MINDFULNESS Do I have a way of focusing my attention on exactly what I am feeling in the present moment?				
DIET Do I usually eat mostly fresh, unprocessed food every day?				
SUPPORT Do I have friends I can call when I am down, friends who really listen?				

continued

TABLE 5.7 GOAL SETTING TO BUILD PERSONAL RESILIENCE *(continued)*				
SUPPORT Can I honestly ask them for help when I need it?				
CLARITY Do I have a clear sense of what is happening in my life and work, including a sense of my future?				
MANAGING STRESS Do I know the skills and attributes I have that can assist me to manage in times of stress?				
MEANINGFULNESS Am I clear about why I do what I do, about what gives me satisfaction in my work and life?				
SELF-KINDNESS Do I forgive myself when I make a mistake?				
GENERAL HEALTH Do I see a healthcare provider for a physical exam yearly?				

needs of suffering accumulate (Antanaitis, 2015). For many, empathy is understood as understanding the suffering of another human being often neglecting the reality that, as clinicians, we often do not know how to be with our own suffering. Mindfulness is an area getting much attention in the preparation of healthcare professionals for practice. The capacity to pay attention in the present moment recognizes the reality of our multifaceted lives, and in doing so, addresses all QSEN competencies with the creative intelligence and compassion that are inherent in the nursing profession (Table 5.8). Mindfulness cultivates a stable healing presence that benefits patients and nurses alike. Mindfulness meditation techniques are widely used to manage stress, and are especially effective at reducing the stresses of time pressure and excessive workload that make healthcare delivery so difficult. Learning techniques to be present in the moment stops the nurse from worrying about the future or dwelling on regrets or negative past experiences. Practicing mindfulness reduces rumination and stress while boosting memory and sharpening attention. By adopting and promoting mindfulness stress reduction programs, we can transform ourselves as a profession to be focused, reflective, resourceful, open, creative, efficient, and resilient care providers (Antanaitis, 2015; Wright, 2014).

BOX 5.2 SELF-ASSESSMENT

What is your stress load? How well do you manage your stress? How adaptable are you to stress? How sensitive are you to stress?

Numerous self-assessments are available to help you respond to these questions. Visit the American Institute of Stress at www.stress.org/self-assessment and complete the self-assessments that are of interest to you. What do the results tell you? What are your strengths when it comes to dealing with stress? What could you potentially improve?

TABLE 5.8 REDUCING STRESS IN THE WORKPLACE: RELEVANT QSEN SKILLS

- Demonstrate awareness of own strengths and limitations as a team member (Skill)
- Initiate plan for self-development as a team member (Skill)
- Act with integrity, consistency , and respect for differing views (Skill)
- Acknowledge own potential to contribute to effective team functioning (Attitude)
- Appreciate importance of intra- and interprofessional collaboration (Attitude)
- Assume role of team member or leader based on the situation (Skill)
- Initiate requests for help when appropriate to situation (Skill)
- Clarify roles and accountabilities under conditions of potential overlap in team member functioning (Skill)
- Respect the unique attributes that members bring to a team, including variations in professional orientations and accountabilities (Attitude)
- Communicate with team members, adapting own style of communicating to needs of the team and situation (Skill)
- Initiate actions to resolve conflict (Skill)
- Value teamwork and the relationships upon which it is based (Attitude)
- Assert own position/perspective in discussions about patient care (Skill)

Source: Quality and Safety Education for Nurses Institute. (2014). QSEN competencies. Retrieved from http://www.qsen.org/competencies/pre-licensure-ksas

CONCLUSIONS

The complexity of our evolving healthcare system creates both acute and chronic stress for nurses. Acute or short-term stress can be experienced by the individual nurse as a response to a real or perceived immediate threat such as short staffing, high-patient acuity, or feeling bullied. As the imbalance between the demands and the resources available to cope with these demands increases, so do negative consequences to the individual nurse, interprofessional team, the patient population, and the organization at large. Chronic or long-term stress is often unremitting and insidious in nature, which can result in negative physical and emotional sequelae. Stress affects people in different ways and each situation needs to be considered in relation to the individual, work environment, and personal factors to understand and provide appropriate support. The way the individual nurse handles internal and external work stressors is truly a balancing act. Organizations must be proactive in developing strategies to alleviate stress while turning negative events into positive growth-producing situations. Nurses have the responsibility to practice self-care to ensure that they are both physically and mentally healthy for the demands of their role. With reflection and careful planning, one can learn to handle workplace adversity by enhancing one's personal resilience. Building resilience as a protective factor can heighten self-awareness and help nurses value both their personal and professional identities.

CRITICAL THINKING QUESTIONS AND ACTIVITIES

- What internal and external factors are contributing to stress in your own workplace? Discuss strategies to alleviate the issues.
- Review your personal resilience plan and select three attainable short-term goals; develop a realistic implementation plan to achieve those goals.
- Use the Internet to search for personal inventory tools, occupational stress tools, and self-care plans.
- Explore the NIOSH stress at work research program at www.cdc.gov/niosh/topics/stress/default.html
- Download a free self-care, stress management or stress reduction application on your smartphone.

REFERENCES

American Association of Colleges of Nursing. (2008). *The essentials of baccalaureate education for professional nursing practice*. Washington, DC: Author.

American Association of Colleges of Nursing, QSEN Consortium. (2012). *Graduate-level QSEN competencies: Knowledge, skills and attitudes*. Washington, DC: Author. Retrieved from https://www.aacnnursing.org/Portals/42/AcademicNursing/CurriculumGuidelines/Graduate-QSEN-Competencies.pdf

Antanaitis, A. (2015). Mindfullness in the workplace: Benefits and strategies to integrate mindfulness-based programs in the workplace. *Ontario Occupational Health Nurses Association, 34*(2), 39–42.

Barker, A. M., Taylor-Sullivan, D., & Emery, M. J. (2006). *Leadership competencies for clinical managers*. Sudbury, MA: Jones & Bartlett.

Borkowski, N. (2011). *Organizational behavior in health care*. Sudbury, MA: Jones & Bartlett.

Boyle, D. A. (2015). Compassion fatigue: The cost of caring. *Nursing, 7*, 48–51. doi:10.1097/01.NURSE.0000461857.48809.a1

Centers for Disease Control and Prevention. (2017). Data and injury trends among OHSN-participating facilities. Retrieved from https://www.cdc.gov/niosh/topics/ohsn/newinjury.html

Cronenwett, L., Sherwood, G., Barnsteiner, J., Disch, J., Johnson, J., Mitchell, P., & Warren, J. (2007). Quality and safety education for nurses. *Nursing Outlook, 55*(3), 122–131. doi:10.1016/j.outlook.2007.02.006

Dellve, L., & Wikström, E. (2009). Managing complex workplace stress in health care organizations: Leaders perceived legitimacy conflicts. *Journal of Nursing Management, 17*, 931–941. doi:10.1111/j.1365-2834.2009.00996.x

Gomaa, A. E., Tapp, L. C., Luckhaupt, S. E., Vanoli, K., Sarmiento, R. F., Raudabaugh, W. M., … Sprigg, S. M. (2015). Occupational traumatic injuries among workers in health care facilities-United States, 2012–2014. *Morbidity and Mortality Weekly Report*, *64*(15), 405–410. Retrieved from https://www.cdc.gov/mmwr/preview/mmwrhtml/mm6415a2.htm

Gulavani, A., & Shinde, M. B. (2014). Occupational stress and job satisfaction among nurses. *International Journal of Science and Research*, *3*, 733–740. Retrieved from https://www.researchgate.net/publication/265784831_Occupational_Stress_and_Job_Satisfaction_among_Nurses

Harris, C., & Griffin, M. T. (2015). Nursing on empty: Compassion fatigue signs, symptoms, and system interventions. *Journal of Christian Nursing*, *32*(2), 80–87. doi:10.1097/CNJ.0000000000000155

Hunter, B., & Warren, L. (2014). Midwives' experiences of workplace resilience. *Midwifery*, *30*, 926–934. doi:10.1016/j.midw.2014.03.010

Jacelon, C. S. (1997). The trait and process of resilience. *Journal of Advanced Nursing*, *25*, 123–129. doi:10.1046/j.1365-2648.1997.1997025123.x

Jackson, D. F., Firtko, A., & Edenborough, M. (2007). Personal resilience as a strategy for surviving and thriving in the face of workplace adversity: A literature review. *Journal of Advanced Nursing*, *60*, 1–9. doi:10.1111/j.1365-2648.2007.04412.x

Jenkins, B., & Warren, N. A. (2012). Concept analysis: Compassion fatigue and effects upon critical care nurses. *Critical Care Nurse Quarterly*, *35*(4), 388–395. doi:10.1097/CNQ.0b013e318268fe09

Jones, J. R. (2012). Manage workplace chaos by building your resilience. *Nursing Standard*, *27*(3), 63. doi:10.7748/ns.27.3.63.s59

Khamisa, N., Oldenburg, B., Peltzer, K., & Ilic, D. (2015). Work related stress, burnout, job satisfaction and general health of nurses. *International Journal of Environmental Research and Public Health*, *12*, 652–666. doi:10.3390/ijerph120100652

Lachman, V. D. (2016). Compassion fatigue as a threat to ethical practice: Identification, personal and professional workplace strategies. *Medical Surgical Nursing*, *25*, 275–278. Retrieved from https://www.nursingworld.org/~4af2bc/globalassets/docs/ana/ethics/compassionfatigue.pdf

Lambert, V. A., & Lambert, C. E. (2008). Nurses' workplace stressors and coping strategies. *Indian Journal of Palliative Care*, *14*(1), 38–44. doi:10.4103/0973-1075.41934

Lambert, V. A., Lambert, C. E., & Yamase, H. (2003). Psychological hardiness, workplace stress and related stress reduction strategies. *Nursing and Health Sciences*, *5*, 181–184. doi:10.1046/j.1442-2018.2003.00150.x

Lee, K. J., Forbes, M. L., Lukasiewicz, G. J., Williams, T., Sheets, A., Fischer, K., & Niedner, M. F. (2015). Promoting staff resilience in the pediatric intensive care unit. *American Association of Critical-Care Nurses*, *24*, 422–430. doi:10.4037/ajcc2015720

McCance, K. L., & Huethe, S. E. (Eds.). (2014). *Pathophysiology: The biologic basis for disease in adults and children*. St. Louis, MO: Mosby.

Pines, E. W., Rauschhuber, M. L., Norgan, G. H., Cook, J. D., Canchola, L., Richardson, C., & Jones, M. E. (2011). Stress resiliency, psychological empowerment and conflict management styles among baccalaureate nursing students. *Journal of Advanced Nursing*, *68*, 1482–1493. doi:10.1111/j.1365-2648.2011.05875.x

Pipe, T. B., Buchda, V. L., Launder, S., Hudak, B., Hulvey, L., Karns, K. E., & Pendergast, D. (2010). Building personal and professional resources of resilience and agility in the healthcare workplace. *Stress and Health*, *28*, 11–22. doi:10.1002/smi.1396

Polk, L. V. (1997). Toward a middle range theory of resilience. *Advanced Nursing Science*, *19*(3), 1–13. doi:10.1097/00012272-199703000-00002

Quality and Safety Education for Nurses Institute. (2013). QSEN Competencies. Retrieved from http://qsen.org/competencies/pre-licensure-ksas

Scott, L. D., Hwang, W. T., & Rogers, A. E. (2006). The impact of multiple care giving roles on fatigue, stress, and work performance among hospital staff nurses. *Journal of Nursing Administration*, *36*(2), 86–95. doi:10.1097/00005110-200602000-00007

Selye, H. (1950). Stress and the general adaptation syndrome. *British Medical Journal*, *1*, 1383–1392. doi:10.1136/bmj.1.4667.1383.

Sergeant, J., & Laws-Chapman, C. (2012). Creating a positive workplace culture. *Nursing Management*, *18*(9), 14–19. doi:10.7748/nm2012.02.18.9.14.c8889

Sullivan, E. J., & Decker, P. J. (2005). *Effective leadership management nursing*. Upper Saddle River, NJ: Pearson.

Tugade, M. M., & Fredrickson, B. L. (2004). Resilient individuals use positive emotions to bounce back from negative emotional experiences. *Journal of Personality and Social Psychology*, *86*(2), 320–333. doi:10.1037/0022-3514.86.2.320

Tusaie, K., & Dyer, J. (2004). Resilience: A historical review of the construct. *Holistic Nursing Practice, 18*(1), 3–10. doi:10.1097/00004650-200401000-00002

Wagnild, G., & Young, H. M. (1990). Resilience among older women. *Image Journal of Nursing Scholarship, 22*, 252–255. doi:10.1111/j.1547-5069.1990.tb00224.x

Wright, K. (2014). Alleviating stress in the workplace: Advice for nurses. *Nursing Standard, 28*(20), 37–42. doi:10.7748/ns2014.01.28.20.37.e8391

6

SETTING PRIORITIES AND MANAGING TIME

BONNIE HAUPT • AUDREY MARIE BEAUVAIS

LEARNING OBJECTIVES

After completion of this chapter, readers will be able to

- Describe the strategies for establishing goals and priorities.
- Identify ways to manage time efficiently and reduce time wasters.
- Analyze various time management techniques to determine their usefulness in one's specific situation.

Effective nurse leaders create well-defined goals for themselves. They do this as goals help them manage their lives, obtain maximum results, stay focused, and make good decisions. In your current role as an associate's degree nurse, you most likely have many competing priorities in your professional as well as personal life. As you continue your education and develop in your leadership skills, you will benefit from learning how to set goals and priorities as well as to manage your time. Undoubtedly, you already have many natural abilities, but you can attempt to maximize your highest level of efficiency for performing tasks (Taylor, 1911). One such way to maximize your level of efficiency is through time management. If time is managed effectively, stress will be reduced and goals will be accomplished. Time is a limited and valuable commodity. Therefore, you need to continually learn ways to optimize time to best accomplish your goals. This chapter presents a framework for the establishment of goals and priorities as well as numerous time management techniques to improve your efficiency.

QUESTIONS TO CONSIDER BEFORE READING ON

Have you ever thought about what you want out of life? Or do you prefer to go where life takes you? What values do you hold near and dear to your heart? Do you have personal goals? Do you have professional goals?

SETTING GOALS AND PRIORITIES

The self-assessment in Box 6.1 is intended to help you identify and reflect on your values. Your values are the things that you cherish the most. Your values should provide the basis for setting your goals and priorities. We begin by talking about setting goals. By establishing goals that align with your values, you are ensuring that you are spending time working on things that are most important to you. Taking the time to develop well-written goals will help you to remain focused and organized. Consider the five principles noted in Table 6.2 as you create and attempt to achieve your goals (Locke & Latham, 1990).

In addition to the principles noted in Table 6.2, goals should be documented (handwritten or on the computer). Documenting your goals with identified time frames for completion will help your commitment. If you don't set a time frame, it can prevent completion of the goal and decrease your motivation and morale. Use Table 6.3 to begin crafting some goals.

Table 6.3 will not only help keep your goals in the forefront of your mind but also help you track and manage your goals.

Once you have established your goals, you need to prioritize them. As you attempt to decide which goals should take precedence, review the value that is linked to each goal as this will help you to focus on the important items that will make a real difference for you. On a daily basis, you should attempt to perform activities that will support your priority goals. Develop a system to categorize your goals. The system can be as simple as using stars or a numbered list. Or you can make it more involved by developing categorizes such as (a) most important goals, (b) complete only after the most important goals are completed, and (c) complete only after (a) and (b) are done.

BOX 6.1 SELF-ASSESSMENT

In Table 6.1, list five of the most important aspects of your personal life as well as five of the most important aspects of your professional life. As you formulate your answer, carefully consider what you value most in these areas of your life.

TABLE 6.1 IMPORTANT ASPECTS OF YOUR PERSONAL AND PROFESSIONAL LIFE
Most important aspects of my personal life
1. (Examples: my significant other, staying healthy, traveling)
2.
3.
4.
5.
Most important aspects of my professional life
1. (Examples: lifelong learning, service to my profession, service to my patients/community)
2.
3.
4.
5.

QUESTIONS TO CONSIDER BEFORE READING ON

How much time do you spend on activities directly related to your top priority goals? Are you able to complete your goals in a timely manner? Are you frequently interrupted during your work day preventing you from accomplishing your goals? Can you think of time management techniques you could use to help you meet your goals?

TIME MANAGEMENT TECHNIQUES

To achieve your goals, it will be essential to manage your time.

Your time should be filled with activities that help you reach your priority goals. Effective time management skills are critical in handling day-to-day situations to reduce stress and ensure high-quality outcomes for you and your patients.

Read the case scenario in Box 6.2 and think about time management.

What time management techniques are John using? What other time management techniques might be helpful to John?

Although life is filled with many competing priorities, the good news is that there are techniques to help you manage your time. We present a few techniques in this chapter that we hope you will find helpful. Before we do so, complete the self-assessment of your time management skills provided in Box 6.3.

TABLE 6.2 FIVE PRINCIPLES FOR GOAL SETTING

Principle for Goal Setting	Description
Clarity	Set clear and concise goals. Develop goals that are **S**pecific, **M**easurable, **A**chievable, **R**elevant, and **T**ime-bound (SMART goals; Doran, 1981)
Challenge	Consider using challenges as a means to propel you toward your passions. Challenges can drive you to accomplish and complete your goals.
Commitment	Commitment is an essential ingredient for accomplishing your goals. If you (and your team) are not committed to reach a goal, it will likely fail.
Feedback	On your path to completing your goal(s), feedback should be solicited. Feedback can be received internally or from others involved in the process. Feedback will guide you in your process and make you aware of any necessary changes that must be made to keep your goal on track.
Task complexity	Task complexity relates to the time required to attain a goal. Less complex short-term goals may require only 1 hour to 2 years of your time; whereas more complex long-term goals may take over 2 years to complete. The more complex the task, the more important is the use of time management techniques.

TABLE 6.3 TEMPLATE FOR GOAL SETTING AND GOAL MANAGEMENT

Identify SMART goals: **S**pecific, **M**easurable, **A**chievable, **R**elevant, and **T**ime-bound	What **value** is linked to this goal? (Refer to Box 6.1 where you identified what you value.)	**Time frame** needed to complete goal:	**Complexity:** (If applicable, identify the steps needed to complete the goal.)	**Goal completion:** (Place a check in this cell when you have completed your goal.)
1.			**1.** **2.** **3.** **4.**	
2.			**1.** **2.** **3.** **4.**	

BOX 6.2 CASE SCENARIO

John is an associate's degree nurse who works at a long-term care unit. He values lifelong learning and improving patient care. John is working on supporting these values with a priority goal of obtaining his BSN degree. He has started his BSN course work but finds it difficult to manage his time with work, school, and family. As far as work goes, several of John's colleagues have been out on extended leave. As a result, they have been working short staffed and his employer is asking that he pick up extra shifts. With regards to John's home life, he is married with two children. John's wife works full time. Their two children are of school age and have numerous afterschool activities. As for school, John is in his second semester of classes for his BSN degree. He finds it difficult to keep up with the readings and numerous assignments given his other responsibilities. John has started keeping an agenda/calendar that has daily to-do lists. He also realized that he can get uninterrupted school work done if he wakes up an hour earlier. Despite these techniques, he is finding it difficult managing the home (grocery shopping, laundry, dinner preparation, providing transportation for the children's school/activities), school, and work activities.

ACTIVITY LOGS

Do you ever wonder how an entire day has passed yet you did not complete many items on your to-do list? On what were you spending your time? One useful technique to help answer these questions is creating and maintaining activity logs. Activity logs help give you an accurate representation of how you are investing your time. In addition, the log will help you to determine if you are spending time on activities that will assist you in reaching your goals. Pay attention to what time of day you do each task. Some of us do our best work in the morning, whereas others are more productive in the evening hours. Save your more mundane tasks for your lower energy times. Consider completing an activity log like the one shown in Table 6.4 for 3 to 5 days to assess how you spend your time. Do not make any changes to your normal routine while completing this exercise. Try to be as honest as you can in your recordings. This activity log can be used for work, school, and personal pursuits.

Once you have completed this log, take time to evaluate the results. Are you spending time on high-value activities that will help you reach your goals or on less productive activities? If you are spending time on tasks that are not part of your job description or do not help you meet your goals, then eliminate or delegate these activities. Consider scheduling your most difficult activities for the time of day when you have the most energy. What other changes can you make to boost your productivity?

BOX 6.3 SELF-ASSESSMENT OF TIME MANAGEMENT SKILLS

Answer the following questions with a Yes or No to obtain an assessment of your present time management skills.

- Are you spending time on high-value activities that will help you reach your goals?
- Do you prepare a to-do list for your day?
- Are you organized?
- Do you handle information (e.g., emails) just once (rather than go back to it several times before resolution)?
- Do you assess challenges and barriers throughout your day?
- Do you prevent time wasters from distracting you?
- Are you able to prioritize and delineate between urgent and not high-priority activities?
- Do you complete tasks on time?
- Are you able to complete assignments without feeling rushed?
- Are you satisfied with your use of time?

If you answered No to any of these questions, you may have an opportunity to try some of the techniques offered in this chapter to improve your time management skills.

Sources: Chapman, S. W., & Rupured, M. (2008). *Time management: Ten strategies for better time management*. Athens: The University of Georgia Cooperative Extension: Colleges of Agricultural and Environmental Sciences & Family and Consumer Sciences. Retrieved from http://www.fcs.uga.edu/docs/time_management.pdf; Dodd, P., & Sundheim, D. (2005). *The 25 best time management tools and techniques: How to get more done without driving yourself crazy*. Ann Arbor, MI: Peak Performance Press.

TABLE 6.4 ACTIVITY LOG

Date/Time/ Duration	Describe Activity	Is the Activity Related to Your Goals (If So, What Goal)?	Value of the Activity (High, Medium, Low, None)
Example: 6/12 from 7:00 to 7:30 a.m.	Bedside report with off-going nurse	Yes—related to goal of service to my patients/patient safety	High

For those of you who prefer more tech-savvy options, there are many apps available on your smartphone such as the following:

- ATracker PRO—daily task and time tracking
- Now Then Pro—time tracker and timesheet
- Activity Log Classic—time manager

One of these apps even offers a reporting feature! New apps are being created each day. See if you can find some other app options that may work for your situation.

DEVELOPING A TO-DO LIST

As an associate's degree nurse back in school for your BSN, I am guessing there are times when you feel overwhelmed by the amount of work you have to complete. You may occasionally miss a deadline or forget to do something. This is where a proper to-do list can come in handy. This technique will benefit you now and as you develop in your leadership role.

The list will help ensure that you do not overlook anything important, as well as help you to prioritize your tasks noting what needs immediate attention and what can wait until later. Table 6.5 provides a template that can be used to create your to-do list.

Begin completing Table 6.5 by writing down each task you need to complete, along with the due date, priority, and needed time frame. Some tasks may need to be broken down into smaller steps. You can combine your personal and professional to-do lists or keep them separate depending on what works best for your situation. Once you have completed the table, review your due dates and the priorities of each item making sure that not all of your items are written as a level 1 (very important) priority. If this is the case, take a moment to review your list to see if you can decrease the priority of some of

TABLE 6.5 TO-DO-LIST TEMPLATE

Due Date	Task	Priority (1: Very Important; 2: Important; 3: Not important)	Time Frame Needed to Complete

your less important tasks. Tackle the tasks that are listed as level 1 priority and have impending due dates first followed by those of lesser priority and later due dates. As you complete each task, cross that item off your list. At the end of each day, take a few minutes to review and reorganize your list (Loder, 2014).

Similar to the activity log, the to-do list can be created and managed using apps on your smartphone. Consider exploring one of the following options:

- To Do List+: to-do list for organizing work and errands
- Any.do: to-do list, calendar, reminders, and tasks
- Wunderlist: to-do list and tasks
- Swipes: to-do and task list; plan and achieve goals

MINIMIZE MULTITASKING

As a nurse, you are required to multitask at times. However, our brains are not able to switch between tasks efficiently which can affect our productivity (Drinon, 2012; Lohr, 2008). It takes less time to complete activities if you focus on one task at a time rather than multitasking (Drinon, 2012; Lohr, 2008). Hence, when possible, it is suggested that you remain focused and concentrate on your priority activities to maximize the use of your time. Save multitasking for your smaller and less important tasks that you need to accomplish throughout the day.

MANAGE TIME WASTERS

Your time at work and home may be affected by external influences imposed by other individuals and things. Being mindful of these time wasters and implementing the suggestions noted in Table 6.6 can help you gain back valuable time. Although there are many time wasters, we focus on those that are more likely to be relevant to your nursing role and home life.

QUALITY AND SAFETY EDUCATION for NURSES (QSEN) CONSIDERATIONS

QSEN competencies target the knowledge, skills, and attitudes that nurses need to develop in order to continuously improve the safety and quality of healthcare. The category of "safety" is directly related to the content presented in this chapter. Review the excerpt from the following "safety" competency and determine if you meet the competency or need to develop it further. If you need additional development, identify an action plan to help meet the competency.

Safety: Minimize the risk of harm to patients and providers through both system effectiveness and individual performance.
Knowledge: Discuss effective strategies to reduce reliance on memory.
Skill: Use appropriate strategies to reduce reliance on memory (e.g., checklists).
Attitudes: Appreciate the cognitive and physical limits of human performance.

TABLE 6.6 TECHNIQUES TO MANAGE TIME WASTERS

Techniques to Manage Time Wasters in Your Professional and Personal Life	Description
Choose your committee work wisely	Depending on your work setting, you may be asked to attend committee meetings. Meetings can be very effective and highly productive when they are conducted with a strong leader and a clear agenda. However, if there is not a clear agenda, chances are they will be a serious time waster. Try not to waste your time on meetings like this as your time is too valuable.
Limit how often you check email	Try not to check your email more than three times a day (morning, noon, end of the day). You may want to silence the email notification so you do not get tempted to view messages as they are delivered. If possible, clean out your email box each day.
Limit your web-surfing/ social media use	It is easy to lose track of time when surfing the web or browsing social media. Set a timer for 15 minutes so you do not waste too much time.
Set aside one day a week for errands	Keep a running list of what errands need to be accomplished. Plan your day by starting at the furthest errand location first and working your way back to home.
Deal with incoming papers	Depending on your nursing role, you may not have many papers to deal with at work. However, the same may not be true at home. Whether you have incoming papers coming from work or home, it is a good idea to set up a system to manage. Take 5 minutes to evaluate your incoming papers and determine what needs to be done with them. Set up a file for items that need your immediate attention and a file for those that need to be handled at a later date. The remaining items should not be needed and can be tossed in the circular file (garbage can).
Learn to say No	Learn to say No to the things that are not of high value to you and/or do not meet your goals (refer to Box 6.1 and Table 6.2). Naturally, make sure you say No in a respectful manner.
Avoid gossip	Gossip is not a productive activity and can negatively impact teamwork. Gossip will not help you reach your goals and will waste your time.
Avoid interruptions	It is difficult to avoid interruptions when you are a nurse. However, when you are performing high-priority tasks, it is crucial that you take measures to avoid interruptions.

Source: MindTools. (2017). Overcoming procrastination. Retrieved from https://www.mindtools.com/pages/article/newHTE_96.htm

CONCLUSIONS

As you develop your leadership skills, it is essential that you understand your personal and professional values. Those values are used as a foundation for your goal-setting activities. Developing well-written goals that align with your values will help ensure that you are spending time on what matters most to you. Those goals need to be prioritized in the order of importance. Implementing the time management strategies noted in this chapter will help you achieve your goals and maximize the use of your time. Effective time management skills require planning and practice. Commitment to enhancing and using time management strategies will increase your chances of successfully achieving your goals.

CRITICAL THINKING QUESTIONS AND ACTIVITIES

- Write down 12 things you did when you were last at work. On a separate piece of paper, write down the four topics that you expect to be discussed at your next performance review. Evaluate both lists and mark all the items on the first list that are directly linked to the second list. What can you determine from your results? Are you spending time on important activities or on tasks that have little value?
- Search the Internet for app and online tools to help with time management that might meet your needs. Consider exploring the following: Rescue Time (www.rescuetime.com), Remember the Milk (www.rememberthemilk.com), My Life Organized (www.mylifeorganized.net)

REFERENCES

Doran, G. T. (1981). There's a S.M.A.R.T. way to write management's goals and objectives. *Management Review, 70*(11), 35–36.

Drinon, R. (2012). Maintaining focus, multitasking, and managing time. Retrieved from https://www.kscpa.org/writable/files/DrinonsLeadershipExpress/dle_8_article.pdf

Locke, E. A., & Latham, G. P. (1990). *A theory of goal setting and task performance.* Englewood Cliffs, NJ: Prentice-Hall.

Loder, V. (2014). Five best to-do list tips. *Forbes.* Retrieved from https://www.forbes.com/sites/vanessaloder/2014/06/02/five-best-to-do-list-tips

Lohr, S. (2008). Slow down, brave multitasker, and don't read this in traffic. *New York Times.* Retrieved from http://www.nytimes.com/2007/03/25/business/25multi.html?_r=2&ref=technology&pagewanted=print

Taylor, F. W. (1911). *The principles of scientific management* (pp. 5–29). New York, NY: Harper Bros.

7

EFFECTIVE COMMUNICATION IN LEADERSHIP AND MANAGEMENT ROLES

SHERYLYN M. WATSON

LEARNING OBJECTIVES

After completion of this chapter, the reader will be able to

- Review effective communication styles, skills, and stages.
- Assess one's own communication style.
- Discuss how effective communication promotes quality and safety in nursing practice.
- Discuss how communication and behaviors differ in healthy versus unhealthy organizational environments.
- Apply effective communication strategies to promote a healthy working environment within an organization.
- Apply strategies to overcome roadblocks to effective communication.
- Explain how generational and cultural influences affect communication.
- Discuss how technology impacts communication.

As a member of the interprofessional healthcare team, a nurse's ability to communicate effectively is integral to patient safety, a healthy work environment, and an effective teamwork and collaboration (American Association of Colleges of Nursing [AACN], 2008; Quality and Safety Education for Nurses [QSEN] Institute, 2014). Communication styles and behaviors are dynamic and responsive to situations, environments, and personal experience (Morgan, 2010). Even with good communication skills, challenges will continue to arise when working with diverse cultures and generations, as well as when using different modes, such as face to face, audio, email, and texting to communicate. Appreciating differences among people's styles and modes of communication is necessary to function in today's healthcare environment.

As a registered nurse, you may have already witnessed or have been a part of unhealthy communication styles in the workplace and have seen the outcomes these styles and behaviors have created. However, while moving forward in your professional development, you will find that understanding factors that influence communication in the organization, such as negative behaviors, generational and cultural differences, and communication roadblocks will assist you in appreciating the issues and forming a more effective communication style when addressing roadblocks.

This chapter discusses how effective communication is critical to the development of leadership and management roles in nursing. The principles of effective communication and how to overcome negative styles are discussed and illustrated in case studies. You will be able to reflect on your current communication style and integrate new communication techniques to improve your leadership skills to promote a healthy work environment.

QUESTIONS TO CONSIDER

As you read the following case scenario, ask yourself:

- Would you choose the same method of communication that Sadie did to disseminate the hospital's decision?
- Recall a time when you were frustrated with a peer, would you have addressed the issue the same as the staff nurses in this scenario or a different way?

BOX 7.1 THE CASE SCENARIO

Sadie, the critical care unit (ICU) nurse manager of 6 months, communicated in an email to the staff about the new hospital policy of no approval of overtime for completing documentation or other end-of-shift activities. Time management concerns would be documented in their annual evaluation if the staff were not leaving on time. The email read:

Dear Staff,

The hospital administration has decided that there will be no approval of overtime for end-of-shift activities that should be completed within the shift, such as documentation or lengthy shift reports. I apologize for this new policy. If I could ask, please use the time clock when starting and ending your shift.

Warmly,

Sadie, RN

(continued)

BOX 7.1 CASE SCENARIO *(continued)*

The week following the announcement, Sadie received multiple complaints by the staff that Alana, an RN who has been working in the ICU for 22 years, is chronically late by 30 minutes, which prevents them from completing their bedside report and generates overtime. The staff nurses left curt messages on Sadie's voicemail informing her when Alana arrived each day. Sadie also received a formal letter signed from the nurses that they refuse to stay late anymore and that they will leave written report for Alana. Sadie emailed the nursing staff who complained that this would be addressed; however, written report was not best practice nor an approved method in the ICU.

COMMUNICATION: PROCESS, STYLE, AND BASIC SKILLS

A widely accepted method to explain the stages of communication is the basic process that explains verbal communication (Blais & Hayes, 2011; Boynton, 2016; Murray, 2017). The communication process is outlined through six steps: sender, encoding, message, decoding, receiver, and feedback. Each phase is important for effective communication to occur, requiring the right sender to select clear, concise, and respectful words to deliver the message. Then, the receiver has to decode the message correctly. To determine that these stages of the communication process occurred accurately, the sender should solicit feedback. The last phase is critical in effective communication, soliciting feedback to ensure that the message was received accurately with the intended message. For nurses, communication is an essential part of the profession and sending or receiving is critical to patient safety as well as their own careers.

Another principle that is important when understanding communication process is formal and informal communication practices. "Formal communication" is defined as a type of communication where information is sent through predefined channels within an organization. This type of communication is practiced in the workplace as it follows a hierarchical chain of command and is typically used to disseminate important information. On the contrary, "informal communication" occurs when information is shared freely, without structured confines. Informal communication is when people have casual discussions about personal or professional issues and share opinions. Formal communication is considered the official communication, whereas informal communication is thought to be gossip and personal opinions.

How do these two communication practices differ in their impact in the organization? Formal communication is the official statements of the organization and employees are expected to follow the chain of command and statements. Traditional formal communication statements are not open for further discussions and have potential to impact employee practices and satisfaction. The impact of formal communication on the organization has advantages and disadvantages. Two advantages are that employees have a clear understanding of expectations and information is accessible to everyone, creating an equal opportunity workplace. Disadvantages include employees' inability to speak openly about their concerns, resulting in dissatisfaction, and the time for the communication takes longer. Informal communication can influence the organization at times more so than formal communication. Although informal communication practices open channels between individuals within the hierarchical chain of command and relationships are built stronger, the potential negative influences that informal communication has on organizations is significant. Informal communication practices foster rumors, inaccurate information, and hurtful gossip, which results in confusion, frustration, and dissatisfaction at a workplace. Morale can be significantly lowered if the informal communication is not positive; one person's opinion could begin a ripple effect that changes the entire unit's teamwork.

In the case scenario, the formal and informal communication practices are identifiable with demonstration of the impact they have on the workplace. The formal communication is Sadie's email to her staff about the change in overtime approval policy. The email served as the official statement and all employees received the same message. Employees did not have the opportunity to discuss their concerns about the change in policy and are expected to follow the new change. The informal communication is how the staff responded to learning of the new policy. When the group of staff nurses wrote the letter, there were informal conversations with each other about the policy and Alana. The impact of the informal communication led to nurses being frustrated with one person, gossiping, and overall workplace dissatisfaction. Informal communication could start with one individual who has influence outside the formal hierarchal chain of command. Although this case scenario shows the negative influence of informal communication, there are many times this type of communication practice can positively impact a change in practice as well.

Although there are several different ways to classify communication styles, two common methods are explored. On the basis of the works of Carl Jung's *Theory of Psychological Types* from 1928, communication styles can be categorized as Thinkers, Feelers, Sensors, and Intuitors (Jung, 1928/2014). The other typical communication style classification method uses the four categories: assertive, passive, aggressive, and passive aggressive. Communication styles are learned behaviors from one's own values and beliefs, previous experiences, and current circumstances (Boynton, 2016). Essential to becoming an effective communicator, nurses should recognize each style and reflect on their own practice to foster professional and personal growth.

All individuals have primary and secondary communication styles that are associated with behavioral patterns. When analyzing yourself or others using the four categories of Thinkers, Feelers, Sensors, and Intuitors, positive and negative attributes are associated with each. Individuals who are classified as Thinkers function in a logical manner, analyze information before making objective decisions, value accuracy, communicate with brevity, and remain focused. Information communicated by Thinkers tends to be logical, well written, but without infliction. These individuals review all information and contemplate before making decisions. However, the drawback of this type of personality is that colleagues perceive this individual as indecisive, critical of others, and impersonal in conversations.

Individuals who are classified as Feelers relate through their response of feelings and emotional reactions to understanding the experience. Feelers tend to be very perceptive and aware of others and situations, resulting in good communication and listening skills. In the workplace, Feelers build relationships to create harmony and are naturally friendly. Their style of communication is best when face to face and tends to be most effective with oral communication. The negative attributes of this style are the over personalization of professional relationship, spending too much time socializing, disorganization, and difficulty in making objective decisions. Thinkers and Feelers could be seen as opposites and without appreciation for each other's strengths and weakness; miscommunication and frustration in the workplace can easily arise.

The next category is of individuals classified as Sensors. Characteristics that sensor-style individuals possess include being resourceful, practical, and productive. Sensors make decisions swiftly on the basis of facts and previous experiences and focus on action and results. Their communication style is typically very brief in written and oral communication, resulting in abrupt, pointed conversations. However, Sensors could be perceived as impulsive, impatient, poor listeners, and competitive.

The last category in this communication style is of individuals known as Intuitors. Individuals who possess primarily this type of style are inducing, visionary, and quick deep thinkers. Intuitors' strengths are optimized on long-term projects or issues that require creative solutions. They tend to be verbose and complex when communicating in either oral or written form. The drawback for Intuitors is how their communication style is perceived by others, such as being condescending, difficult to read, and being scattered.

Comparing and contrasting these four different types of personality with their unique attributes for communicating in the workplace, there are obvious differences that could generate conflict. The key element to remember when self-analyzing which type you are as well as what type of style your colleagues are is to appreciate each other's differences and capitalize on each person's strengths. For example, if the unit is having difficulty with the scheduling, ask an Intuitor to review the master schedule taking into consideration individual and unit needs to see if there could be a creative long-term solution. See Box 7.1 to appraise which style you possess.

The other classic method to classify someone's communication style is using the four categories of assertive, passive, aggressive, and passive aggressive. Individuals who practice assertive behavior appreciate different viewpoints as well as advocate for their own perspective. Characteristics of the assertive style are:

- Using statements when communicating opinions
- Respecting differing perspectives, "agree to disagree"
- Articulating in a calm, clear, and confident manner
- Respecting verbal and nonverbal language
- Participating as a group member and actively listening to others

Thinking about the case scenario presented earlier (Box 7.1), an example of assertive communication style is when Sadie emailed the nursing staff who complained that their concerns would be addressed and that written report was not acceptable. After each style, let us continue to classify the different styles of communication in the case study.

Individuals who use a passive communication style do not share their opinions, values, or needs as they deem them not as important as others (Boynton, 2016). Characteristics of the passive style are:

- Minimizing one's own needs or opinions within the group
- Assuming that one's own contributions to the conversation or situation would not be valuable
- Exhibiting nervous body language
- Apologizing for one's own actions and for others
- Unable to express one's own needs

In this case scenario, an example of passive communication is how Sadie chose to inform all the staff about the change in policy that affects payroll. Choosing an email method was passive rather than holding a staff meeting as well as the apology for implementing the policy within the email.

Individuals who practice aggressive communication style revere their opinion and needs as more important than others with behaviors described as abusive or bullying. Characteristics of the passive-aggressive style are:

- Consistently interrupting others
- Dominating discussions with one's own opinions, discounting other perspectives
- Exhibiting nonverbal cues that show disrespect or negative judgment of others
- Using language that is condescending and humiliating
- Articulating in a loud, rude, and overt manner

In the case scenario, an example of aggressive communication style is when the nurses leave terse voicemails informing Sadie when Alana arrives each day. Sadie would be aware of the exact time Alana would arrive as she is required to clock into a system.

Individuals who practice passive-aggressive communication style believe their opinions are the most important; however, they do not openly show aggression toward others. Characteristics of the passive-aggressive style are:

- Excluding others from participating in an activity
- Gossiping about others behind their backs, harboring resentment
- Indirect hostility toward others through procrastination or not following through on assignments
- Complaining about being underappreciated and treated unfairly
- Undermining change or positive outcomes

One example of passive-aggressive communication style in the case scenario is whoever wrote the anonymous letter to Sadie about Alana. Anonymous letters are not taking accountability for one's own thoughts or actions. Furthermore, you can surmise that the staff nurses were gossiping about the new policy and the chronic tardiness of Alana while not speaking directly to Alana or Sadie, which are also examples of passive-aggressive communication styles.

Assertive communication is the most professional and respectful style. Nurses should practice assertive communication in all situations, regardless of how the other parties are responding and act as role models for others. However, these characteristics are easier to espouse rather than practice consistently. Take a moment to honestly appraise your ability to communicate assertively (www.psychologytoday.com/tests/personality/assertiveness-test; Assertiveness test, n. d.). In certain difficult situations, being assertive is challenging, especially when there is a perceived imbalance of power or during a hostile environment. Therefore, assertive communication behaviors require practice, self-reflection, and commitment for personal development.

Apart from the type of communication style a person chooses to use, basic communication skills are categorized as verbal and nonverbal communication, and active listening. Messages are conveyed through words—written or verbal—and nonverbal language, facial expressions, personal space, gestures, posture, and gait. All these elements may impact how the message was delivered and received at any point in the communication stage.

Nonverbal communication is considered more important than the verbal message as the emotions and subconscious information conveyed through eye contact, posture, personal space, body language, facial expressions, and minor gestures may be contradicting the verbal message. Nonverbal communication illuminates the comfort or discomfort of the sender behind the message. When a sender of a message refuses to make eye contact and slouches in the chair, regardless of the words, the sender is sending the message that he or she is intimidated, apologetic, or does not support the message. When the receiver rolls his or her eyes and sits with arms crossed, it is clear that the receiver does not agree with the message. The power of a nonverbal message significantly influences the entire communication process, positively or negatively.

BOX 7.2 THE CASE SCENARIO CONTINUES TO UNFOLD

Sadie asked Alana into the office to explain about the complaints. Sadie inquired if there were any reasons why she was late each day. While sitting across from the desk, Alana shared that there was always traffic and agreed that it was unfair to her peers if she was consistently late. She smiled when leaving, and stated that she would be on time from this point forward. Sadie was relieved that this problem was resolved as Alana agreed to come on time.

The other essential basic skill of communication is active listening, on behalf of the sender and the receiver. Active listening requires the individual to be engaged and not distracted, being present for the conversation. This is a practiced skill of communication, the individual listens by participating in the conversation by responding in a nonjudgmental manner and being aware of nonverbal cues as well as listening to the words. Although these basic skills of communication are identifiable in someone else, a nurse needs to be reflective of one's own communication skills and continue to practice when communicating with patients and members of the team. The case scenario in Box 7.2 highlights communication skills. Once you have read the case scenario, refer to Box 7.3 and complete a self-assessment of your communication style.

QUESTIONS TO CONSIDER BEFORE READING ON

- What type of communication style do you predominantly use?
- Are you an active listener?
- Do you typically solicit feedback when communicating important information from the patient or a healthcare team member?

BOX 7.3 SELF-ASSESSMENT OF COMMUNICATION STYLE

Analyze the answers to the quiz in Appendix A.

Then, take a self-assessment of how you rate as a listener:

www.cengage.com/resource_uploads/static_resources/0324223048/7346/listen_quiz.html

Were you surprised with your self-assessment results? Read further on to learn how to improve your personal style as well as learn how to best interact with others.

FACTORS INFLUENCING ORGANIZATIONAL COMMUNICATION

Organizational culture relates to how things work at an institution, the explicit and implicit rules. Communication practices are interrelated with the organizational culture, influencing each other. The explicit rules are formal policies and guidelines generated from mission and philosophy, professional standards, and culture of safety and quality care. These rules are typically found in employee handbooks, codes of conduct, evaluation tools, and orientation packets. Employees are aware of the expectations and senior administration and managers have the responsibility to enforce these standards and be role models. Explicit communication examples include having honest and respectful communication exchanges, being open to feedback and suggestions, and following chain-of-command when addressing conflict (Hicks, 2011). Expectations for communications such as specific greetings for phone interactions related to customer satisfaction and respectful, professional interaction may be formally assessed on annual evaluations. Effective clear communication practices set forth by the management improve the overall organizational health (Hicks, 2011).

The implicit rules of the culture have at times more influence on organizational culture. Norms and behaviors that are not written but accepted as common practice are embedded in the culture of the organization, shaping the environment as healthy or toxic (Boynton, 2016; Hicks, 2011). When there is effective implicit organizational communication, the cascading effect on retention, employee satisfaction, and patient safety are positive (Portoghese et al., 2012; QSEN Institute, 2014). Communication is built on trust, sharing of ideas, and respect toward others. Unfortunately, if the inherent communications are not aligned with the explicit rules, double messages are being sent, rendering the written policies and rules of the organization ineffective. In an incident when a policy outlines zero tolerance for aggressive uncivil communication, however no disciplinary actions occur when a manager is uncivil toward one of their employees, mistrust and detrimental effects seep into the culture.

Positive factors that influence organizational communication that are essential for a healthy work environment include management role-modeling behaviors, holding all employees accountable for their actions, and communicating clear expectations (Portoghese et al., 2012). Role-modeling is critical to effective communication, as it reinforces positive behaviors and the practices become embedded into the organizational culture. Other critical elements that impact communication within the workplace are allowing the staff time to share their thoughts during debriefing sessions or open forums, conversing during the right time, and using shared language (Kanerva, Kivinen, & Lammintakanen, 2015). Furthermore, each employee should be cognizant of his or her role and responsibilities within the organization. Leadership may set the tone for communicating within the organization; however, everyone should accept fundamentally that organizations function using a hierarchal chain-of-command and there are acceptable professional communication practices. Although individuals have their primary and secondary communication styles as discussed earlier, employees would be remiss not to acknowledge these fundamental organizational principles and how they influence the culture of the organization. Consider when you are addressing an issue related to a very difficult patient situation to your manager, is the right time during shift change or should you plan a 15-minute meeting? Having proper time to debrief about situations on a scheduled basis or scheduling a meeting allows both parties to be present for the discussion. By requiring yourself and others to discuss important topics in a debriefing session or scheduling meetings, this behavior will become a norm for the organization.

QUESTIONS TO BE CONSIDERED BEFORE READING ON

- Case study consideration: Where did the communication breakdown occur?
- Self-reflect: Do I feel I can voice my concerns to my manager and have my thoughts/opinions valued?

ORGANIZATIONAL COMMUNICATION STRATEGIES

Patient safety and delivery of quality care is dependent on effective communication, requiring the organization to make a commitment to foster a culture of open communication. This fundamental principle of effective communication is the bedrock to an organization's health and should be embedded in every aspect of the culture. The QSEN Institute (2014) outlined essential competencies that undergraduate and graduate nurses must possess to function in the healthcare environment (as listed in Table 7.1). These competencies are learned during education; however, the culture of the organization may place value on different aspects or implicit rules may differ. Therefore, nurses should reflect on these competencies in the context of their own behaviors and communication skills to role-model effective communication abilities.

Specific strategies should be adopted to promote effective communication to improve patient safety as well as foster a healthy work environment. Creating a culture of open communication is necessary between staff–staff, provider–staff, and staff–patient. A safe environment for open communication includes promoting an assertive communication style, having a trusting relationship with leadership, providing time for team debriefing, and feeling each person's voice is being heard (Portoghese et al., 2012). During a debriefing time, ideas are shared and there should be no blame placed on team members, focusing, rather, on areas of concern

TABLE 7.1 DEVELOPING EFFECTIVE OPEN COMMUNICATION SKILLS: RELEVANT QSEN COMPETENCIES
Act with integrity, consistency, and respect for differing views (Skills).
Initiate requests for help when appropriate to situation (Skills).
Analyze differences in communication style preferences among patients and families, nurses, and other members of the health team (Knowledge).
Communicate with team members, adapting one's own style of communicating to needs of the team and situation (Skills).
Value different styles of communication used by patients, families, and healthcare providers (Attitudes).
Describe the impact of one's own communication style on others (Knowledge).
Discuss effective strategies for communication and resolving conflict (Knowledge).
Follow communication practices that minimize risks associated with handoffs among providers (Skills).
Appreciate the risks associated with handoffs among providers and across transitions in care (Attitudes).
Assert one's own position/perspective in discussions about patient care (Skills).
Choose communication styles that diminish the risks associated with authority gradients among team members (Skills).

Sources: From Cronenwett, L., Sherwood, G., Barnsteiner, J., Disch, J., Johnson, J., Mitchell, P., ... Warren, J. (2007). Quality and safety education for nurses. *Nursing Outlook*, *55*(3), 122–131. doi:10.1016/j.outlook.2007.02.006; Institute of Medicine.(2003). *Health professions education: A bridge to quality*. Washington, DC: National Academies Press.

and solutions. Attention should be drawn to removing any imbalance of power during team meetings, as nurses, managers, and other professionals share the same goal to deliver safe quality patient care. In addition to team meetings and debriefings, another strategy that promotes patient safety and requires effective communication is interprofessional team rounding. When all members of the healthcare team are included in the daily rounds of the patient in an acute care setting, patient safety and quality healthcare are delivered. Effective communication that fosters respect and open sharing of thought is essential to productive interprofessional team rounding.

The Agency for Healthcare Research and Quality (AHRQ, 2017) developed a set of evidence-based tools that promote teamwork and effective communication in the workplace. Team Strategies and Tools to Enhance Performance and Patient Safety (TeamSTEPPS) is the AHRQ program that healthcare organizations adopt to optimize outcomes and patient safety. Specific skills that are taught to interprofessional teams include briefings, safety huddles, check back, two-challenge rule, and handoff (AHRQ, 2017). All strategies are aimed at improving communication within the team to deliver quality healthcare and mitigate errors and patient injuries.

An approach for creating effective interprofessional communication in an organization is standardizing protocols. When The Joint Commission recommended that nurses be trained in assertive communication skills, attention was given to how best to address the issue of effective communication among team member (The Joint Commission, 2005). Data analysis revealed that errors occurred when vague or unorganized communication between team members happened, specifically during handoffs or critical information report. Adopted from the military and taught in the TeamSTEPPS curriculum, the Identify-Situation, Background, Assessment, Recommendation (I-SBAR) model emerged as a widely accepted method to convey critical information about a patient's condition to another member of the healthcare team. Each individual is accountable for his or her information and followup. By skipping any of the necessary steps, the probability for miscommunication increases. The standardized tools foster assertive communication style, minimizing perceived imbalance of power among the different professionals, and decreasing errors resulting from miscommunication. Other communication tools are found on the AHRQ (2016) website.

An example of a nurse using I-SBAR when calling a healthcare provider about a patient follows:

I—Identify: Identify yourself, the person with whom you are speaking, and the patient. *Hello, Is this Dr. Smith? This is Victoria, the telemetry nurse caring for the patient, Michael Brown.*

S—Situation: Why are you calling? *I am calling because on the telemetry monitor, Mr. Brown began with multifocal PVCs this past hour. His vital signs are P—88, R—16, BP—140/70, O_2 saturation—94% on 2 liters N/C, and GCS of 15. His potassium level is 3.0 and magnesium level is 1.0 from 6 a.m.*

B—Background: What is relevant background? *He is 70 years old who was admitted 1 day ago with congested heart failure. He has been given 40 mg of furosemide IVP BID and 50 mg of Metoprolol daily.*

A—Assessment: What do you think is the problem? *I think his potassium and magnesium are low, causing the PVCs, and they were not corrected from this morning.*

R—Recommendation: What do you want them to do? *I would like you to consider ordering a replacement of the potassium and magnesium prior to administering his afternoon furosemide order. Is there anything else you would like me to do?*

With clear understanding of the situation and recommendation by the nurse and provider, the patient's safety is properly being addressed. This standardized approach is minimizing miscommunication and potential for blaming if an unusual occurrence happens.

Another effective communication tool grounded in evidence from TeamSTEPPS is the structured approach for handoffs. This tool is to be used during transfers of responsibility and accountability of the patient. Time is allotted for the receiver to ask questions, clarify information, and confirm the message. Typically, handoffs are verbal communication that follows a standard approach. TeamSTEPPS has been successfully implemented through the healthcare sector and has contributed to improving patient outcomes significantly.

BOX 7.4 THE CASE SCENARIO CONTINUES TO UNFOLD

Alana approaches several nurses at the shift change to ask if they were the ones who complained to the manager about her being late. She asks, "Why didn't you just say something to me? Now I may lose my job. I am angry." Two nurses deny being involved. The other two nurses apologize for what the group did and quickly leave their shift. Although Alana is not happy with the situation, she feels better that she addressed her feelings with her colleagues.

Another strategy for effective communication is taking accountability for your action. An "I"-statement is a communication strategy that helps the speaker take ownership over his or her concern or question. When starting a statement off as "I believe...," the shifting of blame does not happen, and the focus stays on the sender of the message. The use of "I" statements requires practice though. Strong examples of "I" statements include "I am concerned about Mr. Brown." "I feel patient safety is being compromised when the unit is left short staffed during the night shift." "I am upset with this new policy because..." Take ownership over your feelings.

"I" statements are not effective if used under the veil of a "you" statement. Consider this statement and how you would feel hearing this from a fellow nurse. "I feel like you are upset with me." This statement is putting the receiver of this statement on the defensive. A better option might be to say "I feel there is tension between us." This is taking ownership of the situation as well, not being the victim or communicating through a passive voice. The next time you are concerned about a patient or situation at work and need to address it, practice framing the beginning of the conversation with an "I" statement. Read the case scenario found in Box 7.4. Can you think of "I" statements that could be used in this scenario?

QUESTIONS TO CONSIDER BEFORE READING ON

- Do I role-model effective communication?
- Do I take accountability for my thoughts and feelings at work?

MODES OF COMMUNICATION

During the past decade, how communication transpires has changed significantly because of technology. There are two basic modes of communication in healthcare, person-to-person or computer-mediated communication. The person-to-person communication includes face-to-face communication as well as via telephone. Face-to-face communication allows for the most interaction, as there is an opportunity for both sender and receiver to use nonverbal cues and social context in communicating the message. The instant feedback is a benefit that no other communication mode can offer.

In the healthcare setting, a common practice is to communicate over the telephone to providers and family members who are not able to be present. The benefit of communicating through the telephone is similar to face-to-face communication when other verbal cues beyond the words can be noted by individuals conversing. Although many nonverbal cues are lost, there is still ample opportunity for the individuals to clarify the message and ask further questions.

As many of today's communications occur through the computer-mediated communication (technology) mode, awareness by the sender and receiver on the shortcomings are important to ensure effective communication occurs. Critical information is conveyed through texting or computer-messaging system. Because no nonverbal cues or social context can be gleaned from the message, there is a higher probability for miscommunications to occur. Therefore, nurses are challenged to ensure that the information being sent is clear and concise for patient safety. The last step in understanding any message is feedback that the message was received correctly. This step in using technology to transmit messages is critical to closing the loop and having effective communication.

Videoconferencing is emerging as a new trend for patient care, combining the face-to-face and computer-mediated methods to allow for specialists to have access in several locations. Videoconferencing is occurring with translators, consultations, and families, all important elements in delivering safe and quality care.

Beyond patient care, the mode to transmit an administrative-type message has faced a change as well. Common practice is for managers to send emails to notify staff of important policy changes and ask about an incident (Koivunen, Niemi, & Hupli, 2015). This communication mode is valuable to ensure that everyone will receive the message. Unfortunately, emails have pitfalls, such as the message may not be read, the tone may be misunderstood, and there is no opportunity for instant feedback or questions. Computer-mediated communication should not solely replace face-to-face communication.

ROADBLOCKS TO EFFECTIVE COMMUNICATION

Knowledge and consciousness awareness are warranted for understanding barriers to effective communication. By appreciating the roadblocks, nurses have the potential to improve effectiveness and minimize the effects of these barriers (Table 7.2).

Healthcare professionals themselves have personal barriers that impact their effectiveness in communicating with their patients as well as other members of the team. Negative nonverbal behaviors about which nurses

TABLE 7.2 BARRIERS TO EFFECTIVE COMMUNICATION
Personal—nonverbal behaviors, poor conflict management
Organizational—culture of mistrust, imbalanced of perceived power within members of the healthcare team
Other barriers—linguistic differences, time constraints

Sources: From Bramhall, E. (2014). Effective communication skills in nursing practice. *Nursing Standard, 29*(14), 53–59. doi:10.7748/ns.29.14.53.e9355; Meuter, R. F., Gallois, C., Segalowitz, N. S., Ryder, A. G., & Hocking, J. (2015). Overcoming language barriers in healthcare: A protocol for investigating safe and effective communication when patients or clinicians use a second language. *BMC Health Services Research, 15*(1), 371. doi:10.1186/s12913-015-1024-8; Thomson, K., Outram, S., Gilligan, C., & Levett-Jones, T. (2015). Interprofessional experiences of recent healthcare graduates: A social psychology perspective on the barriers to effective communication, teamwork, and patient-centred care. *Journal of Interprofessional Care, 29*(6), 634–640. doi:10.3109/13561820.2015.1040873

should have self-awareness when talking to others include avoiding eye contact, displaying agitation, speaking in low volume, slouching, standing behind a chair/furniture, and gazing with a blank look. As a nurse, if one of the patients was sending these signals while you were performing an assessment, concern would be raised that the patient is upset, not accepting the diagnosis, or another issue; regardless, followup would be taken. Consider how you may have demonstrated one or more of these behaviors when talking to an interprofessional team member, colleague, or supervisor. Nurses are concerned when a patient exhibits the negative nonverbal cues; however, it is imperative that nurses conduct a self-assessment on their communication practices (Table 7.3). Second, poor conflict management is a barrier to effective communication. Conflict management is discussed in depth in Chapter 11. However, it should be noted that not having the ability to resolve conflict strains effective communication practice. Some individuals have a perception that all conflicts are bad and avoid uncomfortable conversations. Rather, a perspective that promotes a healthy workplace understands that conflict is natural and professionally addressing the issue is best practice.

TABLE 7.3 SELF-ASSESSMENT OF COMMUNICATION STYLE

Think about your communication style and how others perceive you. Reflect on the following questions honestly.

- Do you find it easy or difficult to communicate assertively?
- Do you express your thoughts clearly and concisely? Or are you long-winded?
- Do you find it easy or hard to say "no" to other's requests?
- Do you withdraw from conflict or remain silent?
- Do you "read" others' nonverbal cues? Are you aware of the nonverbal cues that you use in communicating?

Take a moment to assess your communication style using this free online quiz: http://districts.ca.uky.edu/files/communications_self_assessment.pdf.

Source: Communication styles: A self-assessment exercise [PDF]. (2017). Retrieved from http://districts.ca.uky.edu/files/communications_self_assessment.pdf

Harmful implicit organizational communication practices create potential barriers as well. When a culture of mistrust is perpetuated between management and employees, blaming and misdirected anger manifests (Meuter, Gallois, Segalowitz, Ryder, & Hocking, 2015). Furthermore, when the culture tolerates an imbalance of power among different levels of professionals, feelings of not being valued and closed communication occurs. Patient care becomes affected when perceived imbalance of power exists; staff learn to not share concerns (Thomson, Outram, Gilligan, & Levett-Jones, 2015). As this issue mushrooms to all areas of the organization, a commitment by employees and managers for change is essential. Individual nurses can be part of that change by role-modeling assertive behavior and practicing effective communication strategies such as "I" statements. Each encounter strengthens the organizational culture for more effective communication.

Other barriers impact good communication practices that need awareness to make a change. Language barriers between professionals, staff, and patients contribute to medical errors and increase psychological stress (Meuter et al., 2015). Nurses have the responsibility to minimize this roadblock using clear and concise statements and using interpreters, either computer-based or in-person. External environmental roadblocks that exist are lack of time, interruptions, and noise. How does a nurse overcome time constraints when the workload is high? Consciousness awareness about when to have critical conversations with others is part of a solution, as well as not allowing interruptions, and practicing active listening. Responsibilities lie with each person to practice effective communication and bring awareness to the barriers.

QUESTIONS TO CONSIDER BEFORE READING ON

- Think of an issue that you took to your manger or supervisor. Do you believe you sent the appropriate nonverbal cues to support your message? Explain. Would you change this in the future?
- Are there ways that you may have contributed to the roadblocks discussed above within your organization? Explain.

GENERATIONAL AND CULTURAL INFLUENCES

An important element that has to be considered when discussing effective communication is individual or subgroup differences. The diversity of the nursing workforce necessitates a closer discussion related to generational and cultural influences on communication styles to develop a synergy among the team members.

Understanding the perspective of the three generations of practicing nurses today is essential: Baby Boomers (1946–1964), Generation Xs (1965–1976), and Millennials (1977–2000). An overview of Baby Boomers' communication preferences includes being team-oriented, speaking only when addressed, and being taught to be respectful of authority (Outten, 2012). Generation Xs were raised in the era when parents returned to work, technology emerged (e.g., video games and household computers), and focus was placed on being more independent (Outten, 2012). Millennials grew up with instant communication (e.g., text messaging) and were educated to voice concerns and believe their thoughts are valued (Das, 2013). Although these are generalizations, the fundamental principles remain that mixing the different generations and their preferences for communication poses problems for effective communication practices. For instance, if the nurse manger is a generational Baby Boomer, having clinical nurses share their concerns over practice would be seen as being subordinate. Communication through email is seen as more impersonal for Baby Boomers, while long meetings are seen as ineffective by Millennials (Phillips, 2016). The nurse leaders of today have to navigate through the differing intergenerational perspectives to foster effective team communication. Importance should be placed on using a combination of technology and face-to-face modes of communications to address important issues.

Similar to intergenerational differences, cultural diversity impacts communication in healthcare. Nurse-to-patient effective communication strategies are taught in fundamental nursing education, with emphasis on how to be sensitive to different cultures and overcome barriers. However, more attention is needed to address how ethnocultural differences among the nurses and other healthcare professionals have negative effects on communication (Hendel & Kagan, 2014). Although it is too numerous to list the different cultures and the common perceptions about communication styles in this chapter, the understanding should be that not all cultures accept assertive characteristics as a positive attribute. However, sufficient evidence from leading healthcare organizations, such as the American Healthcare Quality and Research, the AACN, the Institute for Healthcare Improvement, the Institute of Medicine, and QSEN, have proven that assertive communication is necessary for delivery of safe, quality patient care. Therefore, a commitment by nurses, managers, and other professionals is needed to bridge the gap of ethnocultural differences and to foster a culture that supports assertive communication.

Nurses should honor generational and cultural differences in communication by being understanding and accepting of others. Effective communication requires sensitivity to these perspectives as they are not modifiable. Best practice is to learn how to appreciate how each one can contribute to the team.

INFLUENCE OF TECHNOLOGY AND COMMUNICATION

Technology is ever present in today's world, especially in healthcare. Nurses have competencies specifically addressing how to integrate technology use with safe patient care (QSEN Institute, 2014). Benefits associated with technology include electronic healthcare records that allow for better management of patient data, standardized documentation, and accessing consultations quickly (Koivunen et al., 2015). Beyond direct patient care impact, technology use in healthcare organizations to transmit administrative information and communication between nursing professionals is most common practice (Koivunen et al., 2015). Technology allows for more information to be disseminated quickly and with less restrictive time restraints. If a nurse is unable to make a staff meeting, the manager can disseminate the information, allowing for the nurse to learn the information or the latest evidence-based practice alerts can be sent to all nurses on the unit for updated information to be accessed. However, disadvantages to overuse of technology exist. Information is only as good as what is input into the system. Information is not helpful if staff cannot access it in a timely manner. If workload demands prevent access to patient records or interruptions block comprehensive documentation, technology has failed for being an effective mode of communication.

Another area to be aware of for technology being a means for communication is that technology decreases social interactions, which are a foundation for building trusting relationships with colleagues. With the knowledge that 80% of people learn most effectively through visual means and technology removes that integral part of communication, nurses face a challenge on how to overcome this barrier (Rosenblatt & Davis, 2009). Email is not always the answer because of information overload and oversaturation (Cohen, 2013). Think about the case study presented at the beginning of this chapter. What might have happened if the manager set the expectations by discussing the zero tolerance for overtime policy during a staff meeting? For starters, there would have been an opportunity to get feedback on the policy and answer inquires. The manager could have observed the staff's verbal and nonverbal body language. A general email sent to staff as a policy alert does not foster open communication. With technology as a mainstay for communicating important information, emphasis has to be placed on how messages may be received, not oversaturating the amount of emails, and fostering opportunity for open dialogue on the issue.

CONCLUSIONS

Communication skills improve with practice and experience. Being consciously aware of one's own behaviors and skills is most important for improving effective communication. Although organizational culture may seem insurmountable to change, patient care and personal satisfaction may be detrimentally affected if roadblocks continue to manifest. Considering how to practice assertive communication style, using technology to enhance conveying messages, and appreciating different perspectives begin to strengthen effective communication for the individual and the organization.

CRITICAL THINKING EXERCISES

- As a new assistant nurse manager on nights for only 2 weeks, the manager convenes an assistant nurse manager meeting to discuss redistribution of staff responsibilities for each shift. The manager decides that the night shift will perform all the daily baths to allow for more time on day shift to make rounds with the healthcare team. The manager informs you that this is your responsibility to make this change happen starting next shift. You are aware that the night shift already perceives they have more work than other shifts and that they have a higher staff–patient ratio.
  - How would you communicate this change to the night shift staff?
  - What communication strategies could you use to address your concerns with the nurse manager?
- During the day shift as a charge nurse, you observe a new nurse giving an I-SBAR report to an older physician. Halfway through the report, the physician holds up his hand and says "Stop right there, I know the patient and I don't need your recommendation. I will order what I want." The nurse apologizes and walks into a different patient's room. The physician begins to write the new patient orders.
  - How would you address this situation?
  - Would you feel comfortable in your current organization to introduce SBAR as a communication tool?
  - What could the new nurse have done differently in this scenario to promote the use of SBAR with this physician?

REFERENCES

Agency for Healthcare Research and Quality. (2017). TeamSTEPPS 2.0. Agency for Healthcare Research and Quality. Retrieved from http://www.ahrq.gov/teamstepps/about-teamstepps/index.html

American Association of Colleges of Nursing. (2008). *The essentials of baccalaureate education for professional nursing practice*. Washington, DC: Author.

Assertiveness test. (n. d.). Psychology Today. Retrieved from https://www.psychologytoday.com/tests/personality/assertiveness-test

Blais, K., & Hayes, J. S. (2011). *Professional nursing practice: Concepts and perspectives* (6th ed.). Boston, MA: Pearson.

Boynton, B. (2016). *Successful nurse communication: Safe care, health workplaces, & rewarding careers*. Philadelphia, PA: F. A. Davis.

Bramhall, E. (2014). Effective communication skills in nursing practice. *Nursing Standard, 29*(14), 53–59. doi:10.7748/ns.29.14.53.e9355

Cohen, S. (2013). Talk it and walk it: Staff communication. *Nursing Management, 44*(6), 16–18. doi:10.1097/01.NUMA.0000430411.73206.bc

Communication styles: A self-assessment exercise [pdf]. (2017). Retrieved from http://districts.ca.uky.edu/files/communications_self_assessment.pdf

Cronenwett, L., Sherwood, G., Barnsteiner, J., Disch, J., Johnson, J., Mitchell, P., … Warren, J. (2007). Quality and safety education for nurses. *Nursing Outlook, 55*(3), 122–131. doi:10.1016/j.outlook.2007.02.006

Das, R. (2013). Special issue: Audiences: A cross-generational dialogue. *Communication Review, 16*(1-2), 3–8. doi:10.1080/10714421.2013.757162

Hendel, T., & Kagan, I. (2014). Organizational values and organizational commitment: Do nurses' ethno-cultural differences matter? *Journal of Nursing Management, 22*(4), 499–505. doi:10.1111/jonm.12010

Hicks, J. M. (2011). Leader communication styles and organizational health. *Health Care Manager, 30*(1), 86–91. doi:10.1097/HCM.0b013e3182078bf8

Institute of Medicine. (2003). *Health professions education: A bridge to quality*. Washington, DC: National Academies Press.

The Joint Commission. (2005). *The Joint Commission guide to improving staff communication*. Oakbrook Terrace, IL: Author.

Jung, C. G. (2014). Theory of psychological types. In G. Adler, M. Fordham, & H. Read (Eds.), *The collected works of C. G. Jung: Complete digital edition*. Princeton, NJ: Princeton University Press. (Original work published 1928.)

Kanerva, A., Kivinen, T., & Lammintakanen, J. (2015). Communication elements supporting patient safety in psychiatric inpatient care. *Journal of Psychiatric & Mental Health Nursing, 22*(5), 298–305. doi:10.1111/jpm.12187

Knock Out Networking, LLC. (n.d.). *Communication styles*. Jackson, NJ: Author. Retrieved from http://knockoutnetworking.com/wp-content/themes/buildingblocks/pdf/STIF-Assessment.pdf

Koivunen, M., Niemi, A., & Hupli, M. (2015). The use of electronic devices for communication with colleagues and other healthcare professionals- Nursing professionals' perspectives. *Journal of Advanced Nursing, 71*(3), 620–631. doi:10.1111/jan.12529

Meuter, R. F., Gallois, C., Segalowitz, N. S., Ryder, A. G., & Hocking, J. (2015). Overcoming language barriers in healthcare: A protocol for investigating safe and effective communication when patients or clinicians use a second language. *BMC Health Services Research, 15*(1), 371. doi:10.1186/s12913-015-1024-8

Morgan, B. (2010). What are the characteristics of a leader? *Dynamics, 21*(1), 17–19.

Murray, E. (2017). *Nursing leadership and management: For patient safety and quality care*. Philadelphia, PA: F. A. Davis.

Outten, M. K. (2012). From veterans to nexters: Managing a multigenerational nursing workforce. *Nursing Management, 43*(4), 42–47. doi:10.1097/01.NUMA.0000413096.84832.a4

Phillips, M. (2016). Professional issues: Embracing the multigenerational nursing team. *MEDSURG Nursing, 25*(3), 197–199.

Portoghese, I., Galletta, M., Battistelli, A., Saiani, L., Penna, M. P., & Allegrini, E. (2012). Change-related expectations and commitment to change of nurses: The role of leadership and communication. *Journal of Nursing Management, 20*(5), 582–591. doi:10.1111/j.1365-2834.2011.01322.x

Quality and Safety Education for Nurses Institute. (2014). QSEN competencies. Retrieved from http://qsen.org/competencies

Rosenblatt, C. L., & Davis, M. S. (2009). Effective communication techniques for nurse managers. *Nursing Management, 40*(6), 52–54. doi:10.1097/01.NUMA.0000356638.41458.e4

Thomson, K., Outram, S., Gilligan, C., & Levett-Jones, T. (2015). Interprofessional experiences of recent healthcare graduates: A social psychology perspective on the barriers to effective communication, teamwork, and patient-centred care. *Journal of Interprofessional Care, 29*(6), 634–640. doi:10.3109/13561820.2015.1040873

Appendix A

SELF-ASSESSMENT OF COMMUNICATION STYLES

COMMUNICATION STYLES

Please respond to these sets of statements describing your behavior or thinking. For each set of statements, circle the "A" or "B" response that is the more characteristic of you. In some instances, neither the "A" nor the "B" may be typical for you. If this is the case, select the response that would be *more* like you.

1	**A.** I get right to the point.	**B.** I like to analyze the facts before I answer.
2	**A.** I like to propose original ideas.	**B.** I like working with people.
3	**A.** I like to deal with practical people.	**B.** I get excited about new concepts.
4	**A.** My feelings often guide my actions.	**B.** I usually evaluate things before I act.
5	**A.** I am a no-nonsense kind of person.	**B.** I like having some fun at work.
6	**A.** I use lots of data to help make decisions.	**B.** I can be very creative.
7	**A.** I like colleagues who are sincere.	**B.** My ideas are a little far out.
8	**A.** I use step-by-step analysis to make decisions.	**B.** I think long-range planning is a waste of time.
9	**A.** My intuition is often pretty accurate.	**B.** I appreciate fully documented procedures.
10	**A.** I am pretty sensitive to the feelings of others.	**B.** I usually focus on immediate needs.
11	**A.** I am usually logical/consistent in my actions.	**B.** I often help friends solve their problems.
12	**A.** I like to deal with abstract ideas.	**B.** I like to get things done.
13	**A.** I am concerned with getting the work out.	**B.** I like to assess all alternatives before acting.

(continued)

14	**A.** I can be too intellectual for some people.	**B.** I try to analyze why people do things.
15	**A.** I am a practical and realistic person.	**B.** I am a "big picture" person.
16	**A.** I can be too quick to express my feelings.	**B.** I can be impersonal and detached.
17	**A.** I like short meetings with solid objectives.	**B.** I like to socialize during meetings.
18	**A.** I am known as being levelheaded.	**B.** I sometimes base decisions on a strong hunch.
19	**A.** I sometimes get too emotional.	**B.** I am great at ideas but poor at implementation.
20	**A.** I like to read reports backed up by analysis.	**B.** I get bored reading reports.
21	**A.** I like brainstorming sessions.	**B.** I dislike people with "half-baked" ideas.
22	**A.** I base my thinking on how I feel at the moment.	**B.** I like to take immediate action on problems.
23	**A.** I do not like to change my proven methods.	**B.** I am concerned about changes that affect morale.
24	**A.** I daydream about the future.	**B.** I am concerned about today's problems.
25	**A.** I accomplish much in a given amount of time.	**B.** I like to take my time and get all the facts.
26	**A.** My imagination sometimes gets carried away.	**B.** I am known as a good problem solver.
27	**A.** I am impressed by results.	**B.** I am impressed by the potential of ideas.
28	**A.** I am impressed by people who have good social skills.	**B.** I am impressed by people who are well organized.
29	**A.** I am primarily concerned primarily about today.	**B.** I often reflect upon my past experiences.
30	**A.** I am concerned about the past, present and future.	**B.** I often think about future events.
31	**A.** I am occasionally seen as too sensitive.	**B.** I am occasionally seen as being "out in leftfield."
32	**A.** I like facts rather than theories.	**B.** I like to complete projects that I start.

Source: Adapted from Jung, C. G. (2014). Theory of psychological types. In G. Adler, M. Fordham, & H. Read (Eds.), *The collected works of C. G. Jung: Complete digital edition*. Princeton, NJ: Princeton University Press. (Original work published 1928.)

To manage and ultimately communicate with prospects, clients, centers of influence, and even friends effectively, it is important that a sales leader be aware of his or her personal style, as well as those of others. This survey is designed to provide an agent or broker with a simple psychological framework or four styles that might be encountered within a networking or sales scenario. This instrument is designed to be only suggestive, rather than predictive, of the actual behavior.

COMMUNICATION STYLES

Circle the letters that reflect your statement selections. Be careful when scoring.

	Sensor	Thinker	Intuitor	Feeler
1.	A	B		
2.			A	B
3.	A		B	
4.		B		A
5.	A			B
6.		A	B	
7.			B	A
8.	B	A		
9.		B	A	
10.	B			A
11.		A		B
12.	B		A	
13.	A	B		
14.			A	B
15.	A		B	
16.		B		A
17.	A			B
18.		A	B	
19.			B	A
20.	B	A		

(continued)

	Sensor	Thinker	Intuitor	Feeler
21.		B	A	
22.	B			A
23.		A		B
24.	B		A	
25.	A	B		
26.			A	B
27.	A		B	
28.		B		A
29.	A			B
30.		A	B	
31.			B	A
32.	B	A		
Total circled per column				

SENSOR

Suggested strengths:

Action-oriented—acts quickly; a doer

Decisive—makes quick decisions and without hesitation

Impulsive—can make decisions out of impulse, without thinking about consequences or chooses to deal with the consequences later

Suggested limitations:

Poor planner—often does not take the time to sit and plan

Compulsive—may act by a compulsion or obsession

THINKER

Suggested strengths:

Detail-oriented—the small things matter and are noticed

Rational—likes things based on reason or logic; needs to know the facts and consequences

Objective—makes decisions based on fact, not subjectively based on feelings

Suggested limitations:
- **Nitpicking**—picks up on every minute detail
- **Unemotional**—may be seen as insensitive by other styles

INTUITOR

Suggested strengths:
- **Idea generator**—has visions that affect the future
- **Conceptual**—creates new things out of imagination
- **Creative**—has an artistic nature

Suggested limitations:
- **Total dreamers**—visions of great things to come, may be unrealistic
- **Trendy**—tends to like the latest fashion, technology, and so on.

FEELER

Suggested strengths:
- **People-oriented**—a total "people person"
- **Perceptive**—exhibits perception (feeling, anticipating, and reading between the lines)
- **Persuasive**—has such a good feel for people that he or she knows how to persuade people to do things

Suggested limitations:
- **Poor listener**—thinks he or she already has all the answers; seen as asking questions for which he or her does not wait to get answers (works the room)
- **Manipulative**—knows how to make people do "what they may not normally do."

8

ACCOUNTABILITY AND DELEGATION

SUSAN A. GONCALVES

LEARNING OBJECTIVES

After completion of this chapter, the reader will be able to

- Define delegation.
- Discuss why professional nurses need to learn how to effectively delegate.
- Describe the principles of accountability applicable to effective delegation.
- Describe the four steps of the delegation process.
- Identify and describe the "five Rights of Delegation."
- Describe the correct process to ensure safe effective delegation.
- Identify common pitfalls and challenges that prevent effective delegation.
- Discuss tasks and responsibilities that RNs can and cannot delegate.
- Discuss the differences in accountability and delegation between leaders and managers.

Registered nurses (RNs) are accountable to the general public for the provision of culturally competent, safe, effective, quality care for patients in a variety of settings across the continuum of healthcare today (American Nurses Association [ANA], 2012). These settings may include hospitals, short- and long-term healthcare facilities, assisted living homes, community as well as public health centers, home health agencies, schools as well as residential and home settings.

According to the National Council of State Boards of Nursing (NCSBN®) and the ANA, the number of licensed nurses is often limited in healthcare agencies, thus requiring RNs to work with a variety of unlicensed assistive personnel (UAP). Therefore, RNs need the knowledge and skills to assign, delegate, supervise, and evaluate UAP (ANA & NCSBN, 2006). RNs have the authority and ultimate responsibility and accountability for their nursing practice (ANA, 2010).

"Delegation" is the act of assigning a specific task or a set of tasks to another individual while maintaining overall accountability for the outcome (Schub & Cabrera, 2016). Effective delegation is a critical competency for all RNs. However, depending on your educational background and clinical experiences, you may or may not have learned the knowledge and skills you need to effectively delegate. You most likely have had both positive and negative experiences by observing others delegate, or delegating yourself in your nursing practice. Delegation requires critical thinking skills and sound clinical judgment. As a nurse, you already have developed some level of delegation skills that have brought you to where you are today.

This chapter discusses how delegation is a core competency for the nursing profession. The key principles and five steps of the delegation process are explored. Common pitfalls/challenges and both positive and negative outcomes resulting from delegation errors are discussed. Through reflective thinking and delegation activities using guidelines and algorithms, you can further strengthen your confidence and skill set. Further development and proficiency in delegation will continue throughout your commitment to lifelong learning and your experiences.

QUESTIONS TO CONSIDER BEFORE READING ON

- Do I really have to delegate as part of my professional practice as an RN?
- Is it easier to do it myself than to delegate?

DELEGATION: BACKGROUND/HISTORY

Delegation has always been an essential function for the RN; however, the breadth and scope of the art of delegation and the variety of tasks that the RN can delegate have changed dramatically over the past few decades. Many organizations embrace the team model approach to the delivery of care in which you, the RN, responsible for the coordination and planning of patient care, will find yourself faced with the need to delegate work to others.

Historically, there have been varying definitions for delegation among both the ANA and the NCSBN. As healthcare began to change with an increase in unlicensed personnel delivering direct patient care, the ANA and NCSBN (2006), in an effort to support nurses in this critical skill of safe and effective delegation, issued a Joint Statement on Delegation. This Joint

Statement on Delegation (2006) was developed to highlight and reinforce that delegation is an essential nursing skill. Furthermore, to support the practicing nurse in decision-making related to delegation, the ANA and NCSBN developed resources that provide clarity in the delegation process. The ANA and the NCSBN (2006) jointly developed the "ANA Principles of Delegation" (see www.ncsbn.org/Delegation_joint_statement_NCSBN-ANA.pdf) and the NCSBN's "Decision Tree on Delegation" (see www.ncsbn.org/Delegation_joint_statement_NCSBN-ANA.pdf) that defines the four steps of the delegation process. Each of these are discussed in detail later in the chapter.

The ANA, the NCSBN, 2009, and the International Council of Nurses (ICN, 2012) assert that safe and effective delegation is considered an essential and core skill for professional nursing practice on an international level. Learning effective delegation skills requires you to know and understand the Nurse Practice Act for the state in which you practice. In addition, it is the opinion of the ANA and NCSBN that mastery of the art of delegation is an essential step of the journey to nursing excellence, of which many organizations are in pursuit as they seek Magnet® designation. When nurses use the skill and process of delegation accordingly, safe and effective nursing care is the end result and organizations can reap positive fiscal rewards as well.

In 2015, the NCSBN convened two panels of experts representing education, research, and practice areas with the goal of developing national guidelines based on current evidence-based research to once again facilitate and standardize the delegation process. These guidelines are seen in www.ncsbn.org/NCSBN_Delegation_Guidelines.pdf and provide clarity to nurses, delegates, leaders, and the entire organizations.

Since this Joint Statement on Delegation was developed in 2009, the healthcare arena has continued to transform dramatically. This makes the skill of effective and safe delegation even more critical and one with which you must feel comfortable and embrace each and every day you walk in and out of your workplace. Let us take a moment and think about the type of delivery care model with which you are working today. Box 8.1 depicts a typical clinical scenario you may encounter.

QUESTIONS TO CONSIDER BEFORE READING ON

- In what type of healthcare setting are you working?
- Who is part of your team?
- What is your complement of nurses/other team members?
- Are you working with any UAP?
- Do you delegate tasks to other individuals?

BOX 8.1 CASE SCENARIO

As you read this case scenario, think about how Nicole can handle her workload. Where should she begin? Can any of the items listed be delegated to others?

Nicole has been an RN for 1 full year working on a very busy medical–surgical unit, but today is her first day being in charge on the 7 a.m. to 3:30 p.m. shift. She arrives at work to discover the following:

- Three RNs and two UAP have called out sick.
- Two portable nurse phones are broken.
- Narcotic counts are off––with a dose of Dilaudid and Ativan being off.
- Mrs. Smith in Room 704 is infuriated about her care in the overnight shift and wants to see the charge person.
- The toilet in the locker room is overflowing and leaking out onto the floor.
- A 24-year-old is verbalizing suicidal ideation.

The thought that Nicole has to single-handedly manage all the events with which she is faced is untrue. Delegation is an essential aspect of the daily work performed by nurses. Care is coordinated to meet patient needs, but it is imperative that the RNs delegate some aspects of the work to other members of the healthcare team (Finkelman & Kenner, 2016). A single RN or team member cannot possibly do everything that is required for a position or for a patient. There must be an effective use of all resources as well as everyone's expertise and time management.

Through effective time management, some of the above problems that Nicole is facing can be delegated to those best suited to handle them. For example, another nurse can call the staffing office and see if there are any other staff available; a clerical team member can call another unit and ask to borrow phones; the environmental worker can be alerted and take care of the toilet overflow; Nicole's night staff can be directed to investigate and resolve the narcotics issue; members of the nursing team can sit down and speak with the disgruntled patient; and Nicole and/or another appropriate member of the nursing team can collaborate and deal with the patient having suicidal ideation, which is the top priority. There is absolutely no reason to feel overwhelmed or afraid.

DELEGATION: KEY TERMS

Delegation and the delegation process is multifaceted (NCSBN, 2017). In addition to the definition of delegation stated in the introduction, we review some basic key terms and their definitions according to NCSBN. These include:

Delegator—the person (RN) delegating the task

Delegatee or delegate—the person receiving the delegation and accepting the task

Delegation—"transferring to a competent individual the authority to perform a selected nursing task in a selected situation. The nurse retains accountability for the delegation" (NCSBN, 2005, p. 39)

Supervision—"the provision of guidance or direction, oversight, evaluation and follow-up by the licensed nurse for accomplishment of a nursing task delegated to nursing assistive personnel" (NCSBN, 2005, p. 40)

Accountability—the act of "being responsible and answerable for actions or inactions of self or others in the context of delegation" (NCSBN, 2005, p. 39)

Unlicensed Assistive Personnel (UAP)—"any unlicensed personnel [regardless of title] to whom nursing tasks are delegated" (NCSBN, 2005, p. 40).

QUESTIONS TO CONSIDER BEFORE READING ON

- Who is responsible for the delegation process?
- Have you ever delegated a specific task to another person of your team? How did you feel? What was that communication like?

The delegation process starts with your administration at your organization and trickles down to you and the staff responsible for delegating and includes oversight and evaluation (NCSBN, 2017). Effective communication and empowerment for staff members making the decisions based on their clinical judgment is required. It is critical that staff members receive support from all levels within the organization. What exactly does this mean? It means you are not alone. Whether you are the organization itself, the leader, the manager, the staff nurse (delegator), or the UAP (delegate), everyone, regardless of their role, has specific responsibilities within the delegation process (NCSBN, 2017; see delegation model in www.ncsbn.org/1625.htm).

ACCOUNTABILITY

Healthcare organizations as a whole also play a part and are accountable for delegation. Nurse managers and leaders have responsibilities and are accountable for the provision of a safe environment that supports this delegation process (ANA, 2015). This translates into the fact that healthcare organizations also play a part and are accountable for delegation. Organizations' accountability encompasses the responsibility to provide sufficient resources for nurses and other members of the healthcare team to provide nursing care in a safe and effective manner (ANA & NCSBN, 2006, p. 3). These resources include but are not limited to:

- Adequate staffing patterns (nurse to patient ratios) as well as appropriate staff mix

- Established core competencies for all team members providing direct patient care
- Development of organizational policies specifically related to delegation and the delegation process
- Active shared governance councils involving all nurses
- Acknowledgment that delegation and the delegation process is a professional right and responsibility

DELEGATION: LEADERSHIP AND MANAGEMENT ROLES

As a professional nurse and a leader, you will be accountable for the provision of a safe environment that supports the delegation process (ANA, 2015b). Your *leadership* role could require you to do the following to support the delegation process:

- Function as role model, mentor, and resource person
- Maintain patient safety as the guiding principle during the delegation process
- Become an informed and active participant in the development of local, state, and national efforts surrounding scope of practice issues for both nurses and UAP
- Encourage delegation as a process that supports best practice and fiscal responsibility

As part of your *management* functions, you may be required to do the following to support the delegation process:

- Develop clear and concise scope of practice guidelines, job descriptions, and mandatory core competencies required for both RN and UAP roles in accordance with local, state, and national governing bodies and jurisdictions
- Develop and institute a review process (annual or more frequent as required) that includes the assessment and evaluation of personnel and essential job functions
- Know the legal aspects of issues surrounding the delegation process

Irrespective of whether you are a nursing leader, manager, or staff nurse, it is *your* responsibility to be knowledgeable and aware of what is permitted in your own state Nurse Practice Act as well as any specific rules, regulations, policies, and procedures. In the process of delegation, you as the RN must always comply with *your* own state's nurse practice act as well as any regulating bodies and organizational policies and *you* are accountable for the quality of nursing care that is provided. The American Association of Colleges of Nursing (AACN, 2008) clearly notes "nurses are accountable for their professional practice and image as well as the outcomes of their own and delegated nursing care" (p. 9). This is not meant to frighten you, but to emphasize the importance of your professional role as an RN. *You* as the RN are accountable for the decision to delegate and for the tasks that are delegated to others. Therefore, it is imperative that you are familiar with the steps of the delegation process and are proficient in delegating care effectively.

QUESTIONS TO CONSIDER BEFORE READING ON

- Do you have a favorite family member or friend who makes things look so easy when throwing a party or planning an event? What is their secret to making it look so easy?
- Are they delegating some tasks to others? Skills used to plan a successful party in your personal life may be transferable to the work setting.
- Let us now reflect on your professional life. Do you ever feel you are going to have a good (or bad) shift due to which colleagues are scheduled with you?
- What is it about the colleagues that helps make the shift run smoothly? Could a key factor be delegation?

FOUR STEPS OF THE DELEGATION PROCESS

The NCSBN has identified delegation standards and described the delegation process. The NCSBN (2006) defines delegation as "transferring to a competent individual authority to perform a selected nursing task in a selected situation. The nurse retains the accountability for the delegation." This very simply translates into the following:

- RN identifies a nursing task
- RN may delegate elements of care but does not delegate the nursing process itself
- RN (delegator) transfers this task to a competent person who within their scope of practice is allowed to perform such task (e.g., bed bath)
- RN gives the delegate the authority to complete the task
- UAP (delegate) must complete assigned task

As mentioned earlier, the ANA in its joint statement with the NCSBN (2006) defines the principles for delegation. There are four steps in the process of delegation. These are:

STEP 1—PLANNING AND ASSESSMENT

During the assessment and planning step of the delegation process, the nurse carefully outlines patient care and specifies the knowledge, skills, and attitudes (KSAs) required to complete the task based on patient needs and available resources (ANA & NCSBN, 2006). If all criteria are met and both environment and patient are stable, then the nurse plans the implementation of care with the patient/family keeping safety as the guiding principle at all times.

STEP 2—COMMUNICATION: "SECRET INGREDIENT OF DELEGATION"

The one ingredient that, if missing from the delegation process, can strongly impact quality outcomes, basic operations, fiscal bottom line, and patient safety is *effective communication* and the concept of *mindful communication*. Sounds like common sense, right? No, not every nurse is comfortable and proficient at delivering effective communication. Effective communication is critical to the success of the delegation process and it must consist of a two-way process.

Anthony and Vidal (2010) describe "mindful communication" as the process by which individuals engage in communication that is timely, meaningful, and that is in constant motion, responding to unfolding events. Murray (2017) emphasizes that mindful communication entails one to be an active participant in the dynamic processing of information, which requires the players involved to be focused on the reception, perception, and then in turn, to be responsive to this information. The nurse must assess the delegate's understanding of the expectations delegated, which means you as the nurse may have to verify and validate other's understanding and clarify if required (Murray, 2017). It is important to note that mindful communication allows both delegator (RN) and delegate (UAP) an opportunity to be active participants; it allows an opportunity for questions and clarification to occur; it allows that the UAP must accept the task being assigned.

As discussed in Chapter 7, the I-SBAR method of communication is directed at improving team communication dealing with aspects of patient care that requires attention and action steps.

STEP 3—SURVEILLANCE AND SUPERVISION

Nurses are responsible for all aspects of patient care delivered including identifying the level of supervision and surveillance required. Ongoing assessment of both the patient's status, condition, and the staff effectiveness is needed and could potentially require intervention. At all times, the RN is responsible and must supervise the delegate to ensure compliance within the appropriate scope and standards as well as organizational policies and procedures (ANA & NCSBN, 2006).

STEP 4—EVALUATION AND FEEDBACK

The final step is that of both evaluation and timely feedback. During this step, the RN assesses the completion of the task assigned to the delegate, collaborates with the patient/family, determines if the plan of care needs to be revised, and provides the delegate or UAP with feedback regarding the successful completion or next steps if necessary to complete the task originally assigned.

THE FIVE RIGHTS OF DELEGATION

The "Five Rights of Delegation" are a guide for an RN to use to clarify the key elements of the delegation and decision-making process. They clearly illuminate the fact that the RN must always ensure that the **right task** is assigned under the **right circumstances** to the **right person** with the RN him or herself providing the **right direction/effective communication** and the **right supervision/evaluation** (ANA & NCSBN, 2006). RNs must use both critical thinking skills and professional sound judgment when following the Five Rights of Delegation.

1. **Right Task**
2. **Right Circumstances**
3. **Right Person**
4. **Right Direction/Effective Communication**
5. **Right Supervision/Evaluation**

Furthermore, it is important to note that the Five Rights of Delegation delineate accountability for *all nurses* at *all levels* within the organization from bedside to boardroom. This is evident in Delegation Principles nursing practice poster illustrated from Texas Health and Human Services and Texas Board of Nursing (2017) in Figure 8.1.

QUESTIONS TO CONSIDER BEFORE READING ON

- Recall a time when you delegated or chose not to delegate certain tasks to members of your healthcare team and at the end of the day things were not completed or not completed correctly. How did your delegating/not delegating influence patient/family/staff satisfaction? How did delegating/not delegating influence time management (i.e., did it result in saving time, overtime, etc.).

DELEGATION PRINCIPLES

The following "Five Rights of Delegation" delineate accountability for nurses at all levels from nursing service administrators to registered nurses.

NURSING SERVICE ADMINISTRATOR

RIGHT TASK

- Identify appropriate delegation activities in unlicensed assistive person (UAP) job description/role delineation.
- Describe expectations of and limits to organizational policies, procedures and standards.

RIGHT CIRCUMSTANCES

- Assess the health of the client community, analyze the data and identify collective nursing care needs, priorities and necessary resources.
- Provide appropriate staffing and skill mix, identify clear lines of authority and reporting, and provide sufficient equipment and supplies to meet the nursing care needs.
- Provide appropriate preparation in management techniques to deliver and delegate care.

RIGHT PERSON

- Establish organizational standards consistent with applicable law and rules that identify educational and training requirements and competency measurements of nurses and UAP.
- Incorporate competency standards into institutional policies; assess nurse and UAP performance; perform evaluations based upon standards; and take steps to remedy failure to meet standards, including reporting nurses who fail to meet standards to Board of Nursing.

RIGHT DIRECTION/COMMUNICATION

- Communicate acceptable activities, UAP competencies and qualifications, and the supervision plan through a description of a nursing service delivery model, standards of care, role descriptions, and policies or procedures.

RIGHT SUPERVISION/EVALUATION

- Ensure human resources, including time and supervision, to ensure care is adequate, meets clients' needs.
- Identify by position, title and role delineation the licensed nurses responsible for providing supervision needs.
- Evaluate outcomes of client community and use information to develop quality assurance and to contribute to risk-management plans.

The Five Rights of Delegation, identified in the National Guidelines for Nursing Delegation (Journal of Nursing Regulation, 2016) from the National Council of State Boards of Nursing, can be used as a mental checklist to assist nurses from multiple roles to clarify the critical elements of the decision-making process.

STAFF NURSE (RN/APRN)

RIGHT TASK

- Identify appropriate delegation activities are for specific client(s).
- Identify appropriate activities for specific unlicensed assistive person (UAP).

RIGHT CIRCUMSTANCES

- Assess health status of individual client(s), analyze the data and identify client-specific goals and nursing care needs.
- Match the complexity of the activity with the UAP and competency with the level of supervision available.
- Provide for appropriate monitoring and guidance for the combination of client, activity and personnel.

RIGHT PERSON

- Instruct and/or assess, verify and identify the UAP's competency on an individual and client-specific basis.
- Implement own professional development activities based on assessed needs; assess UAP performance; evaluate UAP based upon standards; and take steps to remedy failure to meet standards.

RIGHT DIRECTION/COMMUNICATION

- Communicate delegation decisions on a client-specific and UAP-specific basis. The detail and method (oral and/or written) vary with the specific circumstances.
- Situation-specific communication includes:
  - Specific data to be collected and method and timelines for reporting.
  - Specific activities to be performed and client-specific instruction and limitation.
  - The expected results or potential complications and timelines for communicating such information.

RIGHT SUPERVISION/EVALUATION

- Supervise performance of specific nursing activities or assign supervision to other licensed nurses.
- Provide directions and clear expectations of how the activity is to be performed:
  - Monitor performance.
  - Obtain and provide feedback.
  - Intervene if necessary.
  - Ensure proper documentation.
- Evaluate the entire delegation process including the client and the performance of the activity.

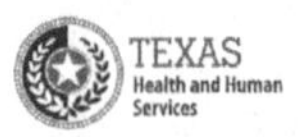

www.dads.state.tx.us/providers/qmp/index.cfm

For more information, visit **www.bon.texas.gov**

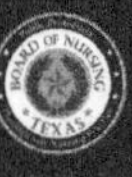

Nursing Practice poster 3 of 6

FIGURE 8.1 The Five Rights of Delegation for staff nurse/administrator.

Source: Texas Board of Nursing. (n.d.) Delegation principles [Poster]. Retrieved from http://www.bon.texas.gov/pdfs/delegation_pdfs/Delegation-fiverights.pdf (reprinted with permission from Texas Health and Human Services & Texas Board of Nursing)

After recalling some of your own experiences, let us dive into this scenario that follows.

COMMON DELEGATION PITFALLS AND CHALLENGES

Delegation is not an easy task or process for the professional nurse. As mentioned earlier, it is a critical leadership skill that evolves over time and is part of lifelong learning. Box 8.2 depicts a clinical scenario that portrays principles of delegation and common challenges you may encounter. Effective delegation that influences both financial and clinical outcomes focused on patient-centered care is paramount to safe, effective, quality patient care. Delegation, not unlike other nursing competencies, is a highly specialized skill that lends itself to error during the planning and implementation (Standing & Anthony, 2008). There are three major very common delegation themes that occur when

BOX 8.2 CASE SCENARIO

As you read this case scenario, reflect on the following questions:

- What obstacles or pitfalls do you think contributed to James's lack of success?
- Do you think James overdelegated? underdelegated? and/or improperly delegated?
- Did James follow the five delegation principles? If not, which one(s) did he omit?
- What could or should James have done differently?

James has been a nurse for 4 years now. He works 3 a.m. to 11:30 p.m. on a very busy 32-bed medical–surgical unit. Census is 32; however, there were eight discharges during the day shift and eight new admissions have been steadily arriving to the floor mostly around the change of shift.

Staff morale and the sense of teamwork are low with coworkers upset with each other when the admission history, medication reconciliation, and plan of care are not completely done prior to leaving the shift.

Four patients have gone for procedures early in the evening and were stable but required frequent vital signs. James has asked the two UAP to take vital signs on the patients. He also asked a transporter to bring in a cup of medications for Mr. Smith because he was on isolation and the transporter was already going in the room.

At the end of the shift, upon reviewing the vital signs to give report to the oncoming nurse, he noticed just one set of vitals were taken for each patient instead of q1 hour as ordered. Upon final rounding for the evening, he also noticed that Mr. Smith's cup of medications was on his bedside and not taken.

In addition, these patients were nothing by mouth (NPO) prior to the diagnostic tests and both patients and families are upset because they never received dinner and now the kitchen is closed. James is upset.

we speak about errors in the skill and process of delegation. These are **under-delegation, overdelegation**, and **improper delegation.** Box 8.3 provides you with different scenarios and an opportunity to identify whether they exhibit underdelegation, overdelegation, or improper delegation.

UNDERDELEGATION

There are a variety of different reasons that underdelegation errors can occur. Underdelegation can occur as a result of the RN's lack of experience or lack of confidence in delegating. Delegators could be afraid that

BOX 8.3 CASE SCENARIOS

Read the following three brief case scenarios. Determine what type of delegation (i.e., improper, underdelegation, or overdelegation) is depicted in each of the three scenarios.

CASE 1

Peter has been a nurse for 3 years. He is a conscientious, caring professional who takes pride in providing quality care to all of his patients. Having worked as a certified nursing assistant (CNA) before becoming a nurse, he is comfortable with providing all of the necessary care for everyone on his assignment. Peter works as a nurse in the same unit where he was a CNA and is hesitant to assign tasks to his coworkers. As a result, he gets behind schedule during morning rounds.

- Why do you think Peter is hesitant to assign tasks to his coworkers?

CASE 2

Linda works in the same unit as Peter and has been a nurse for 10 years. She especially enjoys caring for postsurgical patients when they return to the unit. If an admission arrives while Linda is caring for another patient, she will frequently ask Peter to perform her assigned initial assessment.

- What advice would you give Peter?
- What advice can you offer Peter in his response to Linda's request?

CASE 3

Although Linda is caring for a patient, a postsurgical admission arrives to the unit and is very restless and complaining of severe abdominal pain. Because Linda is busy, she asks the UAP to go see the patient and assess the pain.

- How should the UAP respond to Linda's request?
- What would you do as a member of the team who witnesses Linda's request to the UAP to go see the patient and assess the pain?

they will be perceived as bossy and no one will like them if they delegate. Underdelegating could also be the result of some mistrust or the need to be in total control and persons can do that only if they perform all tasks themselves. Time delay and waiting too long can also contribute to underdelegation. Underdelegating is irresponsible as the nurse who is paid at a higher wage level is now performing specific tasks that could be completed at a lesser rate of pay by a qualified UAP. This does not mean that it is completed better or with a higher degree of quality or caring and compassion. It could actually be viewed as irresponsible because it is fiscally wasteful and it is taking the RN away from other activities he or she could be doing when specialized training and education are required.

OVERDELEGATION

Overdelegation can also occur for a variety of different reasons. Sometimes it is because of the nurse/patient staffing ratios, patient acuity, and/or workload issues. Other times it could be the delegator's lack of experience with a specific task or his or her own poor time management skills. Still other causes could be lack of proper prioritization or fear of safety concerns that lead to over or improper delegation.

IMPROPER DELEGATION

Improper delegation results oftentimes from inexperience or faulty thinking. In Table 8.1, you can see some statements you have probably said to yourself or heard others say when faced with the task to delegate or not. "Will people like me?" "Will they think I am lazy?" "Will it cause conflict?" If so, "I would rather do it myself" and "I am not sure they know how to do it" "What if they do it wrong?" When a nurse does not or will not delegate tasks appropriately to UAP, several outcomes both positive and negative can occur.

OUTCOMES

NEGATIVE OUTCOMES

Negative outcomes resulting from underdelegation, overdelegation, and improper delegation range from unnecessary overtime, fiscal irresponsibility, lack of professional development, poor staff satisfaction and retention, low patient satisfaction rates, adverse medical events reaching the patient/family, and causing harm.

TABLE 8.1 DELEGATION CHALLENGES AND OUTCOMES

Delegation Themes	Common Pitfalls/ Errors	Outcomes
Underdelegating	Mistrust Fear of conflict Lack of confidence Lack of supervision Time delay Faulty thinking "It is easier to do it myself" "People will think I am lazy if I ask them to do something" "People won't like me" "People will think I'm too bossy" "I am responsible for the overall outcome, so what if they do it wrong?" "They won't do it the way I want them to, so if you want something done, you might as well do it yourself"	Unnecessary overtime Budget deficits Unfair workload issues Lack of growth opportunity for other staff members Lack of feeling needed by other staff Poor communication and collaboration of team Erosion of team
Overdelegating	Failure to use critical thinking skills Lack of self-confidence in a skill Lack of prioritization of patient safety Poor time management skills	Unfair workload issues Erosion of team Poor communication and collaboration of team
Improper delegating	Lack of supervision Time delay Lack of self-confidence in a skill Failure to use critical thinking skills Lack of prioritization of patient safety Ineffective communication	Unnecessary overtime Budget deficits Unfair workload issues Lack of feeling needed by other staff Erosion of team Poor communication and collaboration of team Lack of growth opportunity for other staff members Increase or decrease in adverse patient safety events

(continued)

TABLE 8.1 *(continued)*

Delegation Themes	Common Pitfalls/ Errors	Outcomes
	Failure to supervise/ surveillance Failure to evaluate Faulty thinking	High or low RN turnover/retention rates High or low UAP turnover/retention rates Effect on quality outcomes which include but are not limited to falls, HAPU, CAUTI, CLABSI, patient/ family satisfaction Positive or negative employee satisfaction survey results Fiscal responsibility and cost containment

CAUTI, catheter-associated urinary tract infection; CLABSI, central line-associated bloodstrem infection; HAPU, hospital-acquired pressure ulcer; UAP, unlicensed assistive personnel

POSITIVE OUTCOMES

On the contrary, when delegation is carried out and accomplished correctly, the outcomes can be positive and benefits can range from a unit and organization being fiscally responsible to positive budget savings, high staff productivity, low recruitment and high retention rates, low overtime, high morale, high employee satisfaction rate, professional growth and development of employees, and positive patient/family quality indicators and satisfaction.

PATIENT SAFETY DEPENDS ON EFFECTIVE DELEGATION SKILLS AND QSEN COMPETENCIES

The Institute of Medicine's (IOM) landmark report *To Err Is Human* was a wake-up call for healthcare. It highlighted the fact that between 44,000 and 98,000 patient deaths per year were because of medical error. This report recommended that interprofessional team training programs should be implemented in hospitals and academic programs to improve the communication and coordination of care to reduce preventable medical errors (IOM, 2000). The IOM report highlights that nurses and other members of the interdisciplinary healthcare team need to develop and maintain proficiency in five core areas: delivering patient-centered care, working as a part of interdisciplinary teams, practicing evidence-based medicine, focusing on quality improvement, and using information technology.

In response to the IOM recommendations, nurse leaders leapt into action and in 2005, responded to their urgent call for action to improve the quality and safety of healthcare across the country with the establishment of the Quality and Safety Education for Nurses (QSEN) Initiative funded by the Robert Wood Johnson Foundation (QSEN Institute, 2014). This initiative focused on the development of both quality and safety competencies that serve as a blueprint for nursing faculty to integrate and infuse these competencies into the nursing education RN-BSN curriculum.

There are six QSEN competencies that were developed for prelicensure and graduate nursing programs: patient-centered care, teamwork and collaboration, evidence-based practice (EBP), quality improvement (QI), safety, and informatics. This initiative has now evolved into what is known as the QSEN Institute and encompasses not only undergraduate nursing student education but also education focusing on quality and safety for all nurses both pre- and postlicensure. The bottom line and focus of QSEN is to address the challenge of assuring that all nurses possess the KSAs required to adequately and continuously seek to enhance and improve the quality and safety of the patients, families, and healthcare systems in which they work each and every day (Dolansky & Moore, 2013).

SIMPLE TRANSLATION—4Cs

Caring, communication, collaboration, and coordination of care are essential elements in the QSEN competencies that help develop and strengthen your delegation skills. These specific KSAs associated with the patient/family as well as teamwork and collaboration are presented in Table 8.2.

Nurses must recognize the patient or designee as the source of control and full partner in providing compassionate and coordinated care based on respect for the patient's preferences, values, and needs. In addition, working collaboratively as part of an interprofessional team is a core competency that nurses must possess.

SELF-ASSESSMENT OF CURRENT DELEGATION SKILLS

Let us take a pause and perform a self-assessment presented in Table 8.3 on your own current status, comfort level, and ability to delegate in your role as a professional nurse.

DELEGATION WITHIN THE NURSING PROFESSION

It is important to end this chapter with one final note to emphasize how much growth there has been within the profession of nursing. You are part of this growth with your commitment to learning! Delegation does not occur

TABLE 8.2 DELEGATION SKILLS AND QSEN COMPETENCIES

Patient-centered care:

- Describe own strengths, limitations, and values in functioning as a member of a team (Knowledge)
- Integrate understanding of multiple dimensions of patient-centered care; coordination and integration of care (Knowledge)
- Examine nursing roles in assuring coordination, integration, and continuity of care (Knowledge)
- Communicate patient values, preferences and expressed needs to other members of healthcare team (Skills)
- Communicate care provided and needed at each transition of care (Skills)
- Value seeing healthcare situations "through patients' eyes" (Attitudes)

Teamwork and collaboration:

- Describe scopes of practice and roles of healthcare team members (Knowledge)
- Describe own strengths, limitations, and values in functioning as a member of a team (Knowledge)
- Describe strategies for identifying and managing overlaps in team member roles and accountabilities (Knowledge)
- Recognize contributions of other individuals and groups in helping patient/family achieve health goals (Knowledge)
- Discuss effective strategies for communicating and resolving conflict (Knowledge)
- Identify system barriers and facilitators of effective team functioning (Knowledge)
- Function competently within own scope of practice as a member of the healthcare team (Skill)
- Assume role of team member or leader on the basis of the situation (Skill)
- Initiate requests for help when appropriate to situation (Skill)
- Integrate the contributions of others who play a role in helping patient/family achieve health goals (Skill)
- Communicate with team members, adapting own style of communicating to needs of the team and situation (Skill)
- Solicit input from other team members to improve individual, as well as team, performance (Skill)
- Follow communication practices that minimize risks associated with handoffs among providers and across transitions in care (Skill)
- Acknowledge own potential to contribute to effective team functioning (Attitude)
- Value the perspectives and expertise of all health team members (Attitude)
- Respect the unique attributes that members bring to a team, including variations in professional orientations and accountabilities (Attitude)

Source: Quality and Safety Education for Nurses Institute. (2011). Delegation: A collaborative, patient-centered approach. Retrieved from http://qsen.org/delegation-a-collaborative-patient-centered-approach

only with unlicensed personnel but within the varying levels of nursing licensure that exist, such as APRN, RN, and LPN/VN. *You* yourself may be asked to perform a task of which you are unsure whether you are allowed to do so within your scope of practice.

In 2015, the Tri-Council for Nursing, consisting of the AACN, the ANA, the American Organization of Nurse Executives (AONE), and the National League for Nursing (NLN), in collaboration with the NCSBN, determined that a uniform scope of practice decision-making tree tool was needed. This collaboration resulted in a current tool that can be adopted and tailored by individual

TABLE 8.3 DELEGATION SELF-ASSESSMENT
Were you familiar with the Five Rights of Delegation prior to reading this chapter?
How often do you delegate tasks to others during your shift?
Are you comfortable when delegating tasks to others? If so, why?
Are you uncomfortable when delegating tasks to others? If so, why?
Do you feel you underdelegate?
Do you feel you overdelegate?
Can you recall a time when you felt you improperly delegated? Why? What were the circumstances?
Do you verify and validate that the person to whom you are delegating has accepted the task? Understands the task being assigned?
Do you offer an opportunity for questions/clarification if the delegate is unsure of what you are asking from him or her?
Have you ever been in the position where you were the delegate? How did it make you feel? Were you comfortable with the task being assigned?
If as the delegate, you were uncomfortable with the task being assigned and you knew it was not within your scope of practice, what did you do? Did you feel empowered to stop the line and decline the task?
Does your workplace support staff to question inappropriate delegation practices if they were to occur?

state boards of nursing and organizations as an educational tool only to help nurses determine specific tasks and interventions according to a nurse's level of education, licensure, competence as well as specific state jurisdictions (Ballard et al., 2017; see www.ncsbn.org/decision-making-framework.htm).

CONCLUSIONS

Delegation is a complex skill that is an essential and core component for professional nursing practice today. Delegation requires nursing knowledge regarding your specific state's nurse practice act, critical thinking skills, and final accountability for overall patient care. It is important to remember that nurses at all levels, from the bedside to the boardroom, and in all types of healthcare settings, are obligated to actively participate in the delegation process that encompasses assigning and delegating tasks to other healthcare team members as well as the appropriate supervision and evaluation of these tasks that were delegated. Effective delegation is critical to the delivery of safe quality care and results in positive quality outcomes when executed correctly, having positioned the nurse at the appropriate place and time reflective of nursing expertise. Organizations must embrace, elevate, and equip all levels of the nursing leadership team in efforts and strategies to coordinate, delegate, supervise, and evaluate care within each team member's appropriate scope of practice as needed to ensure all care is safe, effective, and patient centered.

CRITICAL THINKING QUESTIONS AND ACTIVITIES

- To delegate or not to delegate? Refer to the basic delegation principles, the four steps of the delegation process, your own state's Nurse Practice Act and/or the NCSBN decision tree algorithm (www.ncsbn.org/Delegation_joint_statement_NCSBN-ANA.pdf) to determine which of the tasks in Table 8.4 you would delegate to a UAP. This activity can be completed either individually or in a group. Once completed, discuss in small groups. Did you all agree?
- Read the article titled *Helping new nurses with the fine art of delegation* found on the webpage link: www.strategiesfornursemanagers.com/content.cfm?content_id=233639&oc_id=602#

  Have you ever delegated a task to UAP and were unsure if they understood what you were asking them to do? If so, what did you do?

  Do you agree that the delegation process is not complete until the delegate accepts responsibility? What does this look like? How can you ensure a proper understanding and acceptance of the task?

  At the completion of the article, you should be able to list common tasks that you could delegate to UAP and recognize potential obstacles to effective delegation. Complete the two delegation activities (case studies). They describe how, when, why, and to whom the task can be delegated. What happens next? Is this the end of the process? What is the final step? What will you do differently the next time you delegate? Will you feel more comfortable and confident the next time you delegate?

TABLE 8.4 DELEGATION OF NURSING TASKS

Tasks	Appropriate to assign to UAP	Inappropriate to assign to UAP
1. Performing a bed bath	2.	3.
4. Assisting a patient out of bed for the first time after gall bladder surgery	5.	6.
7. Emptying urine from a Foley catheter bag	8.	9.

(continued)

TABLE 8.4 *(continued)*

Tasks	Appropriate to assign to UAP	Inappropriate to assign to UAP
10. Tracheostomy care	**11.**	**12.**
13. Admission history and assessment	**14.**	**15.**
16. Routine pain assessment	**17.**	**18.**
19. Nasogastric tube insertion for gastric decompression	**20.**	**21.**
22. Neurological evaluation status poststroke	**23.**	**24.**
25. Neurological evaluation status postcraniotomy	**26.**	**27.**
28. Medication administration	**29.**	**30.**
31. Peritoneal dialysis	**32.**	**33.**
34. Foley insertion	**35.**	**36.**
37. Colostomy care	**38.**	**39.**
40. Post mortem care	**41.**	**42.**
43. Wound vacuum application and maintenance	**44.**	**45.**
46. CBI status post-TURP	**47.**	**48.**
49. Monitor limb with deep vein thrombosis	**50.**	**51.**
52. Placing telemetry monitor leads on patient's chest	**53.**	**54.**
55. Monitoring intravenous fluids	**56.**	**57.**
58. Measuring intake and output	**59.**	**60.**

CBI, continuous bladder irrigation; TURP, transurethral resection of the prostate; UAP, unlicensed assistive personnel.

REFERENCES

American Association of Colleges of Nursing. (2008). *The essentials of baccalaureate education for professional nursing practice*. Washington, DC: Author.

American Nurses Association. (2010). *Nursing's social policy statement: The essence of the profession* (3rd ed.). Silver Spring, MD: Author.

American Nurses Association. (2012). *Principles for delegation by registered nurses to unlicensed assistive personnel (UAP)*. Silver Spring, MD: Author. Retrieved from https://www.scribd.com/document/236757515/Principles-of-Delegation

American Nurses Association. (2015). *Nursing scope and standards of practice* (3rd ed.). Silver Spring, MD: Author.

American Nurses Association & National Council of State Boards of Nursing. (2006). Joint statement on delegation. Retrieved from https://www.ncsbn.org/Delegation_joint_statement_NCSBN-ANA.pdf

Anthony, M. K., & Vidal, K. (2010, May 31). Mindful communication: A novel approach to improving delegation and increasing patient safety. *Online Journal of Issues in Nursing, 15*(2), Manuscript 2. doi:10.3912/OJIN.Vol15No2Man02

Ballard, K., Haagenson, D., Christiansen, L., Damgaard, G., Halstead, J. A., Jason, R. R., ... Alexander, M. (2017). Scope of nursing practice decision-making framework. *Missouri State Board of Nursing Newsletter, 19*(1), 5, 7. Retrieved from https://www.sehcollege.edu/~/media/files/college/missouri-2017-board-of-nursing-newsletter.pdf?la=en

Dolansky, M. A., & Moore, S. M. (2013, September 30). Quality and safety education for nurses (QSEN): The key is systems thinking. *Online Journal of Issues in Nursing, 18*(3). doi:10.3912/OJIN.Vol18No03Man01

Finkelman, A., & Kenner, C. (2016). *Professional nursing concepts: Competencies for quality leadership* (3rd ed.). Sudbury, MA: Jones & Bartlett.

Murray, E. (2017). Nursing Leadership and Management for Patient Safety and Quality Care. Philadelphia, PA: F.A. Davis.

National Council of State Boards of Nursing. (2005). *Working with others: A position paper*. Retrieved from https://www.ncsbn.org/Working_with_Others.pdf

National Council of State Boards of Nursing. (2006). Decision tree-delegation to nursing assistive personnel. Retrieved from https://www.ncsbn.org/Delegation_joint_statement_NCSBN-ANA.pdf

National Council of State Boards of Nursing. (2017). Delegation. Retrieved from https://www.ncsbn.org/1625.htm

Quality and Safety Education for Nurses Institute. (2011). Delegation: A collaborative, patient-centered approach. Retrieved from http://qsen.org/delegation-a-collaborative-patient-centered-approach

Quality and Safety Education for Nurses Institute. (2014). Competencies. Retrieved from http://qsen.org/competencies

Schub, E., & Cabrera, G. (2016). *Delegation of authority: Delegating tasks to assistive healthcare personnel*. Glendale, CA: CINAHL Nursing Guide.

Standing, T. S., & Anthony, M. K. (2008). Delegation: What it means to acute care nurses. *Applied Nursing Research, 21*(1), 8–14. doi:10.1016/j.apnr.2006.08.010

Texas Board of Nursing. (n.d.) Delegation principles [Poster]. Retrieved from http://www.bon.texas.gov/pdfs/delegation_pdfs/Delegation-fiverights.pdf

9

BUILDING AND LEADING TEAMS

DAVID M. DEPUKAT ● KARRI DAVIS

LEARNING OBJECTIVES

After completion of this chapter, the reader will be able to

- Discuss the concept of teams.
- Explain approaches to develop strong teams.
- Describe considerations to have when building teams including roles and experiences.
- Describe team development processes from formation to completion.
- Describe the elements of successful teams including a shared vision and project charter.
- Explain how factors such as incivility, bullying, and workplace violence inhibit team workflow.
- List approaches that a team leader can use to address incivility.
- Describe how to measure the success of teams through both formative and summative evaluation.

Effective teams are essential in healthcare. Consider the delivery of patient care. Each patient has a complex team that works collaboratively to achieve safe, high-quality, and efficient care. The team is composed of registered nurses, physicians, pharmacists, therapists, and many others. Although each profession has key responsibilities, such as physicians prescribing therapies and nurses managing actual and potential human responses to health problems, the team must collaborate and coordinate efforts to deliver its key objective: patient care. However, effective teams are needed in healthcare to address issues beyond the bedside of the patient. For example, teams may be pulled together to improve high rates of adverse events such as hospital-acquired infections, low patient satisfaction scores, or operational metrics such as time for a patient to get a follow-up appointment. Each team, on the basis of its objective, is and should be unique in a variety of ways. As organizations continually strive for improvements and continue the journey toward high reliability, these teams will become more essential. Nurses, in particular, are well-suited to provide leadership to these teams. This chapter focuses on how teams are built, how teams move, progress, and are evaluated.

You have likely been a member of many teams in your experience as a registered nurse. At the very least, you have been a member of a care team, which aimed to provide excellent, safe, and quality care to a patient or a patient population. In this chapter, you will explore an evolving case scenario involving Madelyn, a registered nurse, who will be forming and leading her first team. Box 9.1 introduces this scenario. As healthcare's complexity continues to expand, your roles in improvement teams, beyond the delivery of care to an individual patient, will likely expand. To build upon these experiences, Table 9.1 describes the Quality and Safety Education for Nurses (QSEN) competencies addressed in this chapter related to building and leading teams. Before starting this chapter, take a moment to complete the TeamSTEPPS Teamwork Attitudes Questionnaire (T-TAQ) by the Agency for Healthcare Research and Quality (AHRQ; available online at www.ahrq.gov/teamstepps/instructor/reference/teamattitude.html). After completing this questionnaire, consider the following questions:

- Were there any items that surprised you or that you did not consider when thinking of teams?

BOX 9.1 CASE SCENARIO

As you read this case scenario (Box 9.1), reflect on the following questions:

- What characteristics would make Madelyn successful as a leader?
- Whom do you think Madelyn would need on her team? Think beyond nursing.
- Simply stated, what do you think the objective of Madelyn's team should be?

Madelyn is a registered nurse who recently completed her RN-to-BSN program and provides leadership to a pediatric quality and safety department at a large, academic medical center. During a departmental meeting, the nursing director reviewed each unit's catheter-associated urinary tract infection (CAUTI) rate. Each unit's rate for the previous quarter was above national benchmarks for similar units (higher rate means more CAUTIs). The nursing director asked Madelyn to form a team to investigate any trends and improve the rates. Madelyn had been a nurse providing direct patient care in the pediatric intensive care unit for 3 years. She transitioned into this role 2 months ago, and she has minimal experience leading teams.

TABLE 9.1 BUILDING AND LEADING TEAMS: RELEVANT QSEN COMPETENCIES

Knowledge	• Describe scopes of practice and roles of healthcare team members • Describe strategies for identifying and managing overlaps in team member roles and accountabilities • Discuss effective strategies for communicating and resolving conflict • Describe examples of the impact of team functioning on safety and quality of care • Identify system barriers and facilitators of effective team functioning • Examine strategies for improving systems to support team functioning
Skills	• Clarify roles and accountabilities under conditions of potential overlap in team member functioning • Demonstrate commitment to team goals • Participate in designing systems that support effective teamwork
Attitudes	• Appreciate importance of intra- and interprofessional collaboration • Value the perspectives and expertise of all health team members • Value the influence of system solutions in achieving effective team functioning

QSEN, Quality and Safety Education for Nurses.

Source: American Association of Colleges of Nursing. (2012). *Graduate level QSEN competencies: Knowledge, skills, and attitudes*. Washington, DC: Author.

- Were there any items that you rated as "disagree" or "strongly disagree"? Reflect on those items. What were some previous events in your professional life that influenced your answer?
- Within each section, which items do you think are most important? Limit your consideration to two or three. Why did you think that?

BUILDING TEAMS

According to Frankel and Leonard (2017), a "team" is "a group of people who work together in a coordinated way, which maximizes each team member's strengths, to achieve a common goal." In healthcare, teams take many forms. The most common team in healthcare focuses its attention on the patient, which Frankel and Leonard (2017) term "care teams." These teams leverage the strengths and roles of each discipline—physicians, advanced practice providers, registered nurses, and others—to achieve the mutually developed patient goals. Other teams focus on larger goals or objectives beyond direct patient care, or "improvement teams," on which this chapter focuses. However, different groups may be called different things. "Councils," for example, are typically high-level decision-making bodies with ongoing objectives that may not be quantifiable. For example, a quality council may be the ultimate decision-making body and authority for all quality matters. "Committees," which are usually smaller teams under a council but may exist independently, have focused, measurable, and objective goals. Like councils, the work of committees typically extends beyond meeting short-term goals. As committees and councils develop over time, goals are revised or new goals are made. A team, such as one focused on central-line associated bloodstream infections, would be classified as a committee. A "task force" is a team assembled to address a key deliverable or objective; once the goal or goals are completed, the team disbands. Sometimes, healthcare professionals assemble to discuss various topics but do not have a specific goal. These teams are called "groups." In healthcare, journal clubs or other information-shared venues are examples of groups. Table 9.2 shows the different types of teams and their purposes.

COMPOSITION OF TEAMS

Teams are composed of many different members with different levels of expertise. A team's leader, who provides operational leadership to the team, balances a purposefully considered membership with a manageable team size, such as five to seven for a task force and less than 15 for a council. For example, a team of two members lacking in content expertise will present challenges. Similarly but with different challenges, a team of 20 individuals would be difficult for a team leader to manage. Generally, the team leader builds a team that balances the members' key characteristics of respect, team player, listener, communicator, problem solver, frustration with current system, creator, innovator, and open to change (U.S. Department of Health and Human Services Health Resources and Services Administration [HRSA], n.d.). Although team members—not the team's leader—would rate "highly" on all of these characteristics, the team leader can balance the team's characteristics to assess the team as a whole. In addition to strategically building teams on the basis of characteristics, other elements exist in determining which members to include. The following sections discuss characteristics of team members as described by the Institute for Healthcare Improvement (IHI, 2017), of which one is a designated "team leader." A team leader may also be referred to as a "project leader" or "committee chair." Table 9.3 summarizes these four positions.

TABLE 9.2 SUMMARY OF TEAM TYPES

Team Type	Purpose
Council	Provides team for broad, organization-wide decision-making
Committee	Provides a team that is subordinate to a council for focused (in scope or scan) decision-making
Task force	Provides a team with focused attention on a single topic or goal, which is disbanded after the topic is addressed or goal is met
Group	Provides an information-sharing team or discussion forum that may not have established goals

TABLE 9.3 SUMMARY OF TEAM MEMBERS AND CHARACTERISTICS

Position	Characteristics	Purpose on the Team
Clinical leader	Formal or informal leader with an understanding of the micro- and macrosystems where the team is taking place	Ensures the changes are actualized
Technical expert	Subject-matter expert either in the clinical issue facing the team or in specific quality improvement methodologies	Provides expertise to develop interventions and implementation strategies
Day-to-day leader	Formal or informal leader with authority to implement changes	Implements the changes recommended by the team
Project sponsor	Executive or other formal leader with authority to remove barriers to implementation and improvements	Oversees team progress and intervenes as appropriate to ensure its success

Clinical Leader

The clinical leader has power—formally given or given through empowerment—to actualize the changes recommended by the team. Although formal leadership positions are considered for clinical leaders, registered nurses at the point of care delivery can be empowered by the project sponsor to assume these responsibilities. According to the IHI (2003), the clinical leader understands the direct and indirect impacts of change, for example both within and outside of the area where change is occurring. The clinical leader is not necessarily the team leader.

Technical Expert

A technical expert has strong knowledge of the objective and the associated topics, and these individuals are often referred to as "content experts" or "subject matter experts." The content or subject matter can be superficially gleaned from the objective statement. For example, an objective statement surrounding fall prevention in an older adult inpatient medical unit would require multiple technical experts. For example, a team leader may seek out experts in the care of older adults and in fall prevention. Although one individual may possess technical expertise in both matters, adding members to the team may add to the diversity of thought and experience. For some teams, technical expertise in quality improvement methods, evidence-based practice, and other topics may be required. Team leaders must not forget to include those healthcare professionals who provide care where the objective is focused. For example, some registered nurse or unlicensed assistive personnel may provide important cultural and practical expertise.

Day-to-Day Leader

After the team develops solutions, such as new interventions to reduce falls in an ambulatory surgical center, members of the team implement the changes. These members are referred to as "day-to-day leaders." These individuals are responsible for ensuring that the changes are practicable for implementation and the changes are adhered to after implementation. Often, these individuals have formal or given authority to ensure that members of the care team are accountable for the recommended changes. In addition, these individuals may collect adherence data through purposeful auditing and behavioral correction when deviations occur.

Project Sponsor

The project sponsor, or simply the sponsor, provides executive leadership with abilities to provide necessary resources or remove barriers. Such barriers may exist among departments or with individual persons that cannot be resolved by the team leader or members of the team. The sponsor ensures the direction of the team is correct and ensures the team is accountable for its objectives, goals, and deliverables. Unlike other members of the team, the sponsor is often not involved in the operations of the team and does not attend most meetings. Instead, the designated team leader reviews progress with the project sponsor intermittently and as needed. For example, a sponsor may intervene to influence team members inhibiting progress or ensure adequate resources are available for the team's success.

DIVERSITY AND INCLUSION

Diversity and inclusion have received much attention in nursing and other industries (American Association of Colleges of Nursing, 2017). Diversity extends beyond superficial characteristics such as race and gender. The underlying thought behind diversity and inclusion is that teams can be enriched when the team is heterogenous, or different, in characteristics. Purposefully considering aspects of diversity in team composition will ensure a thorough understanding of the issues associated with the objective as well as innovative ideas for solutions. Two examples of diversity include thought and experience. Inclusion surrounds *purposefully* engaging these individuals when they may not have been considered for their content expertise or leadership experience. Diversity without inclusion is like being invited to a party but not being asked to dance (Sherbin & Rashid, 2017).

Diversity of thought integrates individuals who think differently. Although it may be easiest to form teams with individuals who think similarly or have the same ideas to address issues, it is not necessarily the best approach for the leader to take. If diversity of thought is not considered when composing a team, ideas and innovations may be lost. A complete understanding of the objective's or problem's dimensions may be missed. Excluding members of the clinical care team or interprofessional partners could miss issues of practice that nurse leaders may not recognize. A team leader must purposefully consider and include team members who may think differently. Diversity of experience also enriches a team. Experience does not pertain to one aspect such as time as a registered nurse. Rather, diversity of experience is multifactorial and includes some of the following, albeit not comprehensive:

- Experience in the patient care population
- Experience in the organization
- Experience in the objective (albeit not in the population)
- Experience in leading teams

In Box 9.2, Madelyn will evaluate her team's composition, including aspects of diversity and inclusion.

BOX 9.2 THE CASE SCENARIO CONTINUES TO UNFOLD

As you read this case scenario, consider the following questions:

- Review the matrix of team members given in Table 9.4, which is based on the team composed by Madelyn in the case scenario of Box 9.1. Which team members are the strongest in terms of being respected within the pediatric department? Which members are the most resistant to change? For those members resistant to change, what roles may they take?
- Notice each team member has a similar summative score. What do you think this implies about the team? Is this a strength or a vulnerability of the team?

In the scope of the team, Madelyn composed both a purpose statement and an objective statement that are clear and measurable. The purpose of the team is to improve the CAUTI rates on pediatric units. Although this goal provides general direction, the objective statement provides specific direction and the measure of success: Improve the CAUTI rates on all pediatric units to below 1.5 for 3 consecutive months, within 12 months. She formed a committee as the team's purpose and objective will outlast the primary goal, and she included the following:

- M: Madelyn as the team leader
- D: The director of the pediatric department
- F: The medical director of pediatrics
- T: A pediatric urologist
- K: A nurse providing care in the pediatric critical care unit
- S: A nurse providing care in a general pediatric surgical unit
- E: A nurse manager of a general pediatric medical unit
- C: An infection preventionist who is knowledgeable about CAUTIs with experience in adult populations

TABLE 9.4 SAMPLE MATRIX OF TEAM MEMBERS

	Team Members' Initials							
Characteristics	M	D	F	T	K	S	E	C
Respected	3	4	4	4	2	2	3	4
Team player	4	4	1	2	2	3	4	2
Listener	4	2	1	2	4	3	3	2
Communicator	2	2	2	2	1	4	3	3
Problem solver	2	4	4	3	2	4	1	3
Frustrated with current system	3	1	2	4	4	1	4	4
Creative and innovative	2	4	4	1	3	2	1	3
Open to change	4	1	3	4	3	3	2	2
Total score	**24**	**22**	**21**	**22**	**21**	**22**	**21**	**23**

1, does not exhibit the characteristic; 2, sometimes exhibits the characteristic; 3, usually exhibits the characteristic; 4, almost always exhibits the characteristic.

DETERMINING THE OBJECTIVE OF THE TEAM

Effective teams have at least one objective. The objective—or objectives—provides the team with direction whereas a time frame for the objective sets the need for action. Without clear objectives and a time frame to achieve those objectives, teams often fail to successfully mobilize and achieve success (Sirkin, Keenan, & Jackson, 2005). Team objectives should be simple, measurable, and time-limited. Although teams may desire large-scale or far-reaching goals, McCannon, Schall, and Perla (2008) encourage teams to ensure that the team's objectives are achievable by its members. Otherwise, the team will become discouraged with its inability to meet its expectations. Table 9.5 provides examples of objective statements lacking essential components as well as a well-constructed alternative.

QUESTIONS TO CONSIDER BEFORE READING ON

- Consider a team on which you were a member. Were the goals and objectives clear? If the goals were clear, did that help provide the team with vision and success? If the goals were not clear, how did the team function? Did it meet established criteria?

(*continued*)

QUESTIONS TO CONSIDER BEFORE READING ON *(continued)*

- If you were on a team tasked with improving documentation of restraint episodes, review the following goal statement: Improve restraint documentation on the behavioral units to where 75% of restraint episodes have documentation without errors or omissions per policy. If you were asked to provide feedback on the goal, state how would you respond while taking into account:
  - Currently, only 10% of restraint episodes are documented without any errors.
  - Each time a restraint episode has errors or omissions, it presents violations of policy and significant regulatory implications such as from the Department of Public Health.

TABLE 9.5 EXAMPLES OF OBJECTIVE STATEMENTS

Statement	Simple	Measureable	Time-Limited	Comments
Decrease the CAUTI rate	Yes, but missing area(s)	No	No	An objective statement such as this one is vague and lacks direction for a team, although this statement may be aligned with a team's purpose
Decrease the CAUTI rate in the critical care unit by the end of next quarter	Yes	No	Yes	An objective statement such as this one does not quantify the improvement in the specified time frame, which does not set a unified goal for the magnitude of improvement
Decrease the CAUTI rate in the critical care unit by 40%	Yes	Yes	No	An objective statement such as this one does not provide a time-limit, which can cause the team to lose focus
Decrease the CAUTI rate in the critical care unit by 40% by the end of the next quarter	Yes	Yes	Yes	An objective statement such as this one is well written, clear, concise, and provides direction for the team

CAUTI, catheter-associated urinary tract infection.

TEAM MOBILIZATION

With the members of the team considered, the team leader mobilizes the team to address the problem and meet its objective or objectives. The initial meetings of the team focus on creating a shared vision for the team, which provides the team with general direction and a sense of unification around a problem or objective. With a shared vision, a team can be mobilized to "plan forward, reflect back, communicate clearly, and manage risk" to ensure the team's objectives are met (Frankel, Haraden, Federico, & Lenoci-Edwards, 2017).

CREATING THE SHARED VISION

A team is unified through a shared vision of its purpose, direction, and goals (Bibby, Bate, Carter, Robert, & Bevan, 2007; Kouzes & Posner, 2009). The IHI (2003) poses the following three questions to ask in developing a shared vision:

1. What are we trying to accomplish?
2. How will we know a change is an improvement?
3. What changes can we make that will result in improvement?

A shared vision is created, in part, through a background or problem statement as well as a purpose statement, at the very least. These statements should be clear and succinct while providing the basis for the team and direction for the team. For example, the following statements can be used for a team aimed at reducing falls with injury:

- Problem statement: The surgical units had a rate of falls with injury that was above the national benchmark for the previous four quarters.
- Purpose statement: Reduce the rate of falls on surgical units.

Some statements may require additional information because the problem or purpose may not be clear. For example, a team aimed at decreasing length of stay in an intensive care unit would likely be clear to content experts. However, an explanation of how prolonged lengths of stays create a shortage of intensive care unit beds for the emergency department's (ED's) admissions would provide a justification for the problem statement. Of note, the purpose statement and objective statement are closely related. A purpose statement may be simpler to provide the shared vision for the team. The objective statement adds the clear measures of success by which the team would be evaluated. Without an objective statement, the vision may be limited. An objective statement may be: Reduce the rate of falls with injury in surgical units to below the national benchmarks for each unit within two quarters. Although most teams dedicated to improvements in patient safety, McCannon et al. (2008) remind team leaders to review how one's team aligns with broader organizational goals as well as national trends.

DEVELOPING A CHARTER OR AGREEMENT

A team charter or agreement provides the structure for the team. Ideally, a charter is a written document that contains key information about the team. Although a background or purpose statement for the team is not always necessary, it is valuable. A purpose statement is a simple, quite succinct statement that is more abbreviated than an objective statement. Consider the following examples:

- Objective statement: Decrease the CAUTI rate in the critical care unit by 40% by the end of the next quarter.
- Purpose statement: Decrease the CAUTI rate in the critical care unit.

This charter includes the aforementioned goals and deliverables. In addition, this charter defines the scope of the project team in relation to the goals and deliverables, the beginning and end time of the project team, and other ad hoc members. The following points are typical elements of a charter but are not exhaustive.

Team Leader

The team leader owns the project. This individual provides operational leadership to the team in producing its deliverables and meeting its objectives. The role does not require formal authority or power, but the team leader has key leadership attributes.

Sponsor

In healthcare, the team sponsor may be a manager (if unit based), director (if service or department/program based), or member of the executive team (if wide spanning). As described, this individual ensures the team's success by removing barriers and providing resources as appropriate.

Team Members

A project charter lists all the team members who are included. This group should include content experts and others as appropriate. This list ensures all members have clarity of who is involved in the project. In addition, the charter can be shared with other teams to avoid duplication of work or competing efforts.

Measurable Objectives

To provide the team with direction, measureable objectives—in the form of objective statements—are included. Without measurable objectives, the team may become distracted or side-tracked with other goals beyond the scope of the team's initial purpose.

Scope of the Team

When appropriate, the team provides limits to what is within scope of the team and what is outside of the team's scope. Practically, this section of the charter document limits the team's work by focusing on key aspects despite other problems that may arise during the team's process. For example, a team formed to address the rate of falls in an ambulatory oncology setting may discover incomplete documentation during medical record reviews. The scope of the team may not allow for attention to this matter albeit important, because it may detract from the team's progress. When other problems arise, other teams may be more appropriate to manage it, or a task force may need to be formed.

Decision-Making Process

When forming teams, the decision-making process is essential to ensure that the team can determine interventions to implement. Two common decision-making processes are consensus based and majority based. Consensus occurs after thorough discussion surrounding the team members' viewpoints. At the end of the discussion, the team comes to a general agreement that each member can "live with." On the contrary, majority-based decision-making occurs when a certain percentage of a team agrees to the decision. Often, 60% is used, but 51% is considered a majority. A strong charter lists the percentage needed for a majority. Often, these two processes will require a set number or percentage of a team to be present to allow for decision-making, which is referred to as a "quorum." If enough team members are not present—where a quorum is not met—decision-making does not occur. Furthermore, an agreement upon this process ensures that the team moves forward and does not become dependent on single individuals. For a team to be successful, a sponsor empowers the team to make decisions but remains available and supportive as needed. Chapter 10 provides additional information about facilitating decision-making in teams.

TEAM PHASES

According to Scholtes, Joiner, and Streibel (2003), teams develop through four predictable phases:

- Stage 1: Forming—The team members come together around their leader and focus on priorities. Anxiety about nebulous expectations and workloads may occur as members learn to engage with and work with each other.

- Stage 2: Storming—The team members begin to better understand the complexity and nature of the team's priorities and objectives. In this stage, anxiety surrounding approaches to address the objectives may arise and effective progress will likely not yet begin. Interpersonal issues such as incivility, bullying, and shows of power may occur.
- Stage 3: Norming—Team members begin to cooperate as they understand the shared vision, and efforts are mobilized to address the team's objectives. This focused energy begins to reveal progress to designing tests of change and achieving the objective.
- Stage 4: Performing—In this stage, team members collaborate and move past key interpersonal issues. Communication problems are resolved, and the team develops a strong synergy to ensure progress toward the outcome.

MANAGING THE TEAM

According to McCannon et al. (2008), "superb planning is nearly meaningless in the absence of superb execution—the end of planning is only the beginning of the improvement process" (p. 13). Therefore, a team leader must be equally attentive to the team's structure as the team's processes. This concept draws on the traditional notion that outcomes are achieved through strong structures and processes (Donabedian, 1988).

CHARACTERISTICS OF SUCCESSFUL TEAMS

To be successful, a team needs a strong leader and support from a team sponsor. In addition to the team leader's responsibilities of forming a team, the leader is responsible for ensuring the operational success of the team. See Table 9.6 for team characteristics and their effect on the team's functioning. The lack of any characteristic will be a barrier to the team's success.

QUESTIONS TO CONSIDER BEFORE READING ON

- Reflect on a team of which you were a member or leader. Did any of the listed characteristics of successful teams interrupt the work of the team?
- In your opinion, which characteristic is most essential to the success of a team and which is least essential? From a team member, which characteristics when lacking frustrate you?

TABLE 9.6 CHARACTERISTICS OF SUCCESSFUL TEAMS

Characteristic	Effect on Team
Clear, shared vision	The team members focus and have attention to the problem
Skills and competencies necessary for the team to function (including leadership skills)	The team members gain confidence about the team's ability to be successful
Reward and motivating factors	The team practices steady change rather than change being slow or nonexistent
Adequate resources (human, time, financial, or material and equipment resources) to develop and implement changes	Team members become inspirited with the organization and the team
Action	The team members see change rather than becoming stagnated in discussion and contemplation

STRATEGIES TO HELP THE TEAM WORK EFFECTIVELY

Team Norms

When a team begins to form, all members should be oriented to clear behavioral expectations. These basic group norms will provide a foundation or framework from which the team can function. Expectations are shared among all members regardless of each member's formal, referential, or other power. The HRSA (n.d.) suggests many different norms such as:

- Start and end the meeting on time.
- Provide an agenda with responsible parties at least 1 week in advance of the meeting.
- Set clear expected outcomes for each meeting.
- Complete follow-up items for which members are responsible.
- Be polite and constructive in feedback provided while maintaining overall positivity.
- Ensure mutually agreeable timelines and responsibilities.
- Be actively engaged during the meeting time and between meetings, including being present (or with designee) at all scheduled meetings.
- Use of cell phones during meetings, unless critical, is discouraged.

Orientation of the Team

As noted by the HRSA (n.d.), a clear and thorough orientation of the team members to the goals and objectives of the project team is essential. The team discusses the goals of the team, the deliverables, the scope of the team, and the expected norms. This meeting provides the team with an opportunity to ask questions, express thoughts and concerns, and begin the work to ensure the success of the team. Written documentation of a charter, including the goals and deliverables, should be shared with the team. The team leader reviews these documents, during that orientation, for a clear understanding.

Meeting Effectiveness

A team's success is dependent on the conduction of effective meetings. The HRSA (n.d.) recommends many strategies to ensure success and includes using an agenda to plan meetings. A strong agenda will include discussion of follow-up business, new business with a representative named to lead or introduce items, and other discussion items. The agenda provides guidance to participants to prepare for the meeting. The responsibility of the team leader is to create the agenda and deliver it prior to the meeting to allow everyone time to read and prepare their questions and statements for the agenda. All agendas should include a copy of the previous meeting minutes which each member can review. These minutes will then be approved with any corrections members identify. Therefore, the principal method to ensure the success of the team will be the use of a structured agenda and meeting minutes to ensure everyone is provided a clear picture of what was discussed and decided and what needs to be discussed and decided at the next meeting. An example of an agenda is provided in Table 9.7.

TABLE 9.7 SAMPLE AGENDA

CAUTI Improvement Committee Administrative Conference Room January 11, 2018 0900–0945			
Time*	**Item**	**Preparation**	**Speaker(s)**
0900–0905	Review of previous meeting minutes	Review minutes	D. Depukat
0905–0915	Quality practices audit	Review attached data presentation	D. Depukat
0915–0935	Discussion: urine culture practices	None	K. Davis
0935–0940	Decision: 2018 educational plan	Review discussion in previous minutes as needed	K. Davis
0940–0945	Any remaining business, closure	None	D. Depukat, K. Davis

*Time may be adjusted based on conversational needs.

CAUTI, catheter-associated urinary tract infection.

Reviewing the progress of the committee is an essential activity to ensure the team's success. The review of objectives renews a focus to the aim of the team. This may incorporate a review of the team charter, such as the scope of the project team and progress toward deliverables. These conversations ensure that the team remains accountable to itself, because the review of these performance measures—whether outcome, process, or balancing—reorients the team. The result of these conversations, as well, can inform subsequent agendas, expose internal progresses that are lagging, and ensure the success of the project team. Additional information surrounding the team's evaluation—both formative and summative—is described later.

Team Communication

AHRQ developed TeamSTEPPS, in partnership with the U.S. Department of Defense, to improve patient safety through teamwork and collaboration. TeamSTEPPS is an educational teamwork system that focuses, mostly, on clinical care delivery. These elements of this framework include team structure, communication, leading teams, situation monitoring, mutual support, change management, and implementation. These concepts—especially communication—are generalizable to all types of teams. Communication occurs between a source and a receiver whereby a message is sent from the source to the receiver, and the receiver provides feedback to the source in receipt of the messages. AHRQ (2014) describes good, effective communication as clear, brief and concise, timely, and complete. However, communication in teams can break down quickly, for a variety of reasons such as distractions, fatigue, assumptions, workload, personalities, conflict, and different communication styles. Therefore, teams must be sensitive to these communication challenges by ensuring that communication is clear, concise, timely, and accurate. After all, communication within a team is essential to its success. The forms of communication can vary from interpersonal communication during and outside of meetings, electronic through email or other platform, or being memorialized in meeting minutes or agendas. Regardless of the form, the team leader oversees the communication and provides prompt feedback when appropriate to ensure that strong, effective communication occurs. Moreover, effective communication is the responsibility of each team member.

ISSUES WITHIN TEAMS

The American Nurses Association (ANA, 2015a) calls for nurses and all healthcare professionals to create and act within a civil and kind culture, which is associated with positive teamwork and high-quality patient care. Incivility and its associated behaviors directly impact the performance of care and improvement teams, and patient safety and clinical quality suffers (American Psychiatric Nurses Association [APNA], 2008; The Joint

Commission, 2008). As described by ANA (2015b), civility is demonstrated through the following actions among team members:

- Use respectful communication in all forms: verbal, nonverbal, electronic, written, and others.
- Treat each member of the healthcare team with respect and courtesy.
- Avoid the start and spread of rumors by using facts and information from the source rather than second-handed.
- Offer assistance to members of the team.
- Collaborate to ensure teamwork.
- Take responsibility for uncivil behaviors including those that are accidental.
- Listen to others respectfully and attentively.
- Demonstrate and request mutual respect for all members regardless of experience, role, gender, or other characteristic.

Unfortunately, teams are often impacted by issues such as incivility, bullying, and workplace violence due to a variety of possible reasons. In the arena of healthcare, authority gradients apply to perceived hierarchical relationships due to traditional roles rather than an interprofessional notion, which often leads to conflict. For example, an authority gradient often exists between physicians and nurses, nurses and unlicensed personnel, novice and expert nurses, and others. Consider an example that may happen during a nurse's orientation in the emergency department (ED). A car accident victim is admitted to the department, and the orienting nurse finds the patient's heart sounds to be muffled. The preceptor dismisses the findings as novice ears. Dismayed, the orienting nurse does not speak up when assessing distended neck veins. Unfortunately, the authority gradient, in this hypothetical case, could cause a breakdown in communication that could lead to an acute event related to cardiac tamponade. Generational and cultural differences may influence authority gradients or impair communication. A team leader must be prepared to address issues that may arise. Although these issues are discussed within the context of the team, they represent a much wider issue beyond the scope of this chapter.

Incivility

Incivility takes the form of disruptive and hurtful behaviors such as making derogatory comments, starting or spreading rumors, publically criticizing, using a condescending tone, venting in a negative manner, among other behaviors (ANA, 2015b). These behaviors do not need to be verbal or overt. Rather, eye-rolling or ignoring can be viewed as uncivil behaviors. Although some behaviors, such as venting or criticizing, may not be directed at a single individual and viewed as "harmless," these behaviors can lead to more significant behaviors such as bullying and workplace violence (ANA, 2015a). Regardless, the effects of incivility may extend beyond the recipient or target;

other members of the team can be influenced by the negativity and emotional toll imparted by the incivility and associated behaviors. According to Thomas (2003), incivility decreases worker satisfaction and meaning in the work done. Even small exhibitions of incivility must be addressed by the team leader both quickly and swiftly. After all, incivility aims to disrupt team processes.

Bullying

Persisting incivility leads to bullying. According to ANA (2015b), "bullying is repeated, unwanted harmful actions intended to humiliate, offend, and cause distress in the recipient" (p. 3). These behaviors may also be used to control an individual's actions. Bullying and incivility can be differentiated by the directness, intensity, and severity of the incivility, which leads to significant emotional or psychological impacts on the target of the bullying (APNA, 2008). Furthermore, bullying may be done by a single individual or a group of individuals. In the latter form, known as "workplace mobbing," the group targets an individual—often who thinks or acts differently than the group—using bullying behaviors to control or intimidate an individual (Griffin & Clark, 2014). Regardless of the source of bullying, a team leader must be prepared to address bullying consistent with how he or she addresses incivility. However, bullying may require additional intervention including, but not limited to, engaging the team's sponsor or human resources department (APNA, 2008).

Workplace Violence

In the continuum starting with incivility, workplace violence is the most significant. This form of violence is demonstrated through "physically and psychologically damaging actions" (ANA, 2015a, p. 4). These behaviors often border on criminal actions and are intentionally designed to harm individuals while at work. According to the APNA (2008), workplace violence significantly contributes to detrimental effects on emotional and psychological well-being. Verbal threats and assaults are not routinely considered to be "violence," but team leaders (as well as administrators) must be aware of acts consistent with workplace violence to address these unacceptable behaviors immediately.

Managing Incivility in Teams

Issues of incivility, bullying, and workplace violence decrease productivity (ANA, 2015b) and have lasting effects on an individual's psychological well-being (ANA, 2015a; APNA, 2008), so team leaders must quickly and swiftly address issues associated with these behaviors (The Joint Commission, 2008). Each nurse—and member of the interprofessional team—is accountable for addressing incivility, bullying, and workplace violence through direct action and escalation using organizational policies and procedures for reporting (American Association of Colleges of Nursing, 2008; ANA, 2015a). Unfortunately, Wolf, Delao, and Perhats (2014) have found that workers come to accept the prevalence of incivility and associated behaviors and come to expect it. The overall management of incivility, bullying, and workplace violence requires a multifaceted approach beyond the scope of this text. However, Table 9.8 offers possible responses to incivility as offered by Griffin (2004) and the APNA (2008). Additional resources include "Civility Tool-kit: Resources to Empower

TABLE 9.8 RESPONDING TO INCIVILITY

Action	Responses (APNA, 2008, p. 53)
Nonverbal innuendo	I sense (I see from your facial expression) that there may be something you wanted to say to me. It's okay to speak directly to me.
Verbal affront	The individuals I learn the most from are clear in their directions and feedback. Is there some way we can structure this type of situation?
Undermining activities	When something happens that is "different" or "contrary" to what I understood, it leaves me with questions. Help me to understand how this situation may have happened.
Withholding information	It is my understanding that there was (is) more information available regarding the situation, and I believe if I had known that (more), it would (will) affect how I learn.
Sabotage	There is more to this situation than meets the eye. Could you and I meet in private and explore what happened?
Infighting	Always avoid unprofessional discussions in nonprivate places. This is not the time or the place. Please stop (physically walk away or move to a neutral spot.)
Scapegoating	I don't think that's the right connection.
Backstabbing	I don 't feel right talking about him/her/the situation when I wasn' there or don't know the facts. Have you spoken to him/her?
Failure to respect privacy	It bothers me to talk about this without his/her permission. I only overheard that. It shouldn't be repeated.
Broken confidences	Wasn't that said in confidence? That sounds like information that should remain confidential. He/she asked me to keep that confidential.

Sources: American Psychiatric Nurses Association. (2008). Workplace violence: APNA 2008 position statement. Retrieved from http://www.apna.org/files/public/APNA_Workplace_Violence_Position_Paper.pdf; Griffin, M. (2004). Teaching cognitive rehearsal as a shield for lateral violence: An intervention for newly licensed nurses. *Journal of Continuing Education in Nursing, 35*(6), 257–263.

Healthcare Leaders to Identify, Intervene, and Prevent Workplace Bullying" (Adeniran et al., 2015) and *Ending Nurse-to-Nurse Hostility: Why Nurses Eat Their Young and Each Other* (Bartholomew, 2014).

QUESTIONS TO CONSIDER BEFORE READING ON

- Have you ever experienced incivility, bullying, or violence in the workplace? What impact did this have on the team? How was the behavior handled by colleagues and leadership, if it was?
- What is an example of how a care team or improvement team was disruptive by generational issues?
- How have authority gradients affected you? Consider when you were a newly graduated nurse. Was there a gradient between you and the experienced nurses? Does a gradient exist among different members of the healthcare team (e.g., physician to nurse or nurse to unlicensed personnel)?

TEAM EVALUATION

Teams are evaluated over time to ensure their success; this evaluation is done through both formative and summative assessments. Borrowed from education, these assessments allow teams to be evaluated both during their working phase and at the conclusion of the team's time-limited objective. Formative assessments occur throughout the team's mobilization. The team leader uses these assessments to judge the team's progress toward meeting its objective(s). As necessary, the team may need to design and implement additional improvement interventions, sustain previous gains, or engage other stakeholder and content experts. For well-crafted teams with project charters, the team leader may use a run chart to assess progress. The same run chart can be used for summative evaluations. In addition, team leaders may use additional tools to assess teamwork and collaboration toward improvements such as the IHI's (2004) Assessment Scale for Collaboratives, which is summarized in Table 9.9. Team evaluation can also be done based on performance. In Box 9.3, Madelyn evaluates the success of her team.

SELF-ASSESSMENT

How effective are you and your team at teamwork and team building? Visit the website www.mindtools.com/pages/article/newTMM_84.htm to complete a self-assessment. Calculate your total score and interpret your results. On the basis of this information, what strengths do you identify? What improvements can be made?

TABLE 9.9 ASSESSMENT SCALE FOR COLLABORATIVES

Assessment	Description
1.0	Forming team
1.5	Planning for the project has begun
2.0	Activity, but no changes
2.5	Changes tested, but no improvements
3.0	Modest improvement
3.5	Improvement
4.0	Significant improvement
4.5	Sustainable improvement
5.0	Outstanding sustainable results

Source: Institute for Healthcare Improvement. (2003). *The breakthrough series: IHI's collaborative model for achieving breakthrough improvement. IHI Innovation Series white paper.* Boston, MA: Author.

BOX 9.3 THE CASE SCENARIO CONTINUES TO UNFOLD

Madelyn is reviewing her team's objective: Improve the CAUTI rates on all pediatric units to below 1.5 for 3 consecutive months, within 12 months. Figure 9.1 offers an example of how a run chart can be used to assess progress monthly (formative) as well as at the project's conclusion (summative). With October's data used as baseline data (to inform the problem), formative assessments in November, December, and January imply the team has work to continue. By February, the team's objective is met for the first month. Therefore, February and March data are formative assessments whereby the team moves to sustainment interventions. With April's data being below the objective, the team can have a summative assessment as successful. Madelyn is proud that she has successfully led a team to reduce the rate of CAUTIs in the pediatric units.

CONCLUSIONS

Healthcare improvements often require—if not *always* require—a team. These teams rely on content and practice expertise of many interprofessional members, including nurses, physicians, pharmacists, and others. Teams working in professional silos often are not successful. Healthcare depends on the team of providers to manage direct patient care. In direct care, the patient provides the centered goal around which the team works. For healthcare improvements, the team objectives, scope, and end points

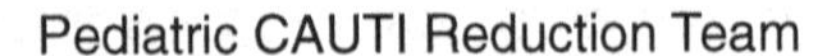

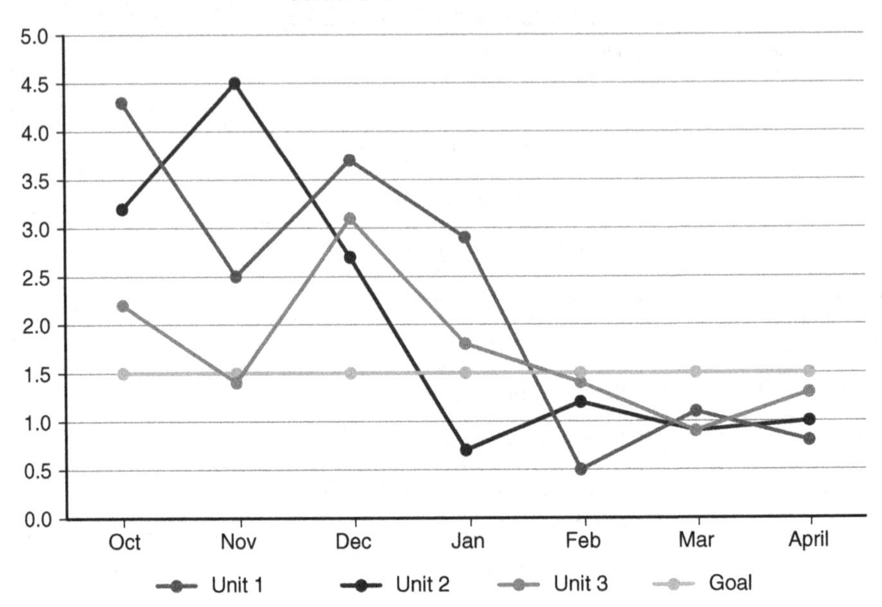

FIGURE 9.1 Improvement team run chart.
CAUTI, catheter-associated urinary tract infection.

may be less tangible at first. However, strong and effective leaders mobilize a team's energy by creating a shared vision of success, which is measured using an objective, time-limited goal. Without such a goal, teams may lose direction or focus on the issue for which the team was formed. Successful teams are composed of members who are purposefully considered for content expertise, stakeholder engagement, and diversity and inclusion. Teams are mobilized after foundational documents, such as a charter, are created. Issues such as incivility and bullying present challenges to any team, but an effective leader is able to provide appropriate feedback to manage these behaviors. Formative and summative evaluations are used to ensure that the team's objectives are met. Teamwork is an essential aspect of healthcare, both surrounding direct patient care and in improving patient care.

CRITICAL THINKING QUESTIONS AND ACTIVITIES

- Answer the following questions considering a practice problem in your area such as prolonged length of stay or high CAUTIs:
  - What would your objective be?
  - What type of team would you need?

(*continued*)

CRITICAL THINKING QUESTIONS AND ACTIVITIES *(continued)*

- Who would be important to have on the team? Consider those necessary for content expertise, stakeholder engagement, and diversity and inclusion.
- What would your greatest concerns be if you had to launch a team in real life?

- In your organization, request a charter or team agreement for an organization-wide decision-making committee or council. What are its objectives? What is the scope of the group? Is the purpose or objective of the team clear? Is anything missing?
- Watch the vignettes in the video developed by Robert Wood Johnson Foundation Executive Nurse Fellows as part of a collaborative called PACERS: "**P**assionate **A**bout **C**reating **E**nvironments of **R**espect and Civilitie**S**": www.youtube.com/watch?v=t8XddfSddzU
  - What are your reactions to these vignettes?
  - Which event(s) have you experienced or witnessed?
  - How did you feel watching these vignettes? Are these events "common" in your work environment?

REFERENCES

Adeniran, R. K., Bolick, B., Cuming, R., Edmonson, C., Khan, B., Lawson, L. B., & Wilson, D. (2015). Civility tool-kit: Resources to empower healthcare leaders to identify, intervene, and prevent workplace bullying. Retrieved from http://www.stopbullyingtoolkit.org

Agency for Healthcare Research and Quality. (2014). TeamSTEPPS fundamentals course: Module 3. Communication. Retrieved from http://www.ahrq.gov/teamstepps/instructor/fundamentals/module3/slcommunication.html

American Association of Colleges of Nursing. (2008). The essentials of baccalaureate education for professional nursing practice. Retrieved from http://www.aacnnursing.org/Portals/42/Publications/BaccEssentials08.pdf

American Association of Colleges of Nursing. (2012). *Graduate level QSEN competencies: Knowledge, skills, and attitudes*. Washington, DC: Author.

American Association of Colleges of Nursing. (2017). Diversity, inclusion, and equity in academic nursing: AACN position statement. Retrieved from http://www.aacnnursing.org/Portals/42/News/Position-Statements/Diversity-Inclusion.pdf

American Nurses Association. (2015a). *Code of ethics for nurses with interpretive statements*. Silver Spring, MD: Nursesbooks.org.

American Nurses Association. (2015b). Incivility, bullying, and workplace violence [Position statement]. Retrieved from https://www.nursingworld.org/practice-policy/nursing-excellence/official-position-statements/id/incivility-bullying-and-workplace-violence

American Psychiatric Nurses Association. (2008). Workplace violence: APNA 2008 position statement. Retrieved from http://www.apna.org/files/public/APNA_Workplace_Violence_Position_Paper.pdf

Bartholomew, K. (2014). *Ending nurse-to-nurse hostility: Why nurses eat their young and each other* (2nd ed.). Danvers, MA: HCPro.

Bibby, J., Bate, P., Carter, E., Robert, G., & Bevan, H. (2007). *The power of one, the power of many: Bringing social movements thinking to health care improvement*. Coventry, England: NHS Institute for Innovation and Improvement.

Donabedian, A. (1988). The quality of care: How can it be assessed? *Journal of the American Medical Association, 260*, 1743–1748. doi:10.1001/jama.1988.03410120089033

Frankel, A., Haraden, C., Federico, F., & Lenoci-Edwards, J. (2017). *A framework for safe, reliable, and effective care* [White paper]. Cambridge, MA: Institute for Healthcare Improvement and Safe & Reliable Healthcare.

Frankel, A., & Leonard, M. (2017). Lesson 1: Why are teamwork and communication important? In L. Fink (Ed.), *PS 104: Teamwork and communication in a culture of safety*. Retrieved from http://app.ihi.org

Griffin, M. (2004). Teaching cognitive rehearsal as a shield for lateral violence: An intervention for newly licensed nurses. *Journal of Continuing Education in Nursing, 35*(6), 257–263. doi:10.3928/0022-0124-20041101-07

Griffin, M., & Clark, C. M. (2014). Revisiting cognitive rehearsal as an intervention against incivility and lateral violence in nursing: 10 years later. *Journal of Continuing Education in Nursing, 45*(12), 535–542. doi:10.3928/00220124-20141122-02

Institute for Healthcare Improvement. (2003). *The breakthrough series: IHI's collaborative model for achieving breakthrough improvement. IHI Innovation Series white paper*. Boston, MA: Author.

Institute for Healthcare Improvement. (2004). Assessment scale for collaboratives. Retrieved from http://www.ihi.org/resources/Pages/Tools/AssessmentScaleforCollaboratives.aspx

Institute for Healthcare Improvement. (2017). Science of improvement: Forming the team. Retrieved from http://www.ihi.org/resources/Pages/HowtoImprove/ScienceofImprovementFormingtheTeam.aspx

The Joint Commission. (2008, July 9). Behaviors that undermine a culture of safety. *Sentinel Event Alert Issue 40*. Oakbrook Terrace, IL: Author. Retrieved from https://www.jointcommission.org/assets/1/18/SEA_40.PDF

Kouzes, J. M., & Posner, B. (2009, January). To lead, create a shared vision. *Harvard Business Review*. Retrieved from https://hbr.org/2009/01/to-lead-create-a-shared-vision

McCannon, C. J., Schall, M. W., & Perla, R. J. (2008). *Planning for scale: A guide for designing large-scale improvement initiatives*. IHI Innovation Series white paper. Cambridge, MA: Institute for Healthcare Improvement.

Scholtes, P. R., Joiner, B. L., & Streibel, B. J. (2003). *The team handbook* (3rd ed.). Union, NJ: Oriel.

Sherbin, L., & Rashid, R. (2017, February 1). Diversity doesn't stick without inclusion. *Harvard Business Review*. Retrieved from https://hbr.org/2017/02/diversity-doesnt-stick-without-inclusion

Sirkin, H. L., Keenan, P., & Jackson, A. (2005, October). The hard side of change management. *Harvard Business Review*. Retrieved from https://hbr.org/2005/10/the-hard-side-of-change-management

Thomas, S. P. (2003). Handling anger in the teacher-student relationship. *Nursing Education Perspectives, 24*(1), 17–24.

United States Department of Health and Human Services Health Resources and Services Administration. (n.d.). Improvement teams. Retrieved from http://www.hrsa.gov/quality/toolbox/508pdfs/improvementteams.pdf

Wolf, L. A., Delao, A. M., & Perhats, C. (2014). Nothing changes, nobody cares: Understanding the experience of emergency nurses physically or verbally assaulted while providing care. *Journal of Emergency Nursing, 40*(4), 305–310. doi:10.1016/j.jen.2013.11.006

10

FACILITATING PROBLEM-SOLVING AND DECISION-MAKING IN TEAMS

AUDREY MARIE BEAUVAIS

LEARNING OBJECTIVES

After completion of this chapter, the reader will be able to

- Identify the similarities and differences of problem-solving and decision-making.
- Discuss the benefits of team problem-solving and decision-making.
- Describe the following three group problem-solving techniques: standard agenda, nominal group technique, and fish bone diagrams.
- While leading a group, describe three techniques to generate solutions.
- Compare and contrast two decision-making strategies (voting and consensus processes).
- Describe the role of the nurse as an effective team member and as an effective team leader in problem-solving and decision-making.
- Recommend how one can incorporate technology in the problem-solving and decision-making processes.

As a nurse, you have already been involved in group problem-solving and decision-making as part of the healthcare team. Healthcare teams gather at times to solve problems and make decisions to promote high-quality, safe care. Effective team problem-solving and decision-making are essential for positive patient outcomes. In this chapter, you learn the leadership skills needed for team problem-solving and decision-making. Problem-solving and decision-making are basic components of leadership. As a nursing leader, you will be expected to use effective communication skills to help facilitate group discussions, assist in information gathering, help group members share their thoughts, and focus the discussion on the group's goal.

PROBLEM-SOLVING VERSUS DECISION-MAKING

Effective problem-solving and decision-making skills are needed to resolve issues encountered by the healthcare team. You may recall from your past education that problem-solving is an analytical approach that involves identifying the problem, gathering facts, developing options, selecting an option, as well as developing, implementing, and monitoring a plan of action. Decision-making is a component of the problem-solving process. Once you have generated possible options, you can make a choice (or a decision) about which option is best to reach the desired result (Keyton, 2005). Decision-making involves reflective thinking and judgments about each potential option suggested to solve a problem. A common pitfall of groups is that they skip to decision-making before they have accurately identified the problem and/or before they have generated enough options (Hicks, 2017). We talk about problem-solving and decision-making in greater detail in the subsequent text. Prior to discussing problem-solving and decision-making in teams, refer to Box 10.1 to complete a self assessment of your individual decision-making skills.

BOX 10.1 SELF-ASSESSMENT

Before we talk about how to facilitate problem-solving and decision-making in teams, complete the self-assessment of your individual decision-making skills found at the following website: www.mindtools.com/pages/article/newTED_79.htm.

How did you score on the assessment given in Box 10.1? Did you notice any common themes?

Think about an individual problem you may have had at work and how you solved it. How you solve problems as an individual might influence how you approach your teamwork problems. Let us look at a basic problem you could encounter at work. Your patient came back from a procedure. The patient's dinner was waiting for her in the room but it is now at room temperature. The patient asks if you can heat up the meal in the microwave. You go to the kitchenette to heat up the food only to discover that the microwave does not work. How do you decide what the problem is? What is the cause of the problem? Is it unplugged? Is there a power outage? Was a fuse blown? Does it have a broken part? The cause of the problem will influence how you choose to solve your problem. If it was unplugged, you could simply plug it in. If the microwave is broken, you will have to generate ideas on how to solve your problem. Will you talk to your charge nurse about getting someone to repair it or suggest buying a new one? The answer might depend on how long the unit had the microwave, if it is under warranty, and the cost to repair versus the cost to buy a new one. Will you go to another floor and ask to borrow their microwave? Will you call the kitchen and ask them to heat the food?

Having self-awareness about how you solve problems and make decisions as an individual will help you in your roles as both a team member and a team leader. The good news is that problem-solving and decision-making are skills that can be enhanced with practice and with the use of problem-solving/decision-making tools and processes that are now presented and explained.

TEAM PROBLEM-SOLVING AND DECISION-MAKING

Do teams solve problems and make decisions better than individuals? Some would argue that teams are much better at handling complex issues because any one individual is unlikely to possess or have access to all the information and resources needed to make sound decisions (Keyton, 2005). In addition, groups often bring increased diversity of perspectives to the situation. This helps to prevent members from becoming focused on a solution that lacks worth. Finally, by involving the group in the process, you are providing an opportunity to evaluate ideas before one is chosen and implemented. This helps foster confidence in the decisions because it puts faith in the group rather than in one individual (Keyton, 2005). Read the case scenario in Box 10.2, highlighting issues around team problem-solving and decision-making.

QUESTIONS TO CONSIDER BEFORE READING ON

Reflect on a recent time when you were involved in a problem-solving activity with a team and answer the following questions:

- What was the problem the team was addressing?
- Did the team brainstorm possible solutions?
- How did the team evaluate the solutions?
- What was the agreed-upon solution?
- Was everyone on the team in favor of this solution?

BOX 10.2 CASE SCENARIO

As you read the case scenario in the subsequent text, reflect on the following questions:

What is the underlying problem? Is it evident how the problem was identified? If you were involved in this team, how would you approach this problem? Are all the necessary disciplines represented at this meeting? Has the team gathered all the important information? What is missing from this problem-solving case scenario that is essential to promote a successful resolution to the problem?

Mary works at Southport Medical Center on a 24-bed medical unit. At the request of her nurse manger, Mary attended a series of quality improvement team meetings. At the first meeting, a facilitator from the Quality Improvement

(continued)

BOX 10.2 CASE SCENARIO *(continued)*

Department welcomed everyone to the group and explained the purpose to the team. The purpose was to address the issue of underreporting of medication errors. The team members all introduced themselves. There were representatives from pharmacy, nursing, and the quality improvement department. Mary was surprised to hear that underreporting was a problem because she was not aware that it was an issue. After the problem was identified, the facilitator explained that the team should try to gather information to understand the cause of the problem and identify ways to overcome the cause. The facilitator used flip charts to capture team members' ideas about causes. A list of contributing factors was identified such as the following:

- Nursing staff's fear of punishment and consequences
- Effect on performance appraisals
- Low self-esteem
- Confusion between what constitutes a medication error and a near miss
- Lack of time
- Lack of education
- Increased workload and less staff
- Increased nursing turnover
- No feedback from pharmacy—not aware of the importance
- Pharmacy short-staffed
- No audits
- No enforcement to report errors
- Ineffective communication
- Fear of losing job
- Lack of standard procedures
- No risk-management program
- No systems in place to monitor policies
- No online system for medication administration/lack of medication tracking

The team sets up regularly scheduled meetings to continue problem-solving the issue of underreporting of medication errors. The team members were given a task to continue to gather additional information and report back to the group as well as to start exploring possible solutions to the problem. At a subsequent meeting, the group discussed potential solutions. They generated ideas and captured them on a master list. Having read the literature, some team members suggested creating a "just culture" and establishing a "high-reliability organization." Other ideas were generated as well such as implementing educational programs compliance with the policy, implementing an online system for medication administration, and improving communication with pharmacy. The group used flip charts posted around the room to display potential solutions. Each member was given five dot stickers and asked to place the dots on the top five solutions that he or she would like to implement.

PROBLEM-SOLVING

Finding and implementing solutions to correct challenges is called the "problem-solving process" (Yazdani & Tavakkoli-Moghaddam, 2012). The purpose is to obtain an answer(s) for a problem. Problem-solving begins with the process of defining the problem:

- Is there a problem?
- What makes you think there is a problem?
- How is this happening?

Once you identify the cause of the problem, you can use several processes and tools to lead others in group problem-solving and decision-making. Several different group problem-solving techniques are highlighted in Table 10.1 (Hartwig, 2010).

In this section, we explain in detail these three problem-solving processes: standard agenda, nominal group technique, and fish bone diagrams. These three problem-solving processes were selected because they are commonly used in healthcare.

STANDARD AGENDA

The standard agenda follows a reflective and linear process to take the group through a process intended to solve a problem (Keyton, 2005). The group intentionally completes each of the following steps (Junior Reserve Officers' Training Corps [JROTC], 2017; Keyton, 2005; Laughlin, 2011; Raison, Lukshin, & Bowen-Ellzey, 2013; Shahbazi, 2014):

- **Identify/define the problem:** What is the fundamental problem? How long has the problem been occurring? Who is impacted by the problem? How are things now in comparison to how you want them to be (Raison et al., 2013)? Determining the problem is often easier if the issue is a pressing issue. However, a problem-solving team meeting can also be conducted to consider preventative solutions to problematic situations that may occur in the future (Meetingsift, 2017). Although it sounds very basic, teams may not recognize that there is a problem. Teams must see and acknowledge that a problem exists and that a decision needs to be made to address the issue. Once a problem is acknowledged, it is imperative that the team accurately identifies what the problem is. One of the most common errors of teams is identifying the wrong problem and identifying the wrong causes of a problem. Erroneous problem identification can lead to the wrong decision. Different team members might have different perspectives on what the problem is (Hicks, 2017).
- **Gather information (facts, assumptions, people's interests):** At this phase in the process, leaders should help gather all available information that pertains to the identified problem. Teams should try to gather all the

TABLE 10.1 SAMPLE GROUP PROBLEM-SOLVING PROCEDURES

Technique	Description	Advantages	Disadvantages
6M analysis	Used for cause and effect analysis. The 6M stands for six aspects to be taken into consideration: manpower, machinery, materials, method, mother nature, and measurement.	Addresses the entire process, not just the final product/outcome Proactive approach	Can create inflexibility. The official procedures can produce delays and curb creativity.
Cognitive mapping	Rather than using linear outlines for examining information, cognitive maps use graphics and show relationships in a visual representation. Main ideas are in the center and related ideas branch outward. Arrows are used to show relationships among the ideas.	Can be used for a variety of different problems Good for use with complex problems	Takes time to learn. Can be a time-consuming process.
Delphi method	A forecasting method that surveys a panel of experts. Several rounds of surveys are administered and the unidentified responses are gathered. These results are shared with the group after each round. The experts are permitted to adjust their responses in each round. This helps to determine what the group feels as a whole.	Reaches a response through consensus	Takes time because multiple surveys have to be sent out to reach consensus.
Devil's advocacy	Group members critique the solution by posing questions about the solution's assumptions and consequences.	Simple approach Takes into consideration many alternatives Effective with larger groups Helps ensure that the group is looking at the assumptions and consequences of the proposed solution Helps control for group think	The approach does not offer an alternative plan. Concentrates on the negatives of the plan and does not offer another solution.

(continued)

TABLE 10.1 SAMPLE GROUP PROBLEM-SOLVING PROCEDURES *(continued)*

Technique	Description	Advantages	Disadvantages
Dialectical inquiry	Two groups are assigned a specific problem and they are responsible to evaluate and determine alternatives. Create plans and counterplans through successive rounds. Different ideas and perspectives are examined. Examine solution from multiple viewpoints.	Numerous possible viewpoints are tested Stimulates creativity Gives equal importance to the positives and negatives of each solution Helps control for group think	Consensus does not always result from this process. Need to be careful that participants do not take on a win–lose attitude rather than concentrating on achieving an effective solution.
Flowcharts	Group creates an easy-to-understand graphic of a step-by-step process. Flowcharts typically use four symbols (elongated circles, rectangles, diamonds, and parallelograms) linked with arrows to indicate the direction of the flow.	Make the process easy to understand at a glance Help to solve a problem and standardize a process	If the process is too complicated, the flowchart can become very complex and messy-looking. If the process is altered, the flowchart might have to be redrawn, which can be time-consuming.
Focus groups	Collect information on the problem and potential solutions from groups of people who would be influenced by the potential decision or change.	Can obtain in-depth and complex responses from group members	Takes more time to do focus groups than individual surveys because of the recruitment needed to get the group members and the time to run the group itself. Some group participants may not want to speak openly about the issues.

(continued)

TABLE 10.1 SAMPLE GROUP PROBLEM-SOLVING PROCEDURES *(continued)*

Technique	Description	Advantages	Disadvantages
Force field analysis	Helps to examine the forces for and against a potential decision or change.	Provides a visual aid (a single graphic) of the forces for and against a change Helps identify potential obstacles The force field diagram provides a visual that can help simplify communication about the subject to the group members	All group members need to actively participate to obtain all the information needed to make an informed decision; otherwise, it will not be possible to get a complete picture of the forces. It can potentially lead to a division in the group because some will support the change and some will be against the change.
Pareto analysis	Helps to focus on the most important issues. The Pareto principles states that 20% of the causes result in 80% of the results. The following steps are used in Pareto analysis: identify problem(s), identify the root cause of the problem(s), score each problem, group problems together by their root cause, add up the scores for each group, and take action.	Relatively simple way to focus on 20% of the issues that are causing the majority of the issues Helps determine the most important problem to solve and provides a score indicating how serious the problem is	Need to make sure scoring is accurate. Might need more than one chart. Once there is more than one chart, there is the risk of losing sight of the causes in comparison to each other.

facts as well as the assumptions. They should perform this step to verify that the problem was defined correctly as well as to develop alternative solutions to the problem. During this phase, the group should try to gather information to understand the cause of the problem and find ways to overcome the cause.

Here is a simple example highlighting the importance of properly identifying the problem, gathering all available information, and including the right people in the discussion of the issue. A medical group has just recently moved into a newly remodeled space. They have gathered the doctors, nurses, and office staff together to address whether there are any remaining issues with the building. One of the nurses identified that the bathroom waste receptacles are often overflowing by 11 a.m. Others concur that this is a problem because of the large number of people using the facilities. The members of the team identify that the new waste receptacles are too small and that larger ones should be purchased. Such a decision will cost additional money but the team feels that it is necessary to solve their problem. Another suggestion was made to have the cleaning personnel make another pickup rather than buying new waste receptacles. Again, this solution will cost additional money. However, the problem was not correctly identified, nor were the right people present to make the decision. No one thought to include the housekeeping personnel in this discussion. If the team had included the head of housekeeping in the discussion of the problem, they would have known that the waste receptacles were large enough but that some housekeeping employees did not realize they had to open the plastic lining properly to hold the waste. Had the team gone ahead with the solutions noted earlier, it would not have solved the issue and would have cost additional money. A simple in-service teaching the housekeeping staff how to load the plastic bags into the new containers would solve the issue.

- **Search for alternatives/solutions/options:** The teams need to explore multiple potential solutions to the problem to engage in effective problem-solving. Try not to accept the first solution. Several ways to generate alternative solutions are presented as follows:

  Brainstorming: Brainstorming is a creative process that encourages team members to propose as many solutions to a problem as possible through noncritical discussion (Laughlin, 2011). Here are a few guidelines to follow when brainstorming (Laughlin, 2011; Mosser & Begun, 2014; Raison et al., 2013):
  - Every team member should be given a chance to verbally suggest ideas.
  - Write down every idea exactly as it is stated on a board or flip chart.
  - Keep a relaxed and open atmosphere explaining that there are no right or wrong ideas.
  - Do not criticize/judge and stay neutral with all the ideas presented. The purpose is to create freewheeling of ideas to generate or stimulate more thoughts or ideas that otherwise may be suppressed.
  - Encourage the group to generate as many solutions as possible.

  Ask questions of your network: Network with colleagues inside and outside of your organization to get their thoughts on the issue. Professional list-serves are a good tool to use for this purpose.

  Investigate: Complete a review of the literature regarding this problem. Go to conferences that address similar problems. See how other industries handle similar issues.

- **Evaluate the alternatives/solutions; analyze and compare:** As you start to evaluate the alternatives, ask the group "What is our goal or desired end state?" and "What will success for solving this problem look like to us?" Then discuss the merits of each potential solution generated by the group and the extent to which it can result in the desired end state. List the pros and cons (advantages and disadvantages) of each solution. As you examine each possible solution, think about the consequences of choosing this alternative. Who will be involved and influenced by this alternative? Does this solution cost money? If so, who pays for it (Raison et al., 2013)? Some teams opt to rank the desirability of each solution on a ranking scale (e.g., on a scale of 1–5) to help choose their top-rated solutions.
- **Select an alternative/solution/option or options:** What is the best solution? Is the solution that has the most advantages and fewest disadvantages the best choice? Often, this is true but not always. The group will need to weigh the importance of each pro and con because there may be occasions when certain pros or cons outweigh others. Objectively and logically analyze each solution against the pros and cons of the others. Also consider what the group's intuition tells them. How do they feel about the choices? The decision-making process is not solely an objective process. Rather, the mind is both rational and emotional, and because the decision-making process is a thought process, it is also both rational and emotional (JROTC, 2017). However, encourage the group not to make decisions solely on the basis of emotions because that is a recipe for disaster (JROTC, 2017). Attempt to find the best solution that is rational and apt to be successful as well as feels good with regards to the team's emotions, standards, and values (JROTC, 2017).

Ask the team to consider combining a number of solutions to potentially get a better result (Hicks, 2017). The final decision should be realistic and should unite the team to move forward. This step involves making a decision regarding what solution to choose, that is, decision-making. We expand on this step further when we discuss decision-making later in the chapter.

- **Develop and document an action plan:** Do not rely on everyone's ability to recall the information (Hicks, 2017). Write down the action plan to help develop all the details and implications (Hicks, 2017). The plan should include who is responsible for each step, when, where, how, and why. Break the action plan down into small steps, with allocated time frames and the name of the person who will be accountable for the completion of the step (Raison et al., 2013). How will those involved measure what is done? How will the group evaluate the implemented plan? Try to anticipate as many "what-ifs" as possible. Be prepared to handle such situations with a contingency plan. See Table 10.2 for a sample action plan template.

TABLE 10.2 SAMPLE ACTION PLAN TEMPLATE

Action Plan

Project and purpose: ____________________

Goal: ____________________

Team members: ____________________

Time frame for completion of goal: ____________________

Action Steps Needed to Complete Goal	Responsible Person for Each Action Step	Necessary Resources (Time/ Materials) for Each Action Step	Target Date for Completion of Action Step	Evaluation/Feedback Mechanism/ Performance Measurements (What Demonstrates That the Desired Outcome Has Been Achieved?)	Adjustments Needed for Successful Completion (What Is Needed to Ensure That the Desired Outcome Has Been Achieved?)
1.					
2.					
3.					
4.					
5.					

What obstacles might interfere with the successful achievement of the goal?

How will the team deal with unanticipated obstacles?

Who else should be communicated with who might also be addressing this problem?

- **Implement the best alternative:** Once the team has chosen the best option and developed a plan, it is time to implement the plan. One essential element to ensure successful implementation is effective communication among all the team members and with those affected by the plan but have been outside of the problem-solving/decision-making process (administrators and other health team members not involved directly in the process). Thus, all stakeholders who could be impacted by the process should be made aware of the plan.
- **Evaluate the outcome:** Once the plan has been implemented, the team needs to reconvene periodically to evaluate the progress toward the goal and to hold individuals accountable for the results that have not been actualized. Teams need to assess whether the plan of action achieved the desired outcomes. Was the plan effective? Did it result in positive outcomes? If not, why? Seek feedback because this is a learning process and helps with team building.

NOMINAL GROUP TECHNIQUE

This technique gathers a team in a structured meeting with limited interaction. The technique involves a six-step process (Keyton, 2005; Laughlin, 2011; Mosser & Begun, 2014):

1. Team members assemble to solve a problem. The leader/facilitator states a particular question. Team members silently and independently write down each idea.
2. Each team member presents one thought to the group. The group is not to discuss the thought. These ideas are recorded on a flipchart by a group leader/facilitator.
3. After each member has presented a thought, the group interacts to evaluate the ideas. Taking one idea at a time, group members discuss each idea for clarification. The leader can ask if any members have a question about the suggestion.
4. Each member individually (and without discussion with other members) ranks the suggestions. This can be done in a number of ways such as by ranking each idea on a scale of 1 to 10 or voting for the top five choices.
5. Group discusses the results of the vote. Members can elaborate on each of the ideas. However, the ideas should be discussed in a random or neutral order so the focus is not on the most popular thoughts to encourage discussion of each item.
6. Repeat steps 4 and 5. Vote again and discuss the ideas that received the most votes. At this point, a final vote is taken and the group selects the idea they like best.

This technique helps foster independent idea generating and equal participation of group members without consideration of status or power. For example, if you are involved in fundraising efforts but the results are not meeting expectations, then this technique could help you develop other ideas for fundraising rather than relying on the ideas of the most powerful of the group. The process has the potential to generate more ideas at a higher quality than other techniques. Members may also feel satisfaction that they helped in the decision-making process. This technique helps when the group is not very cohesive (Keyton, 2005).

FISH BONE DIAGRAM (CAUSE AND EFFECT DIAGRAM)

Team problem-solving can be used to get at the root cause of a problem. One way to capture ideas regarding the causes is through a fish bone diagram. Fish bone diagrams help to visually display the possible causes of a problem. It is called a "fish bone diagram" because the chart will look like fish bones with a circle at the top (the head of the fish) identifying the problem and the back bone identifying the causes. Figure 10.1 shows the template of a fish bone diagram and Figure 10.2 gives an example of how it can be completed to help solve a problem.

The following steps outline how to create a fish bone diagram:

- **Problem statement:** State the problem in the form of a question in the circle at the head of the fish bone. All members of the team should agree with the problem statement. In Figure 10.2, the problem is: Why is Jane late to work?
- **Document the possible causes:** The rest of the fish bone consists of a line across the page that is attached to the circle at the head of the fish with

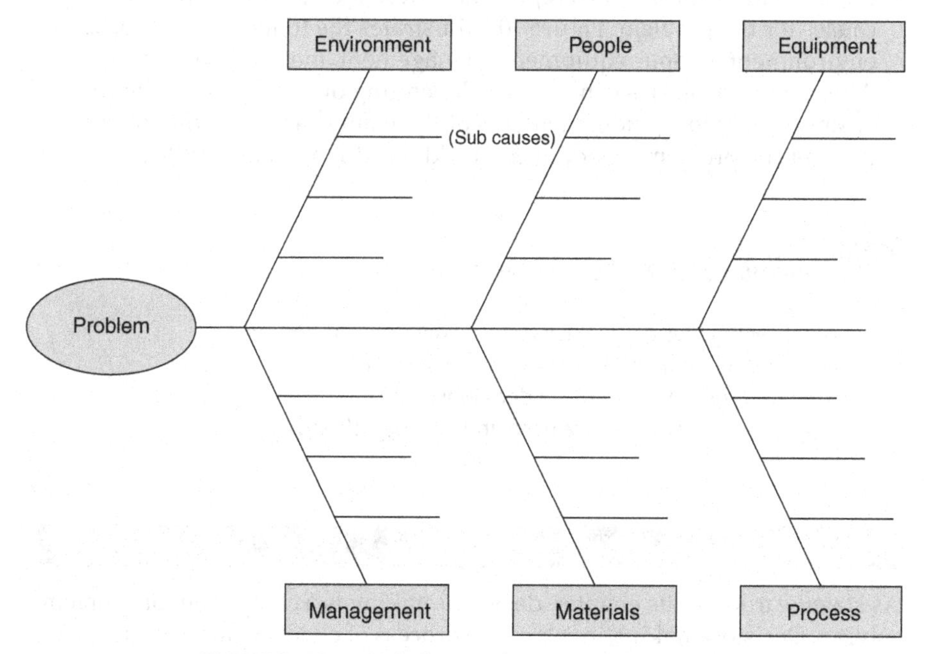

FIGURE 10.1 Fish bone diagram template.

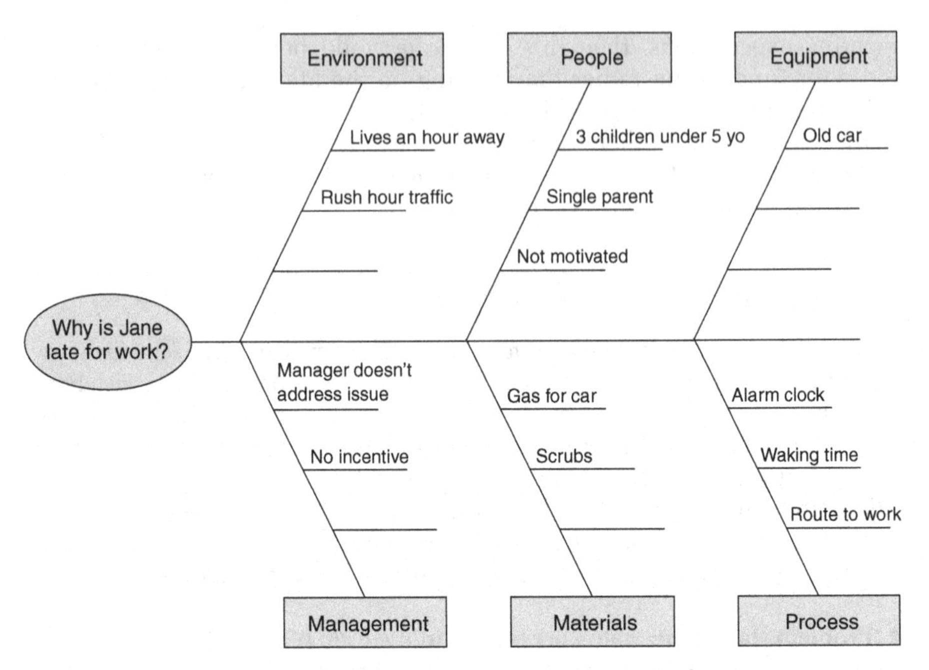

FIGURE 10.2 Fish bone diagram example.

the problems statement. Several lines/bones come out diagonally from the main line. These bones represent different categories of potential causes for the problem. Figure 10.2 illustrates the following categories: environment, people, equipment, management, materials, and process. Alternative categories can be used depending on the problem. On the basis of this information, members of the team share ideas on how to prevent the problem (Yazdani & Tavakkoli-Moghaddam, 2012).

QUESTIONS TO CONSIDER BEFORE READING ON

- What techniques do you use to make decisions at home?
- How are decisions made at your place of work?
- Are teams used to help make decisions?
- If yes, what techniques are used and are they effective?

DECISION-MAKING

As stated earlier in the chapter, decision-making is a component of problem-solving. Decision-making involves the process of choosing among the generated solutions (Yazdani & Tavakkoli-Moghaddam, 2012). That choice should solve the problem and move the organization forward. There are many strategies that can be used to make decisions. We review voting and the consensus process in the subsequent text.

VOTING

The purpose of voting is to make a choice from the generated alternatives (Keyton, 2005; McNamara, 2017). Voting has its advantages because it is a simple, quick way to assess the thoughts of each group member. A disadvantage of the voting technique is that some group members might not be well informed, yet they are voting. Another disadvantage is that people might feel pressure to change their vote because of an influential member trying to sway their decision. The four different types of voting techniques are the following:

1. **Show of hands:** In this technique, the group reviews each alternative on the list. Reviewing one alternative at a time, participants are asked to raise their hands if they support each alternative on the list. The item that receives the most votes represented by a show of hands is the item that is chosen (McNamara, 2017). For example, if your group was deciding what fundraising activity it should implement, then the group members could be asked to raise their hands if they support each of the potential fundraising activities presented. Perhaps five people raised their hands to support a silent auction of gift baskets, four raised their hands for a bake sale, and two raised their hands for a wrapping paper sale. In this show of hands scenario, the silent auction of gift baskets would be the chosen alternative.
2. **Ranking:** Ranking involves selecting the most important or desired solution from the list of items (Keyton, 2005). Members of the group give one distinct value to each of the alternatives to select the best alternative (McNamara, 2017). For example, the group would rank one alternative as 1, another as 2, and so forth. If we use the fundraising example again, then the group might choose a distinct value of 1 (highest value) for the bake sale, 2 for a wrapping paper sale, and 3 for the silent auction. In this ranking scenario, the bake sale would be the chosen alternative.
3. **Rating:** Rating involves selecting a range of the most desired alternatives from the list (McNamara, 2017). With rating, group members assign a value to each alternative to identify ranges of items from the list. Several of the alternatives can have the same value associated with them (unlike the ranking in which each item had its own distinct value). For instance, a rating list could have several alternatives rated as 1. Alternatively, some groups, rather than using a numeric rating system (i.e., 1, 2, 3, etc.) to rate alternatives, might choose some other ways of categorizing the ratings such as high, medium, or low. An example of the "rating" technique can be seen in

the following example. Members of a search committee are asked to evaluate candidates for a nurse manager position. Ten nurse manager candidates have been brought in for evaluation. Group members may be asked to rate each of the candidates individually in one of the following three different categories: "good candidate," "maybe," and "no." The group might end up having three candidates who they feel are "good candidates," two who are a "maybe," and five who are outright "no."

4. **Dot-voting:** In the dot-voting technique, each member of the team receives a set number of dot stickers that can be used to vote for his or her preferred options (McNamara, 2017). Often, people will get dots that correlate to the number of choices that can be made from the list. For instance, if four items can be selected, then each member would receive four dots. Each choice is often written on flip chart paper that is posted in the room. Alternatively, an overall list of items can be made allowing for space for the dots to be placed on the paper. Members of the group then walk up to the flip chart paper (or the overall list) and place their dots on their choices. The choice that has the most dots is the one that is selected.

CONSENSUS PROCESS

The purpose of the consensus process is to arrive at a conclusion that all members can "live with" (Mosser & Begun, 2014). That is not to say that everyone completely agrees with the decision, but that they can tolerate it. The technique is intended to be participative and egalitarian (McNamara, 2017). This technique is desirable with larger groups. A disadvantage of the consensus process is that often times the "squeaky wheels" or more difficult group members are catered to, whereas the more agreeable members are overlooked. Unfortunately, this can reward group members for disagreeing and they might do so out of self-interest and slow down the decision-making process.

There are different ways to reach a consensus. One easy way to build consensus is to suggest a decision to the group. Once the suggestion has been made, in a roundtable fashion, ask each member whether he or she can live with that decision. Each member should be given equal time to share his or her choice and the reason for that decision. The leaders in the group should share their opinions last to promote free expression. Once all members have had a chance to speak, the facilitator of the group shares the choice made by the majority of members and asks all members if they can support that decision. If not, they might have a discussion about the choices and then repeat the process. Another option if there is not an agreement is to get volunteers from the group to serve on a task force to gather additional information and research on the topic. The task force will then present its findings and recommendations back to the group (McNamara, 2017). After this presentation, the group follows the consensus process again. Having read about the group decision-making process, refer to Box 10.3 for an assessment on your experiences with decision-making teams.

QUESTIONS TO CONSIDER BEFORE READING ON

In your personal and professional life, what difficulties have you encountered with problem-solving and decision-making when in a group or team? What can you change to improve your skills to lead a group in effective problem-solving and decision-making?

BOX 10.3 ASSESSMENT OF GROUP DECISION-MAKING SKILLS

This is not a scientific self-assessment but rather is intended to foster reflection. Please answer "yes" or "no" to the following questions. Think about a recent experience being part of a decision-making team.

- Did the group have difficulty staying focused on what needed to be accomplished?
- Did the group have trouble sticking to the agenda?
- Did the group conduct a superficial analysis of alternatives (rather than a detailed analysis)?
- Did the group members show little motivation in resolving the problem?
- Did the group fall into a rut?
- Did the group members become immobilized by conflict?
- Did the group fail to consider all alternatives?
- Did the group fail to compare the alternatives?
- Did the group members fail to analyze the problem at hand but rather go straight to the decision-making process?
- Did the group fail to use its time efficiently?
- Did the group members fail to evaluate each choice along with its merits?

Source: Adapted from Keyton, J. (2005). *Communicating in groups* (3rd ed., pp. 147–175). Oxford, UK: Oxford University Press. Retrieved from http://global.oup.com/us/companion.websites/9780195183436/about/samplechapters/CHAP07.pdf

These questions highlight common problems and limitations that arise with team problem-solving and decision-making. Looking at the results, reflect on how you can improve the process to help improve your team problem-solving and decision-making. What strategies will you try at your next group meeting?

ROLE OF THE NURSE LEADER

Nursing leaders are expected to guide groups to make sound decisions that are accepted and implemented in a timely fashion (JROTC, 2017). The nurse leader helps with facilitating the discussion, gathering information, helping members verbalize their position, and focusing conversations on the group goals. The leader should also encourage members to be open to new ideas and prevent them from becoming immobilized by conflict. Nurse leaders need skills for *climate building* and *conflict management* to help facilitate problem-solving and decision-making in teams.

Climate building: The leader should facilitate a positive, supportive environment to promote effective group problem-solving and decision-making (Keyton, 2005). This climate is created when group members feel valued and their input is welcomed (2005). It is not always easy to create such an environment and this important factor is often overlooked (2005). One technique to promote climate building is through a "check-in." The following example demonstrates how a "check-in" can be used in nursing to promote positive climate building. Members of the nurse management team meet every Thursday with the vice president of nursing. Each meeting begins with a "check-in" exercise in which each manager provides a brief update of his or her units and how he or she is addressing any issues that are arising to ensure positive outcomes. This helps the managers become comfortable as a team. By sharing this information, the managers get to know each other because they learn about the issues on the units as well as learn about the skills of each manager. This also provides an opportunity for each member to see how each unit is functioning and how this will influence activities across the healthcare organization. In addition, this exercise allows each member to speak, which helps to equalize roles and status differences among team members.

Conflict management: As a nursing leader working in teams to facilitate problem-solving and decision-making, you will most certainly have to manage conflict. Conflict is not a bad word. In fact, conflict about ideas can be positive because it promotes better decision-making (Keyton, 2005). Conflict becomes a problem when it is no longer about the ideas but becomes personal and is not managed (Keyton, 2005). The decision-making process can go awry when the struggle between two people becomes personal. Imagine a group of hospital nurses who work in different specialties who are tasked to work on an organizational problem. A seasoned nurse from the maternity ward, Joan, does not like the psychiatric nurses because she feels it is not "real nursing." A younger nurse, Marie, from the psychiatric unit feels that Joan acts superior to others and is "mean." Marie feels that Joan's maternity unit gets everything it requests because it is a revenue-producing unit, whereas the psychiatric unit financially breaks even and is the last to get needed resources and renovations. The feelings of these nurses toward each other can easily cloud their ability to focus on the issue at hand. An effective leader would be cognizant of the dynamics between group members, would try to keep the nurses from making the issues personal, and would focus the members on the problem-solving task at hand. Chapter 11 provides in-depth information on how to analyze and facilitate constructive conflict resolution among staff.

Even if you are not the designated leader, all team members should share responsibility for the leadership of the group (Smith, 2017). In interprofessional teams, the roles of leadership and membership are regarded as equal. Every member of the team should have a vested interest in seeing the team achieve its goals; hence, each team member has an obligation to assist the team in reaching its goals.

USE OF TECHNOLOGY IN PROBLEM-SOLVING AND DECISION-MAKING

Technology can assist in the problem-solving and decision-making processes. For example, technology can be used to collect, organize, and distribute data (Erukulapati & Sinn, 2017). Once you have data, then the technology can aid with analyzing data to help ensure that you are properly identifying the problem (Erukulapati & Sinn, 2017). Technology can also be used to access evidence-based practices in the literature to ensure that staff are using information on the basis of research for problem-solving and decision-making.

In addition, there are collaborative technologies available that are aimed at improving the sharing of information among team members during decision-making (McNamara, Dennis, & Carte, 2011). This is particularly useful because teams need to have all available information that is important to making a decision. There are some instances when team members may withhold information because of their status or worry about how the team might react (McNamara et al., 2011). Using a collaborative technology helps mediate this issue because it allows team members to send messages to each other rather than during a face-to-face meeting. Simple baseline discussion collaborative techniques (e.g., instant messenger) can provide electronic communication with anonymity. Individuals can type comments that are added to a discussion list window that all can see. Although this is one way to share information, sometimes team members ignore certain information or rely on prediscussion preferences.

As a result, there are other technologies that may help address this issue. For example, there are applications that require participants to evaluate each remark they get from the "team comment" window and place it into one of several different categories (e.g., "important," "somewhat important," or "not important" [McNamara et al., 2011]). Sorting the information helps to raise awareness as well as evaluate each comment to help increase integration (McNamara et al., 2011).

There are decision support systems that allow users to interact directly with the computer to help make decisions for solving complex problems. For example, FacilitatePro (facilitate.com) provides software that can help with prioritizing, categorizing, voting, planning, evaluating, surveying, action planning, and documenting. There is even simulation software available (goldsim.com) that assists teams to compare and contrast alternative solutions as well as helps them to develop plans and policies. Having this decision support helps to explain and defend choices to the teams and stakeholders.

QUALITY AND SAFETY EDUCATION FOR NURSES (QSEN) CONSIDERATIONS

As you read the QSEN competencies related to teamwork and collaboration in Table 10.3, ask yourself the following:

- Which of these competencies do I meet and which competencies do I need to develop more fully?
- What plan of action can I take to enhance those competencies in which I am weak and to develop those that I lack at this time?

CONCLUSIONS

Team problem-solving and decision-making are the most crucial and risky components of nursing and healthcare (Shahbazi, 2014). Consequently, being acquainted with team problem-solving and decision-making models and strategies will provide you with a critical skill to help you address problems associated with your work environment. These problems most often involve providing safe, quality care to your patients. There may be times when you are looking to solve problems related to medication errors, readmission rates, and infection rates. Other times, you may be looking to solve problems related to staff turnover, patient satisfaction, and wait times. No matter what the issue, the problem-solving and decision-making opportunities will often involve you working with a team and perhaps even the patients and their families to develop and implement the best alternatives to achieve the desired outcomes and evaluate the effectiveness of your action plan.

TABLE 10.3 QSEN COMPETENCIES

Knowledge	Skills	Attitudes
Describe own strengths, limitations, and values in functioning as a member of a team	Demonstrate awareness of own strengths and limitations as a team member Initiate plan for self-development as a team member Act with integrity, consistency, and respect for differing views	Acknowledge own potential to contribute to effective team functioning Appreciate importance of intra- and interprofessional collaboration
Describe scopes of practice and roles of healthcare team members Describe strategies for identifying and managing overlaps in team member roles and accountabilities Recognize contributions of other individuals and groups in helping patient/family achieve health goals	Function competently within own scope of practice as a member of the healthcare team Assume role of team member or leader on the basis of the situation Initiate requests for help when appropriate to situation Clarify roles and accountabilities under conditions of potential overlap in team member functioning Integrate the contributions of others who play a role in helping patient/family achieve health goals	Value the perspectives and expertise of all health team members Respect the centrality of the patient/family as core members of any healthcare team Respect the unique attributes that members bring to a team, including variations in professional orientations and accountabilities
Analyze differences in communication style preferences among patients and families, nurses, and other members of the health team Describe impact of own communication style on others Discuss effective strategies for communicating and resolving conflict	Communicate with team members, adapting own style of communicating to needs of the team and situation Demonstrate commitment to team goals Solicit input from other team members to improve individual, as well as team, performance Initiate actions to resolve conflict	Value teamwork and the relationships on which it is based Value different styles of communication used by patients, families, and healthcare providers Contribute to resolution of conflict and disagreement
Explain how authority gradients influence teamwork and patient safety	Assert own position/perspective in discussions about patient care Choose communication styles that diminish the risks associated with authority gradients among team members	

Source: Quality and Safety Education for Nurses Institute. (2014). QSEN competencies. Retrieved from http://qsen.org/competencies/pre-licensure-ksas

CRITICAL THINKING QUESTIONS AND ACTIVITIES

Ask your supervisor if you can accompany him or her to his or her next decision-making group as part of an exercise for your leadership course. As you observe the group, ask yourself the following:

- What problem is the group addressing?
- Did the group take time to understand the problem?
- Did the group members agree on identification of the problem?
- Did the group identify and generate a list of ways to address the problem?
- Did the group use any criterion with which to evaluate the alternatives?
- Did the group assess the positive and negative aspects of each of the alternatives?
- How did the group decide to resolve the problem?
- Do you feel that the group's decision-making process was effective?
- What improvements would you suggest?
- What actions did the leader take in facilitating the group problem-solving process?
- What actions do you think may have hindered the group problem-solving process?

REFERENCES

Erukulapati, K., & Sinn, J. W. (2017, September). Better intelligence. *Quality Progress, 50*(9), 34–40. Retrieved from http://asq.org/quality-progress/2017/09/statistics/better-intelligence.html

Hartwig, R. T. (2010). Facilitating problem solving: A case study using the devil's advocacy technique. *Group Facilitation: A Research and Application Journal, 10*, 17–31.

Hicks, T. (2017). Seven steps for effective problem solving in the workplace. Retrieved from http://www.mediate.com/articles/thicks.cfm

Junior Reserve Officers' Training Corps. (2017). Decision making and problem solving. Retrieved from http://www.au.af.mil/au/awc/awcgate/army/rotc_dm_ps.pdf

Keyton, J. (2005). *Communicating in groups* (3rd ed., pp. 147–175). Oxford, UK: Oxford University Press. Retrieved from http://global.oup.com/us/companion.websites/9780195183436/about/samplechapters/CHAP07.pdf

Laughlin, P. R. (2011). *Group problem solving*. Princeton, NJ: Princeton University Press.

McNamara, C. (2017). Guidelines to successful group decision making and problem solving. Retrieved from https://managementhelp.org/groups/group-decision-making.htm

McNamara, K., Dennis, A. R., & Carte, T. A. (2011). It's the thought that counts: The mediating effects of information processing in virtual team decision making. *Information Systems Management, 25*, 20–32. doi:10.1080/10580530701777123

Meetingsift. (2017). How to run problem solving meetings. Retrieved from http://meetingsift.com/problem-solving-meetings

Mosser, G., & Begun, J. W. (2014). *Understanding teamwork in health care*. New York, NY: McGraw-Hill.

Quality and Safety Education for Nurses Institute. (2014). QSEN competencies. Retrieved from http://qsen.org/competencies/pre-licensure-ksas

Raison, B., Lukshin, D., & Bowen-Ellzey, N. (2013). Group problem solving process. Retrieved from https://u.osu.edu/raison/files/2014/02/FACT-SHEET-Group-Problem-Solving-CDFS_13_13-1cqoba2.pdf

Shahbazi, H. M. (2014). The effect of problem solving training on decision making skill in nursing students. *International Journal of Nursing Education*, *6*(1), 15–18. doi:10.5958/j.0974-9357.6.1.004

Smith, P. M. (2017). Shared leadership sustains high performance in teams. Retrieved from https://edgarramirezochoa.wordpress.com/2016/08/15/shared-leadership-sustains-high-performance-in-teams

Yazdani, A.-A., & Tavakkoli-Moghaddam, R. (2012). Integration of the fish bone diagram, brainstorming, and AHP method of problem solving and decision making: A case study. *International Journal of Advanced Manufacturing Technology*, *63*, 651–657. doi:10.1007/s00170-012-3916-7

11

CONFLICT RESOLUTION SKILLS IN PROFESSIONAL NURSING PRACTICE

ROBIN S. KRINSKY

LEARNING OBJECTIVES

After completion of this chapter, the reader will be able to

- Identify the various types of conflict that one encounters in the workplace.
- Discuss conditions that arise that can lead to conflicts.
- Identify the effects conflict can have in the work environment.
- Determine which method of conflict management is appropriate to resolve and prevent conflict from occurring in the future.
- Use proven proactive and reactive conflict management interventions that will normalize the conflict.

Nurses practice in environments that are filled with potential conflicts. Positive, respectful, and collaborative working relationships are needed to provide quality care. Building relationships in an atmosphere that demands shorter length of stays, efficiency of resources, short staffing, better quality outcomes, and transparency of outcomes and scores creates not only a stressful work environment but also an environment that can breed conflict. This is an environment that is a challenge for the novice nurse, the experienced nurse, and the nursing leadership as well. These challenges need to be managed and overcome, so that the well-being of all staff is guaranteed and quality patient care is not negatively impacted. Reducing and mitigating conflict requires one to understand the sources of conflict within the individual and the organization, various approaches to conflict management, and the consequences that conflict has on the individual and organization as well as the impact on both personal and organizational relationships.

You most likely have some working knowledge of conflict given your role as an associate's degree nurse. This chapter helps you further build upon your leadership skills by helping you identify the sources of interpersonal, intrapersonal, and organizational conflicts that can lead to poor patient outcomes, poor working relationships, and poor personnel well-being. Identifying these sources will allow you to foster a work environment that facilitates the mitigation or resolution of conflicts. In addition, this chapter encourages you to think outside of the box, and that conflict is not always negative, because it can be the catalyst to elicit changes. Education on strategies to engage, manage, and reduce conflict is briefly touched upon in nursing school and needs to be offered in the work setting to lead to better outcomes, and to a culture where there are cooperation, positive outcomes, mutual respect for one another, and the well-being of individuals.

WHAT IS CONFLICT?

"Conflict" is an internal and external discord that results from differences in ideas, values, and feelings between two or more people (Marquis & Huston, 2011). It is a disagreement in values or beliefs within oneself or between people that causes harm or has the potential to cause harm. Conflict is a result from the interaction of interdependent people who perceive incompatibility and the potential for interference (Folger, Poole, & Stutman, 2012). This dissension is created when there are differences in economic and professional values, and where there is competition among professionals. If conflict is not addressed and instead is allowed to escalate, people may feel frustrated and upset, and even act aggressively. The major concern for nursing is that when conflict transpires, the result can be the unnecessary anguish and harm that can come to patients. The case scenario found in Box 11.1 highlights a conflicting situation that can occur in healthcare.

QUESTIONS TO CONSIDER BEFORE READING ON

- Recall a time when you questioned why you are working in the job or position you are in. What type of conflict was this?
- Have you ever wondered whether you should stay on your unit when you know that there is no room for advancement? Should you transfer to another unit to expand your knowledge base and become more marketable, even though it may result in changing shifts and leaving friends? What type of conflict is this?
- Have you found yourself in a situation where the healthcare team has decided on one way to treat a patient and you know it is not what the patient or family would have wanted? What type of conflict is this?
- Have your staffing guidelines been tightened so much that you cannot provide the level of care that you have grown accustomed to providing for your patient population? What type of conflict is this?

BOX 11.1 CASE SCENARIO

As you read this case scenario, reflect on the following questions:

- Have you ever found yourself in a conflicting situation with a colleague at work or school?
- Did those conflicts relate to the different work styles of coworkers, staffing shortages, a heavier workload, or cultural differences?

Josh works on a very busy ambulatory unit that prepares outpatients for surgical procedures. The schedule is demanding with patients frequently added on at the last minute. Being efficient on this unit is paramount, because one never knows what can occur at any given moment. Also, patients need to get to the operating room for the start of the schedule so rooms can be turned over efficiently. Arriving to the unit prepared to work on time is very important. Today, just like most other days, Jill has not arrived, and it is 15 minutes into the shift. Josh is preparing his assigned patient for the procedure, whereas Jill's patient, Ms. P, is sitting watching all of the nurses rushing around prepping other patients. Most of the nurses have not even noticed her because they are focused on their work. Jill's lateness has become the norm.

After about 20 minutes of watching this and feeling ignored, Ms. P stops Josh on his way past her and says, "Is anyone coming to get me ready for my surgery? I have been waiting here for a very long time and nobody is taking care of me like all the other patients." Josh looks at her empathetically, then over at his patient, then at the clock, and around the unit but there is no sign of Jill anywhere. He has a host of emotions going on simultaneously in his head, and feeling torn on what is the right thing to do and how he should proceed.

TYPES OF CONFLICT

The recognition that conflict is a part of life in a dynamic setting advocates for conflict mitigation and resolution. Identifying the type of conflict is essential to bringing resolution to it. So, what are the different types of conflict one can have? It is important to establish the type of conflict that exists because the better we can define it, the more likely we can resolve it. There are three comprehensive categories (intrapersonal, interpersonal, and organizational) that we consider when defining conflict, which can occur in isolation or in combination with each other.

Intrapersonal conflict occurs within a person when confronted with the need to think or act in a way that seems at odds with one's sense of self. It can be questioning oneself about values, ethical issues, and priorities, thinking about what lies in the future while working on this particular unit, or trying to implement new evidence-based protocols on this unit and bypassing others to accomplish this. These can produce intrapersonal conflict because it involves professional priorities as well as professional interests.

Interpersonal conflict is the most common type of conflict a nurse encounters because it occurs between patients, families, nurses, other healthcare providers, and members of other departments. It is "a dynamic process that occurs between interdependent individuals and/or groups as they experience negative emotional reactions to perceived disagreements and interference with the attainment of their goals" (Barki & Hartwick, 2004, p. 4). Interpersonal conflict occurs within healthcare teams as individuals seek to achieve organizational goals and meet expectations. Usually, the discrepancies are related to varying opinions, urgency of issues, how to best treat and care for patients, or how to pursue goals. This may be a positive type of conflict because it may fast-track the group to find a solution to the issues that have been long-standing.

Organizational conflict arises when friction exists about policies and procedures, personnel codes of conduct, or accepted norms of behavior and patterns of communication (Marquis & Huston, 2011). This can be related to the organizational structure, role confusion in the department, and overlap of job function. Staffing levels and patterns are a common organizational conflict that is seen between front line staff and nursing leadership. It also occurs when service lines are eliminated, in times of downsizing, and when there is lack of information and communication on organization goals, mission, and vision between upper management and frontline providers.

There are several components associated with the most common type of conflict, interpersonal conflict. They are disagreement, interference, and task conflict. "Disagreement" represents the key cognitive component of interpersonal conflict. When individuals think that there is a departure from values, interests, opinions, needs, or goals, there will be disagreement. However, disagreement in isolation is not adequate for conflict to emerge. When the behavior of one party interferes with or opposes another's attainment of his or her interests and objectives, conflict is said to exist. Many researchers believe that the central process for conflict to manifest is the behavior where one or more individuals encounter another's interests or goals (Wall & Callister, 1995). Although behaviors such as debating, arguing, competing, and backstabbing may be typical attributes of conflict; they do not always indicate the existence of conflict. "Interference" is the "incompatible activities where one person is interfering, obstructing, or in other ways making the behavior of another less effective" (Alper, Tjosvold, & Law, 2000, pp. 627–628). It is where one person gets in the way and needs to be pushed out of the way for one person to succeed. Finally, "task conflicts" are defined as "... a condition in which group members have interpersonal clashes characterized by anger, frustration, and other negative feelings" (Pelled, Eisenhardt, & Xin, 1999, p. 4). The individuals or groups involved feel a sense of frustration, anger, or friction within the relationship.

QUESTIONS TO CONSIDER BEFORE READING ON

- Recall personal conflicts you have had in your own life. How did you respond to those?
- When you were growing up, how was conflict viewed and dealt with in your family unit?

HISTORY OF CONFLICT MANAGEMENT

In the early 20th century, conflict was considered to be an indication of poor organizational management, and it was deemed destructive and avoided at all costs. When conflict occurred, it was ignored, denied, or dealt with immediately and harshly as if it did not exist at all. During the mid-20th century, organizations recognized that worker satisfaction and feedback were important in acknowledging the existence of conflict. Conflict was accepted passively and perceived as normal and expected. Attention centered on teaching managers how to resolve conflict rather than how to prevent it from occurring in the first place. The interactionist theorists of the 1970s recognized conflict as a necessity and actively encouraged organizations to promote conflict as a means of producing growth (Marquis & Huston, 2011). The traditional approaches to conflict in the healthcare field continue to be direct negotiation, litigation, and/or legislation and regulation (Mazadoorian & Latham, 2004). These approaches to dispute management are often costly and time-consuming for both healthcare providers and clients. Organizations can no longer afford to respond to conflict with traditional methods (i.e., to avoid or suppress it), because this has proven to be nonproductive in the long run (Marquis & Huston, 2011).

In an effort to better manage these disputes, the healthcare profession has shown an increased interest in alternative dispute resolution (ADR) practices such as conflict management training, facilitated early settlements, collaborative claims management, mediation, and internal neutral or ombudsman programs (Hetzler, Morrison, Gerardi, & Hayes, 2004). On January 1, 2009, The Joint Commission (TJC) required that healthcare organizations establish policies and procedures for conflict management among leadership groups in an effort to maintain a culture of safety (Schyve, 2009). Specifically, TJC requires that all healthcare organizations have a code of conduct that defines both appropriate and inappropriate behaviors as well as a process where leadership addresses disruptive and intimidating behaviors (TJC, 2017).

The American Nurses Credentialing Center (ANCC) Magnet® Recognition Program Standard number 4 requires that healthcare organizations have systems in place to address patient care and practice concerns

(Pinkerton, 2005). The pathway to achieve this is the dispute mechanism that has been put in place by the designated organization to address patient care and practice concerns without retribution. Silence and poor communication lead to patient safety issues and reduced job satisfaction. In a study by Siu, Spence Laschinger, and Finegan (2008), it was demonstrated that positive work environments enhance nurses' conflict management skills, thus influencing unit effectiveness.

CONFLICT HAPPENS

Conflict is unavoidable in environments in which people are working closely with one another because individuals have differences in goals, responsibilities, needs, desires, perceptions, and ideas. Conflicts happen in all walks of life and may arise in environments because of issues such as personality clashes, differing goals, differences in judgment, uncooperative behavior, and cultural misunderstandings. Nursing by nature is a discipline that works closely with others and has interactions with many individuals on a day-to-day basis to provide for a safe and therapeutic patient care environment in an effort to have positive patient outcome (Cohen & Bailey, 1997). Unresolved conflict among nurses is a major work issue that results in job dissatisfaction, absenteeism, and poorer retention of nursing staff. Patient satisfaction scores have been found to be lower in hospitals in which nurses report higher levels of frustration and burnout, which is a sign of problems in providing quality of care (McHugh, Kutney-Lee, Cimiotti, Sloane, & Aiken, 2011; Wright, 2011).

WHY CONFLICT OCCURS

Conflict occurs because people are different. Individuals see things through different lenses, want different things, and have different thinking styles. Factors such as varying personalities, variable status in the workplace and in personal lives, changing ideological, political, and philosophical differences, different goals, and different approaches to care lead people to disagree. In addition, people are influenced by various factors such as fear, force, fairness, or economic sources. The majority of the research has shown that the most common sources of conflict include lack of emotional intelligence, personality traits, various aspects of the job and work environment, role ambiguity, lack of support from manager and colleagues, and poor communication (Montoro-Rodriguez & Small, 2006).

How conflict begins and is resolved has much to do with people and their personalities, and the factors that exist in the environment. The changing composition of nurses and the demand for nurses have resulted in a workforce that is more diverse than a comparable cohort 10 years ago. As new groups of nurses who are culturally different enter the workforce and move up the organizational ladder, conflicts emanating from class, gender, race, and ethnicity have become more obvious and are more likely to be ignited in the workplace. Society's diversity-based conflicts are imported into organizations and have become a growing concern (Burawoy, 1979; Hearn, Sheppard, Tancred-Sheriff, & Burrell, 1989; Kanter, 1977; Marshall, 1984). These diversity-based conflicts in nursing, such as culture, age, hierarchy, gender, and work environment, can impact conflict development. Our workplaces have paralleled what we see across the globe, which is the increase in a culturally diverse workforce as well as in a population of patients. The diversity of workplace teams and managers has created an opportunity for nurses to become culturally aware. Awareness is an important aspect of understanding how the conflict developed and how it will be resolved (Brett, Behfar, & Kern, 2006).

Age and hierarchy can highly influence conflict. If one employee has a view different from another's view as to what the proper role for a younger worker or subordinate should be, conflict can arise. How do older nurses take direction and instructions from younger superiors? It was found that younger workers tend to be more sensitive to generational issues, such as differences in technical skills, and are more likely to feel that older coworkers do not take them seriously. On the contrary, older workers tend not to spend as much time on cell phones and other technologies, and may take matters such as being late for one's shift more seriously (DiRomualdo, 2006).

There are also gender variations that influence conflict. Brewer, Mitchell, and Weber (2002) concluded that men were more likely to assert themselves in conflict, whereas women more often try to avoid it. In another study, it was found that women were more likely than men to be collaborative in their approach to conflict resolution.

Organizational factors that hospitals and clinical areas possess tend to have specific rules and regulations that govern practice. These rules have a tendency to be very much delineated and when one deviates from these norms, and conflict ensues, having all parties involved coming to a resolution usually means a compromise. Most of these environments do not allow for compromise, and it is difficult because many who share a belief in what is right often view other's beliefs as wrong—hence, the "right is right and wrong is wrong" attitude (Byford, 2006). Read the case scenario in Box 11.2, about Diane's taking a new job, and reflect on on the questions listed.

QUESTIONS TO CONSIDER BEFORE READING ON

Recall an incident where you observed conflict between two people.

- What type of verbal and nonverbal communication was occurring?
- What was the outcome of the conflict? Was it resolved?
- Were there any lingering aftereffects of the conflict between the two individuals?

BOX 11.2 CASE SCENARIO

Consider the following questions as you read this case scenario:

- Have you ever had a mentor, either professionally or personally, with whom you could consult to provide you with direction on various concerns that were discouraging you?
- What attributes did your mentor possess that allowed you to resolve your concerns? How did that person coach you to resolve those concerns?

Diane, a 23-year-old new RN, just relocated to a large metropolitan area where she has taken a position at an academic medical center on a surgical floor. Her preceptor is May, a middle-aged foreign-born surgical nurse who has been working on this unit for 10 years. Diane finds herself becoming impatient with May during this important learning experience. She finds it difficult to understand May because of her very heavy accent and fast-paced speech. In addition, Diane finds May's bedside manner toward the patients very rushed and not personable. When Diane asks a question, May tells her to "look it up." When Diane spends time speaking with patients, May becomes impatient with her. Diane is torn between requesting a new preceptor versus staying with her current preceptor in an effort to not upset the situation.

ANTECEDENTS TO CONFLICT

Conditions that need to be present for conflict to occur can be broken down into three major antecedents. The first is individual characteristics, which can be differing opinions and values that can create the substrate for conflict. Demographic differences, gender, educational preparation, and generational differences in nurses are sources of tension among individuals and are causes of conflict (Jehn & Shah, 1997; Swearingen & Liberman, 2004). Each generation of nurses brings a unique set of values to the work environment where traditional models of hierarchy are challenged depending on which generations are leading or directing and which generations are attempting to follow.

Next are interpersonal factors, such as lack of trust, injustice or disrespect, and inadequate or poor communication. If colleagues trust each other, their disagreements will be less likely interpreted as negative (Mishra, 1996). The way people are treated and how information is provided as well as the rationale behind decision-making is a source of conflict. The style that one communicates can (whether that is verbal, nonverbal, or lack thereof) be interpreted as disrespectful and be the source of conflict.

Organizational factors that can contribute to conflict can be seen by the level of interdependence each individual has on one another. If each individual relies on many other members of the team to accomplish his or her goals, there is more opportunity for conflict to arise because there is more interaction and opportunity for this to occur. If there are changes in structure and shifts in power within the organization, this will manifest itself as conflict between managers and workers (Pondy, 1967). Ambiguous power, conflict of interest, communication barriers, dependence on one party, differentiation in organization, association of the parties, behavioral regulation, performance expectations, competition for limited resources, lack of cooperation, or unresolved prior conflicts can lead to increased occurrences of conflict.

More information on the antecedents and consequences of conflict can be found in an article by Almost (2006) at the following website: http://onlinelibrary.wiley.com/doi/10.1111/j.1365-2648.2006.03738.x

QUESTIONS TO CONSIDER BEFORE READING ON

- Describe a conflict that you have experienced with a patient, the patient's family, or significant other.
- What skills were you able to use to resolve the conflict?
- Did you bring another coworker or another member of the team to help with the situation?

CONFLICT PROCESS MODEL

The Conflict Process Model (Pondy, 1967) has various stages in which the ongoing conflict at hand cycles through. In the first stage, "latent conflict," conditions are ripe for conflict, although no conflict has actually occurred and none may ever occur. For example, unit change and budget cuts almost invariably create conflict. Such events, therefore, should be well thought out so that interventions can be made before the conflicts created by these events escalate. The second stage is known as "perceived conflict." In this stage, the person recognizes it logically and impersonally as occurring. Sometimes conflict can be resolved at this stage before the person or groups begin to internalize it. The third stage, "felt conflict," occurs when the conflict is emotionalized. These felt emotions may include hostility, fear, mistrust, and anger. Next is the fourth stage, "manifest conflict," where some action is taken. The action may be to withdraw, compete, debate, or seek conflict resolution. The final stage is "conflict aftermath." There is always conflict aftermath, or fallout, which can be positive or negative depending on the outcome of the conflict as well as the parties involved (Marquis & Huston, 2011; Pondy, 1967). More information on the conflict process model can be found in an article by Pondy (1967) at the following web address: www-personal.umich.edu/~lroot/ConflictMgtConceptMap/Pondy-Organizational-Conflict-1967.pdf.

CONFLICT IS NOT ALWAYS THE ELEPHANT IN THE ROOM: POSITIVE ASPECTS OF CONFLICT

Organizations without conflict can be characterized as stagnant with no change. On the other hand, too much conflict that occurs frequently can create pure chaos with poor outcomes. In contrast, an optimal level of conflict will generate creativity, a problem-solving atmosphere, a strong team spirit, and motivation of its employees. Conflict in an interdisciplinary team can result in better patient care when collaborative treatment decisions are based on carefully examined and combined expertise (Tschannen et al., 2011). It has been shown that high levels and prolonged conflict can be detrimental to the individual and team. Moderate levels of conflict trigger quality ideas, increase the cohesiveness of groups, increase the feeling of integration of individuals, and strengthen relationships as well as individuality (Tjosvold, 1987).

Filley (1975) claimed that the positive values of conflict included both its functioning as a preventive measure against more destructive outcomes and its promoting the search for facts, new methods, or new solutions to interpersonal problems. The integrative conflict resolution style directs the parties involved to conquer the problem at hand and not conquer each other. Attempts are made to clarify the problem by fact finding and expressing the parties' personal feelings about the situation. Although this can become time-consuming, it allows the opportunity for people to disagree, work on these disagreements with all of the facts, and to achieve a better understanding of each other (Filley, 1975). This approach to conflict resolution is based on certain beliefs and attitudes that provide the foundation for the interpersonal communications skills that must be used. Filley suggested that the following beliefs would be conducive to the problem-solving approach:

- Belief in the availability of a mutually acceptable solution that will achieve everyone's goals
- Belief in cooperation rather than competition
- Belief that everyone is of equal value—no status or power imbalance is involved
- Belief in the view expressed by others as legitimate statements of their position
- Belief that differences of opinion are helpful
- Belief in the trustworthiness of the other member
- Belief that the other party can compete, but chooses to cooperate

As you read in Box 11.3 about Terry's frustrations concerning the time sheet, consider Filley's beliefs and determine which ones could be conducive to Terry's problem-solving.

BOX 11.3 CASE SCENARIO

As you read this case scenario, reflect on the following:

- Supervisors often make decisions on the basis of the needs of the organization. Sometimes these decisions affect our personal lives negatively. What approaches have you used to resolve these decisions that have resulted in a positive outcome for you? What approaches have not yielded positive outcomes?

Terry was checking the new time schedule that Ms. Valarie, her supervisor, posted and noticed that in addition to her requests for certain days off not being granted, she is working three out of the four weekends on the posted schedule. She looked over the weekend schedules of some of her peers and found that nurses with less seniority were assigned only two of the four weekends, and one of the other nurses was scheduled to work only one weekend. She banged the staffing book down at the nurse's station so loud that several staff and visitors turned around and looked over at her. With a loud and harsh tone, Terry said, "This is not fair; I requested certain days off and others with less seniority were granted the days off instead of me. I am so sick of this going on."

MEDIATING AND RESOLVING CONFLICT

In healthcare organizations, there are obstacles such as professional or departmental boundaries that do not allow for effective worker engagement to address conflicts in a face-to-face meeting. In addition, there are time limits, meeting costs, and staffing constraints that do not allow for people to meet together and address their concerns. Usually, conflict is addressed using either a hierarchical or a rights-based (or legal) approach. When one party files an incident/occurrence report or informs a supervisor about a problem, it starts the chain-of-command process, which is based on an order of authority that just passes the conflict for someone else to manage. This usually leads to an investigation, filing of a grievance, or even a lawsuit, and possible disciplinary action, which may or may not be appropriate depending on the situation. It does not give those involved with the conflict an opportunity to mitigate or resolve their issues and this delay can lead to an escalation of the conflict.

TJC accreditation standards and sentinel event alerts highlight the need for conflict management to improve quality of care and protect patient safety. They require a process for addressing conflict and improving communication at several levels within healthcare organizations. A specific standard (LD.02.04.01) of TJC requires that senior leadership develop a process for addressing conflict among themselves. There are many options available for this which can range from formal to informal conflict management, which provides a medium for issues to be addressed earlier and more directly. Unfortunately, the formal process of conflict resolution such as reprimands, formal grievance processes, progressive discipline, peer review, and other legal processes often results in poorer relationships and additional disagreements, and puts more fuel on the conflict (Scott & Gerardi, 2011). In the informal process, engagement of the parties involved can confront the real issues such as trust, respect, miscommunication, hurt feelings, and the collapse of the healthcare team.

Methods that encourage engagement include mediation, coaching, facilitation, dialogue, and collaborative problem-solving. These are different from the formal investigations because they do not involve any legality and focus on rebuilding trust, clarifying misinformation, reinforcing respectful conversation, and making joint arrangements to move on.

SELF-ASSESSMENT

You can begin to determine your conflict resolution approach by answering the following questions:

- What type of conflict resolution style do you feel you use most often?
- Complete the *Conflict Management Styles Assessment* questionnaire found at www.blake-group.com/sites/default/files/assessments/Conflict_Management_Styles_Assessment.pdf and determine what conflict resolution strategy you tend to use. Is it of the same or different style than what you thought prior to doing the questionnaire?
- With what approach do you identify more often: collaborating, competing, compromising, accommodating, or avoiding?

CONFLICT RESOLUTION APPROACHES

Thomas and Kilmann Approach

The Thomas–Kilmann model (1974) was designed by two psychologists, Kenneth Thomas and Ralph Kilmann, to explain the options in handling conflict. There are two dimensions in the model; the first dimension (vertical axis) is concerned with conflict responses on the basis of attempting to get what we want. These are the assertiveness options. The other dimension (horizontal axis) is concerned with responses on the basis of helping others get what they want. Thomas and Kilmann call these the "cooperativeness options." This creates five basic types of responses to conflict resolution. Thomas and Kilmann (1974) identified these *five approaches* to conflict resolution that have proven beneficial in situations where conflict needs to be mitigated. See Table 11.1 which outlines the conflict resolution options and when they could be used.

The first approach is *collaboration*, which creates an environment in which a win–win solution is possible if both parties are willing to be creative. This

TABLE 11.1 CONFLICT RESOLUTION OPTIONS ON THE BASIS OF THE THOMAS–KILMANN CONFLICT MODES

Conflict Resolution Option	When to Use	Advantages	Disadvantages
Competing	When you are in a position of power; have the expertise; when there are emergencies	Effective when the issue is unpopular; immediate direction; viewed as assertive	Disempowers staff; viewed as noncooperating; no feedback considered
Accommodating	When you want to appear reasonable to others	Appear as a peacemaker between people; creates an environment of good will	Can appear as a weak leader, or indecisive; not receptive to change
Avoiding	When you do not want to handle the conflict; want to leave the conflict unresolved	Allows you to address the problem at another time; if a dangerous situation exists, could be ridiculed for decision; receptive to changes	Problems can intensify or erupt and unknown consequences can ensue
Collaborating	When you want to have unity among people; show that you are assertive; engage cooperativeness	Fosters agreement among people; decision is important to both parties	Time-consuming; personal responsibilities can be ignored; one party may feel taken advantaged of
Compromising	When you want to find a middle ground; both sides can claim victory	Mutually acceptable to all parties	Appear to not have firm values; power struggle; confrontations can continue

approach to conflict resolution can be useful in creating a partnership where hostility existed earlier. It is a method of resolving differences between people who worked well with each other earlier. There is mutual attention to the problem and the focus is on solving the problem and not defeating each other. This approach needs the individual or groups to be highly assertive and highly cooperative. However, there are several drawbacks with collaboration; it is very time-consuming, and at any given time either party could go back on its agreement because it is not binding.

The second approach is *compromising*. In this method, both parties in the disagreement have to meet somewhere in the middle. This approach proves of value when the individuals involved are equally committed to their points of view or where they are of similar status within the organization, peers on a unit rather than a frontline employee and a supervisor.

Compromise can increase the rate of the dispute and resolve the conflict sooner than other approaches. In this mode, there is moderate assertiveness and moderate cooperation. There should be a division of the rewards for both parties. A major drawback with this method of resolution is that if one side is truly correct, then compromising is wrong, and should not be the method to use. Also, it can be used only when the exact outcome of the dispute is not as important as achieving resolution.

The third approach is *accommodating*. This is when giving in to one view of the conflict is useful when one side realizes that the issue is more important to the other side, or that he or she is wrong. Accommodating allows for social capital to be built up and used in the future. It helps to maintain working and personal relationships that may be more important than the actual cause of the conflict in the first place. The major drawback with using accommodating is that it can be interpreted as weakness.

The fourth method is *competing*. In this style, the concerns and position of the opposition are ignored. Winning is all that matters. If you are challenged by someone whose viewpoint is incorrect and who is just trying to get his or her way, it may be essential to challenge him or her so as not to set a precedent. Competing may escalate conflict and may not be a wise method to consider when the conflict may become physical in nature. In this mode of resolution, there is high assertiveness and low cooperation. When you use competing, it is an effort to win, regardless of the cost of the conflict.

The final approach is *dodging*. This is a very good short-term strategy when the conflict is not very important or if you are too busy to deal with an issue or you need time to calm down or there is no chance of your winning. There is low assertiveness and low cooperation in this mode. Dodging can make things worse in the long run and may allow the offender to win because you are shirking the issue.

Filley Approach

Filley (1975) identified three basic outcomes for conflict (*win–lose*, *lose–lose*, and *win–win*). The *win–lose* outcome occurs when one person obtains his or her desired ends in the situation and the other individual fails to obtain what is desired. One party exerts dominance, usually by power of authority, and the other party submits and loses. Forcing, competing, and negotiation are techniques likely to be used in the win–lose strategy. Majority rule is another example of this type of strategy. In the *lose–lose* outcome, there is no winner, and the settlement that is reached is unsatisfactory to both sides. The *win–win* outcome is the most desirable. In this strategy; the goal is to meet the needs of both parties. The focus is to solve the problem, not to force, dominate, overpower, or compromise.

PEARLA Approach

Skills that create connection between the parties who are having conflict can be achieved by the approach *PEARLA*, a mnemonic that provides a method to remember the steps. PEARLA stands for **p**resence, **e**mpathy, **a**cknowledgment, **r**eflect or reframe, **l**isten openly, and **a**sk questions. These skills collectively provide a compassionate approach toward engaging the parties and achieving resolution (Gerardi, 2010). They provide a method of de-escalation in an emotional situation; provide some insight by illuminating others' concerns, wants, and needs; allow for trust to be built to proceed to problem-solving; make clear what is possible; and help to realistically move forward.

Creating a connection using the PEARLA approach can often be enough to resolve a situation by providing a forum where concerns are made clear and where people can resolve a problem by themselves. In addition, this connection also creates a foundation for ongoing dialogue when more than one session is needed to resolve complex issues.

QUESTIONS TO CONSIDER BEFORE READING ON

- Recall a time when you were in a conflict with a peer.
- Assess the real cause of that conflict.
- What skills did you use to attempt to resolve the conflict? Was it successful?
- If you could go back to that situation, would you have managed it differently on the basis of what you have learned in this chapter?
- Apply Thomas and Kilmann's model to the situation. Would you use a different conflict management strategy next time in the same situation?

COST OF CONFLICT IN NURSING

Conflict in healthcare environments can cost an organization not only financially but in human resources as well. In 2004, the Institute for Safe Medication Practices (ISMP) linked workplace conflict to medication errors. This conflict took the form of intimidation, condescending language or tone of voice, impatience with questions, and being the recipients of strong verbal abuse or threatening body language (ISMP, 2004). TJC reported that the majority of perinatal deaths and injuries were the result of problems with organizational culture and communication among caregivers (TJC, 2008). The lack of collaboration results in lost productivity, reduced efficiency, increased medical errors, and the compromising of patient care (Almost, 2006; Rowe & Sherlock, 2005). In addition, consistent unresolved conflict is often associated with poorer job satisfaction, higher job turnover, decreased job commitment, absenteeism, an increase in grievances, continual orientation of nursing staff, and considerations of leaving the profession (Almost, 2006; Jameson, 2003; Rowe & Sherlock, 2005). Working in an environment of continued conflict results in stressed employees. Interpersonal conflict has been noted as one of the major sources of stress for nurses (Rowe & Sherlock, 2005). Conflicts that are not resolved and ignored often resurrect at a later time in an escalated form blown way out of proportion. It may appear so distorted that the real cause may not be easily recognized.

In 2016, the American Association of Critical-Care Nurses (AACN) published the second edition of their *AACN Standards for Establishing and Sustaining Healthy Work Environments: A Journey to Excellence* in response to the growing evidence that unhealthy work environments contribute to medical errors, ineffective delivery of care, and conflict and stress among healthcare professionals. The six essential standards for establishing and sustaining healthy work environments are evidence-based and relationship-centered principles of professional performance. A critical element of Standard 1, skilled communication, appeals to the healthcare organization to provide team members with support for and access to interprofessional education and coaching that develop critical communication skills, including self-awareness, inquiry/dialogue, conflict management, negotiation, advocacy, and listening (AACN, 2016).

QUESTIONS TO CONSIDER BEFORE READING ON

Consider a conflict you have had in your clinical area that is continuous and ongoing. Have you consulted with your colleagues who have been on the unit longer than you have?

- How much time can you estimate that you all have spent on this issue?
- What obstacles impede you from resolving this issue?
- Have there been negative effects of this issue such as staff turnover, hostility, or burnout between members of the team?
- Are there any new ideas and actions that you could think of to manage this issue?
- What inhibits you or the group from effectively managing this issue?

QUALITY AND SAFETY EDUCATION FOR NURSES (QSEN) CONSIDERATIONS

As nurses, we work with colleagues from various cultures, with different ages, and in varying roles. It is important that we are aware of how others manage conflict. Effective conflict and conflict management skills are also considered essential QSEN competencies (Table 11.2), for both undergraduate and graduate nurses. As nurses, we are always reevaluating the techniques we use to resolve conflict in both our professional and personal lives because we "Value continuous improvement of own communication and conflict resolution skills" (QSEN competency; Table 11.2). Nurses must have the knowledge to manage conflict as noted in the QSEN competency, "Describe basic principles of consensus building and conflict resolution" (Table 11.2), to work harmoniously in their environment. Review the QSEN competencies related to conflict resolution in Table 11.2. What skills, knowledge, and attitudes do you possess? What skills, knowledge, and attitudes can be strengthened?

TABLE 11.2 DEVELOPING CONFLICT MANAGEMENT SKILLS: RELEVANT QSEN COMPETENCIES
Integrate understanding of multiple dimensions of patient-centered care: patient/family/community preferences, values, information, communication, and education (Knowledge)
Elicit patient values, preferences, and expressed needs as part of clinical interview, implementation of care plan, and evaluation of care (Skills)
Communicate patient values, preferences, and expressed needs to other members of healthcare team (Skills)
Value seeing healthcare situations "through patients' eyes" (Attitudes)
Seek learning opportunities with patients who represent all aspects of human diversity (Attitudes)
Recognize personally held attitudes about working with patients from different ethnic, cultural, and social backgrounds (Attitudes)
Willingly support patient-centered care for individuals and groups whose values differ from own (Attitudes)
Appreciate shared decision-making with empowered patients and families, even when conflicts occur (Attitudes)
Discuss principles of effective communication (Knowledge)
Describe basic principles of consensus building and conflict resolution (Knowledge)
Participate in building consensus or resolving conflict in the context of patient care (Skills)
Value continuous improvement of own communication and conflict resolution skills (Attitudes)
Describe own strengths, limitations, and values in functioning as a member of a team (Knowledge)
Demonstrate awareness of own strengths and limitations as a team member (Skills)
Act with integrity, consistency, and respect for differing views (Skills)
Appreciate importance of intra- and interprofessional collaboration (Attitudes)
Clarify roles and accountabilities under conditions of potential overlap in team member functioning (Skills)
Respect the unique attributes that members bring to a team, including variations in professional orientations and accountabilities (Attitudes)
Analyze differences in communication-style preferences among patients and families, nurses, and other members of the health team (Knowledge)
Describe impact of own communication style on others (Knowledge)
Discuss effective strategies for communicating and resolving conflict (Knowledge)
Communicate with team members, adapting own style of communicating to needs of the team and situation (Skills)
Initiate actions to resolve conflict (Skills)
Value different styles of communication used by patients, families, and healthcare providers (Attitudes)
Contribute to resolution of conflict and disagreement (Attitudes)
Assert own position/perspective in discussions about patient care (Skills)

(continued)

TABLE 11.2 DEVELOPING CONFLICT MANAGEMENT SKILLS: RELEVANT QSEN COMPETENCIES *(continued)*
Choose communication styles that diminish the risks associated with authority gradients among team members (Skills)
Give examples of the tension between professional autonomy and system functioning (Knowledge)
Describe factors that create a culture of safety (e.g., open communication strategies and organizational error reporting systems) (Knowledge)

Source: American Association of Colleges of Nursing. (2012). *Graduate level QSEN competencies; Knowledge, skills, and attitudes*. Washington, DC: Author; Cronenwett, L., Sherwood, G., Barnsteiner, J., Disch, J., Johnson, J., Mitchell, P., ... Warren, J. (2007). Quality and safety education for nurses. *Nursing Outlook, 55*(3), 122–131. doi:10.1016/j.outlook.2007.02.006

CONCLUSION

As nurses, we must never lose sight that the foundation of nursing care is the therapeutic nurse–patient relationship, which contributes to the patient's well-being and health. The therapeutic relationship is threatened whenever there is conflict, with the patient, the patient's family/significant others, or our own colleagues. It hinders our communication, collaboration, and teamwork. Nurses need to remember that they share the responsibility with their employers to create a healthy workplace environment, ensuring that conflict does not negatively impact on patients' health outcomes or the relationships among colleagues (College of Nurses of Ontario [CNO], 2006).

In the healthcare setting, it is important to realize that conflict is inevitable. Conflict between nurses and other providers of care has been identified as a significant issue that can lead to job dissatisfaction, burnout, poor patient outcomes, and safety issues. There are many variables that contribute to conflict and the identification of these is important to the resolution of the conflict. The advent of new technology and ways of communication such as email, social media sites, and texting has decreased face-to-face interaction and previous methods of managing conflict by the traditional face-to-face method have impacted on how we effectively communicate with one another.

The way that leadership manages conflict will in turn determine how other employees manage their conflict with each other. Nurses are held accountable and need to be able to decrease, if not eliminate, conflict in their organization by using blameless communication skills and assisting in facilitating conflict resolution between individuals. Every employee needs to take an active role in building his or her conflict resolution skills to maintain a safe, functional working environment that can have positive outcomes both for patients and for healthcare teams.

CRITICAL THINKING QUESTIONS AND EXERCISES

- Using the website provided, take the Healthy Work Environment Assessment (2015) to evaluate your environment on the basis of standards and not individual groups within a team to isolate specific factors that your organization needs to address to mitigate conflict.
  www.aacn.org/nursing-excellence/healthy-work-environments/aacn-healthy-work-environment-assessment-tool
- Explore your communication skills during conflict by taking this assessment and how you can improve upon your communication.
  https://hbr.org/2015/03/assessment-how-well-do-you-communicate-during-conflict-2
- Visit the following website for a Best Practice Guideline on managing conflict from the Registered Nurses Association of Ontario (2012): http://rnao.ca/bpg/guidelines/managing-conflict-healthcare-teams. After reviewing the guidelines, identify three recommendations that you would consider implementing in your workplace. Take a Massive Open Online Course (MOOC) on conflict management for free at the following websites:
  https://ocw.mit.edu/courses/sloan-school-of-management/15-667-negotiation-and-conflict-management-spring-2001
  www.openlearningworld.com/innerpages/Conflict%20Management.htm

After completing a MOOC, reflect on what information you found useful for your nursing practice. Describe how you will change how you deal with conflict the next time on the basis of what you learned in viewing this MOOC.

REFERENCES

Almost, J. (2006). Conflict within nursing work environments: Concept analysis. *Journal of Advanced Nursing, 53*(4), 444–454. doi:10.1111/j.1365-2648.2006.03738.x

Alper, S., Tjosvold, D. W., & Law, S. K. (2000). Conflict management, efficacy, and performance in organizational teams. *Personnel Psychology, 53*, 625–642. doi:10.1111/j.1744-6570.2000.tb00216.x

American Association of Colleges of Nursing. (2012). *Graduate level QSEN competencies: Knowledge, skills, and attitudes*. Washington, DC: Author.

American Association of Critical-Care Nurses. (2016). *AACN standards for establishing and sustaining healthy work environments: A journey to excellence*. Aliso Viejo, CA: Author.

Barki, H., & Hartwick, J. (2004). Conceptualizing the construct of interpersonal conflict. *International Journal of Conflict Management, 15*(3), 216–244, 335–336. doi:10.1108/eb022913

Brett, J., Behfar, K., & Kern, M. C. (2006). Managing multicultural teams. *Harvard Business Review, 84*(11), 84–91. Retrieved from https://hbr.org/2006/11/managing-multicultural-teams

Brewer, N., Mitchell, P., & Weber, N. (2002). Gender role, organizational status, and conflict management styles. *International Journal of Conflict Management, 13*(1), 78–94. doi:10.1108/eb022868

Burawoy, M. (1979). *Manufacturing consent*. Chicago, IL: University of Chicago Press.

Byford, J. (2006). Right is right, wrong is wrong. *Southeast Farm Press, 33*(18), 17.

Cohen, S. G., & Bailey, D. E. (1997). What makes teams work: Group effectiveness research from the shop floor to the executive suite. *Journal of Management, 23*(3), 239–290. doi:10.1177/014920639702300303

College of Nurses of Ontario. (2006). Conflict prevention and standard of care [Practice guidline]. Toronto, ON, Canada: Author. Retrieved from https://www.cno.org/globalassets/docs/prac/47004_conflict_prev.pdf

Cronenwett, L., Sherwood, G., Barnsteiner, J., Disch, J., Johnson, J., Mitchell, P., ... Warren, J. (2007). Quality and safety education for nurses. *Nursing Outlook, 55*(3), 122–131. doi:10.1016/j.outlook.2007.02.006

DiRomualdo, T. (2006). Geezers, grungers, genXers, and geeks: A look at workplace generational conflict. *Journal of Financial Planning, 19*(10), 18–21.

Filley, A. C. (1975). *Interpersonal conflict resolution*. Glenview, IL: Scott, Foresman.

Folger, J. P., Poole, M. S., & Stutman, R. K. (2012). *Working through conflict: Strategies for relationships, groups, and organizations* (7th ed.). Boston, MA: Allyn & Bacon.

Gerardi, D. (2010). Conflict engagement training for health professionals: Recommendations for creating conflict competent organizations—A white paper for healthcare and dispute resolution professionals. Retrieved from http://www.ehcco.com

Hearn, J, Sheppard, D. L, Tancred-Sheriff, P., & Burrell, G. (Eds). (1989). *The sexuality of organization*. Newbury Park, CA: Sage.

Hetzler, D. C., Morrison, V. L., Gerardi, D., & Hayes, L. S. (2004). Curing conflict: A prescription for ADR in health care. Retrieved from http://www.collaboration-specialists.com/pubs/ABA-Curing%20Conflict.pdf

Institute for Safe Medication Practices. (2004, March). Survey shows workplace intimidation adversely affects patient safety [Press release]. Retrieved from http://forms.ismp.org/pressroom/pr20040331.pdf

Jameson, J. K. (2003). Transcending intractable conflict in health care: An exploratory study of communication and conflict management among anesthesia providers. *Journal of Health Communication, 8*(6), 563–581. doi:10.1080/716100415

Jehn, K. A., & Shah, P. P. (1997). Interpersonal relationships and task performance: An examination of mediating processes in friendship and acquaintance group. *Journal of Personality and Social Psychology, 72*, 775–790. doi:10.1037/0022-3514.72.4.775

The Joint Commission. (2008, July 9). Behaviors that undermine a culture of safety. *Sentinel Event Alert Issue 40*. Oakbrook Terrace, IL: Author. Retrieved from https://www.jointcommission.org/assets/1/18/SEA_40.PDF

The Joint Commission. (2017). *Comprehensive accreditation manual for hospitals (CAMH)*. Oakbrook Terrace, IL: Joint Commission Resources.

Kanter, R. M. (1977). *Men and women of the corporation*. New York, NY: Colophon Books.

Marquis, B. L., & Huston, C. J. (2011). *Leadership roles and management functions in nursing: Theory and application* (7th ed.). Philadelphia, PA: Wolters Kluwer Health/Lippincott Williams & Wilkins.

Marshall, J. (1984). *Women managers: Travelling in a male world*. Chichester, England: Wiley.

Mazadoorian, H. N., & Latham, S. R. (2004). ADR for health care organizations. *Dispute Resolution Magazine, 11*, 8.

McHugh, M. D., Kutney-Lee, A., Cimiotti, J. P., Sloane, D. M., & Aiken, L. H. (2011). Nurses' widespread job dissatisfaction, burnout, and frustration with health benefits signal problems for patient care. *Health Affairs, 30*(2), 202–210. doi:10.1377/hlthaff.2010.0100

Mishra, A. K. (1996). Organizational responses to crisis: The centrality of trust. In R. M. Kramer & T. R. Tyler (Eds.), *Trust in organizations: Frontiers of theory and research* (pp. 261–287). Thousand Oaks, CA: Sage.

Montoro-Rodriguez, J., & Small, J. A. (2006). The role of conflict resolution styles on nursing staff morale, burnout, and job satisfaction in long-term care. *Journal of Aging Health, 18*(3), 385–406. doi:10.1177/0898264306286196

Pelled, L. H., Eisenhardt, K. M., & Xin, K. R. (1999). Exploring the black box: An analysis of work group diversity, conflict and performance. *Administrative Science Quarterly, 44*, 1–28. doi:10.2307/2667029

Pinkerton, S. (2005). AACN standards for establishing and sustaining healthy work environments. *Nursing Economic$, 23*(3), 138–140.

Pondy, L. R. (1967). Organizational conflict: Concepts and models. *Administrative Science Quarterly, 13*, 296–320 doi:10.2307/2391553

Registered Nurses' Association of Ontario. (2012). *Managing and mitigating conflict in health-care teams*. Toronto, ON, Canada: Author.

Rowe, M. M., & Sherlock, H. (2005). Stress and verbal abuse in nursing: Do burned out nurses eat their young? *Journal of Nursing Management, 13*, 242–248. doi:10.1111/j.1365-2834.2004.00533.x

Schyve, P. M. (2009). *Leadership in healthcare organizations: A guide to Joint Commission leadership standards. A Governance Institute white paper winter 2009*. San Diego, CA: Governance Institute.

Scott, C., & Gerardi, D. (2011). A strategic approach for managing conflict in hospitals: Responding to the Joint Commission leadership standard, Part 1. *Joint Commission Journal of Quality Patient Safety*, *37*(2), 59–69. doi:10.1016/S1553-7250(11)37008-0

Siu, H., Spence Laschinger, H. K., & Finegan, J. (2008). Nursing professional practice environments: Setting the stage for constructive conflict resolution and work effectiveness. *Journal of Nursing Administration*, *38*(5), 250–257. doi:10.1097/01.NNA.0000312772.04234.1f

Swearingen, S., & Liberman, A. (2004). Nursing generations: An expanded look at the emergence of conflict and its resolution. *Health Care Manager*, *23*(1), 54–64. doi:10.1097/00126450-200401000-00010

Thomas, K. W., & Kilmann, R. H. (1974). *Thomas-Kilmann conflict mode instrument*. New York, NY: Xicom.

Tjosvold, D. (1987). Participation: A close look at its dynamics. *Journal of Management*, *13*, 739–750. doi:10.1177/014920638701300413

Tschannen, D., Keenan, G., Aebersold, M., Kocan, M. J., Lundy, F., & Averhart, V. (2011). Implications of nurse-physician relations: Report of a successful intervention. *Nursing Economic$*, *29*(3), 127–135.

Wall, J. A., & Callister, R. R. (1995). Conflict and its management. *Journal of Management*, *21*, 515–558. doi:10.1177/014920639502100306

Wright, K. B. (2011). A communication competence approach to healthcare worker conflict, job stress, job burnout, and job satisfaction. *Journal for Healthcare Quality*, *33*(2), 7–14. doi:10.1111/j.1945-1474.2010.00094.x

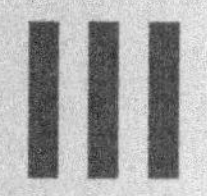

LEADING CHANGE

12

FACTORS THAT INFLUENCE ORGANIZATIONAL CULTURE

KELLY HANCOCK

LEARNING OBJECTIVES

After completion of this chapter, the reader will be able to

- Describe how organizational leadership influences change within an organization.
- Discuss how organizational structure and design influence overall organizational culture.
- Describe tools to assess organizational culture and readiness for strategic planning.
- Describe the complexity of healthcare systems including patient care service and payment models.
- Apply principles of shared governance to empower others in the workforce.

The U.S. healthcare system is embarking on system-wide transformation that is on a magnitude that has never been witnessed before. Many factors are influencing this transformation and a key driver is affordability. The rising costs and increasing demands from both consumers and third-party payers place organizations under significant pressure to reform. The demands of the global healthcare system require improved clinical and patient experience performance for financial success (Luzinski, 2011). The nursing workforce must be included in healthcare reform transformation because it is the largest profession among U.S. healthcare employees today, with over 3 million members. As a registered nurse, understanding the complexities of the healthcare environment will empower you to be an effective healthcare team member.

This chapter provides an overview of concepts that will explain both organizational and systems leadership. This knowledge will enhance your current leadership and communication skills to more effectively provide high-quality nursing care. Describing the organizational culture and design in an organization will enable you to be an active, engaged member of the healthcare team. This engagement will encourage you to participate in patient safety and quality care initiatives aligned with organizational goals. This chapter also discusses key concepts of an organization's professional practice model that supports nursing clinical practice. These concepts support the registered nurse in gaining knowledge to promote and participate in a shared governance model.

QUESTIONS TO CONSIDER

As you read the following case scenario, ask yourself:

- Did Sue take enough of her own initiative to understand the professional practice model of nursing in her new organization?
- Depending on your answer to the previous question, what questions could Sue have asked earlier in her orientation to gain a better understanding?

QUESTIONS TO CONSIDER BEFORE READING ON

- Does your organization have a written mission, vision, and values statement?
- If yes, can you recite those statements? Are those statements well known by the employees?
- If you do not know the statements, obtain a copy of each.

There are a number of terms that can assist nurses in identifying and reflecting on their own organization. When entering into a organization as a new hire, one of the first things to do is to understand the professional practice model of nursing (Box 12.1).

BOX 12.1 THE CASE SCENARIO

Sue is a new baccalaureate-prepared nurse graduate in week 6 of her orientation on a medical–surgical nursing unit. Sue sometimes questions why they adhere to specific clinical guidelines. Carol is one of Sue's primary coaches during the orientation period. During her first week of her new role, Sue learned about the professional practice model of nursing for her organization during the general session of nursing orientation. There was much information shared at that session and it was difficult to understand how that model had a relationship to the care she was going to be delivering to her patients. Sue did not consider it an important aspect of her orientation. It was not until Carol took the time during the unit's daily huddle to pause and explain how the model had an impact on the care they delivered. Sue quickly realized the value of understanding the model because it allowed her to be a more effective member of the healthcare team.

Organizational mission is usually communicated through a written statement. The mission statement of a healthcare organization is usually succinct and precisely describes the purpose of the institution. Mission statements provide clarity around answering the three questions of purpose, defining stakeholders, and methods to achieve the goal.

Vision statements are developed to appeal to commitment and invigorate people, to create meaning in their work, create principles of quality, and bridge the current state to the future.

Values are the framework that supports the mission and vision of an organization. Organizations typically have four to five values that are easy to remember and cite. For example, some healthcare organizations commonly list "excellence, teamwork, collaboration, and respect."

Professional practice model is a system composed of structure and processes that largely refer to nursing practice within a variety of healthcare settings. This model supports the belief in the importance of the autonomy of the registered nurse in the delivery of nursing care to obtain superior clinical outcomes.

Organizational culture can be understood by observing the people who work in and make up the organization and how committed those people are to the shared mission and vision of the organization.

Organizational leadership influences the culture of an organization. The chief executive officer (CEO) of a healthcare organization is responsible for setting the "tone" of the organization. CEOs are identifying, developing, and enabling leaders to build cultures of engagement and accountability. The chief nursing officer (CNO) is responsible for overseeing the development and sustainability of the culture of nursing practice. The CNO, the most senior nurse leader in an organization, is responsible for overseeing nurses, patient care, finances, and strategic planning by professional nurses in the organization. The CNO has a team of nurse leaders who have diverse responsibilities at the macro and micro levels of an organization.

At the micro or unit level of an organization, the nurse leader is typically the nurse manager. The nurse manager oversees the day-to-day operations of a nursing unit and has a large responsibility to influence the culture. Nurse managers have the ability to foster staff empowerment, satisfaction, and creativity so that staff memebrs can in turn provide safe, compassionate care to patients. Organizations that have energetic, transformational-minded nurse managers are well positioned to meet these challenges. In the leadership literature, evidence is growing toward movement away from managing change, and toward transforming change. The ability to lead transformation requires a different set of skills and behaviors of nurse managers than in the past. One of the most critical skills includes the ability to influence change by creating a shared vision. This skill allows the leader to motivate people to adopt the vision as their own and carry it out (Habel & Sherman, 2012). Establishing a relationship with people allows the nurse manager to engage with the people who are doing the work. This skill allows the nurse manager to understand the people's strengths and opportunities so as to align support needed that optimizes their performance.

In 2010, the Institute of Medicine (IOM) released the *Future of Nursing: Leading Change, Advancing Health* report. In this report, nurses were encouraged to step up and prepare for the future. The report included educating leaders at all levels and recommended nurses receive leadership development at every level, to transform the healthcare system.

QUESTIONS TO CONSIDER

As you read the following case scenario, ask yourself:

- How did the nurse manager foster a culture of "speaking up" at her unit?
- What would have happened if Sue did not speak up?

Think of another situation which you have witnessed in your nursing practice when "speaking up" was the right thing to do. Does your practice area have a supportive supervisor who promotes a positive working environment for nurses?

TOOLS TO ASSESS ORGANIZATIONAL CULTURE

Understanding the perspectives of all caregivers in an organization is imperative to fostering a favorable organizational culture. For example, in the case scenario (Box 12.2), Sue clearly felt that the culture at her unit supported her to speak up appropriately when she felt things were not being done the correct way. Promoting patient safety is paramount for all healthcare leaders. Despite this awareness, we still have patients who are harmed due to errors. Healthcare organizational leaders and nurses need to identify where the processes and systems are broken to develop a plan to repair them (Evanoff et al., 2005). The optimal way of improving the culture of safety is to hear feedback from those working in the culture.

BOX 12.2 THE CASE SCENARIO CONTINUES TO UNFOLD

Sue has now completed her 6 months at her nursing unit. She had a patient who required a central line to be placed at the bedside. Prior to the procedure taking place, a time out was performed. During the time out, one of the members of the team was not fully engaged in the time out. Sue was not certain if she should speak up, especially still being a novice nurse. Sue remembered that her nurse manager, Terri, had just reviewed in a staff meeting the importance of having a culture of safety and encouraging the nursing staff to speak up when they felt that safety may be jeopardized. Sue spoke up and asks that everyone focus on the time out so they could ensure it was done safely. Sue's nurse manager, Terri, had heard about Sue speaking up. Terri sought out Sue and recognized her for speaking up and thanked her for ensuring a culture of safety existed at the unit.

One way of measuring the perceptions of members of a healthcare team is using a tool to survey perceptions. Usually, healthcare organizations administer a validated survey on an annual basis to assess the caregiver's perception of the culture that includes safety and one's active engagement in the process. The "culture of safety" best describes caregivers' perceptions, attitudes, and beliefs about risk and safety in their work unit. Once feedback is received, analyzed, shared, and discussed, an action plan is developed at both the unit and organizational levels. The following is a sample of questions on a survey:

- Does your leadership provide a work climate that promotes patient safety?
- Are you involved in decisions that affect your work?
- Can you report patient safety mistakes without fear of punishment?
- Is your organization actively doing things to improve patient safety?

The action plan will be successful if the culture of safety is viewed as a strategic priority by the organization's leadership team. Wide organizational commitment ensures that caregivers are aware that safety standards and behaviors are supported at the individual and team levels. There are a number of characteristics that can assist the caregiver in understanding and practicing the elements of a culture of safety. They include:

- Leadership commitment to discussion of near misses and actual errors
- Use of visual management to track and discuss patient safety
- Encouragement of effective communication among team members
- Use of systems for reporting potential or actual events

The goal of supporting a culture of safety is typically included in the strategic plan of the organization.

STRATEGIC PLANNING PROCESS

The strategic planning process of an organization is about ensuring there is a clear vision to achieve the goals that have been outlined. It allows for those who work in an organization to understand how their contributions align with this process (Box 12.3).

QUESTIONS TO CONSIDER

As you read the following case scenario, ask yourself:

- Why is it important that the CNO ask for the input from frontline nursing staff when developing nursing's strategic agenda?
- Who is responsible for the strategic agenda? How can Sue gather and verify facts to clearly understand the current state?
- What issues can be anticipated if frontline nursing staff does not gain agreement on what the strategy should be?

BOX 12.3 THE CASE SCENARIO CONTINUES TO UNFOLD

Sue had attended a nursing town hall meeting at her hospital, which was led by the CNO of her organization. In this town hall meeting, the CNO provided the audience with the overall goals of the organization, which were established by the hospital's executive team. The CNO shared strategies in which nursing could contribute to meeting those goals. The CNO asked for the frontline nursing staff to provide feedback on specific tactics for those strategies. She shared that the nurse managers of their units would be meeting with them to gather that information.

A strategic plan is a tool for leaders to use in the healthcare setting to communicate a clear vision of goals, priorities, and strategies to caregivers who work in the organization (Table 12.1). The goals and priorities are established by the leadership team using input from staff nurses to meet needs of the stakeholders. The priorities and strategies are created on the basis of feedback provided by the leadership team, nurses, and other applicable stakeholders. The goals are assigned metrics that are measurable. These metrics are reviewed on a regular schedule at the micro and macro levels of the organization. This drives accountability and effective implementation of the strategies supporting the goals. A strategic plan is usually updated on an annual basis with some goals remaining, whereas others may be added or deleted. The shift to value-based models of care and consumerism in today's healthcare market is transforming the way care is delivered in and out of the hospital. Therefore, the need for a solid strategic plan for a healthcare system today is necessary to improve quality and experience, and to provide affordable healthcare.

Nurse leaders who engage with their frontline staff in pursuit of a shared strategic vision have seen significant achievement in reaching overall organizational goals. This pursuit of a shared vision is an effective approach for achieving widespread and fundamental organizational change. Nurses are the largest group of healthcare providers in a hospital. They are closest to the patients and spend most of their time in patient care areas. Leveraging that experience and feedback to inform the nursing strategic agenda in an organization will only foster a culture of empowerment and success of organizational goals.

SELF-ASSESSMENT

Complete the following self-assessment related to your organization's mission and vision statements as well as related to its strategic planning process. Answer "yes" or "no" to the following statements:

- My organization has a clear, succinct mission statement that states its purpose for existence.

(Text continued on page 240)

TABLE 12.1 EXAMPLE OF A STRATEGIC PLAN TEMPLATE

Initiative—the What? Tactic—the How?	Current Performance	Target	KPI Description	Lead	Start Date	End Date	Clinical Enterprise Priority	Key Dependencies
Define major **initiatives** (programs/projects) for each of the five strategic goals (12- to 18-month span in duration) and supporting tactics to achieve targeted performance **Multiyear initiatives:** Use a phased approach to manage scope, resources, and time frame (enter only the work for the current planning year)	Current YTD performance	Planned performance target to achieve	Measure to evaluate the success of the initiative or tactic	Designated person(s) who will own initiative or tactic (two to three maximum)	Estimated timeline for initiative or tactic		Priority that your initiative most significantly impacts (one to three maximum)	Explain dependencies on organizational support functions (i.e., IT, finance, lab support, nursing resources, registration, enterprise initiatives, hospital or institute support)

(continued)

TABLE 12.1 EXAMPLE OF A STRATEGIC PLAN TEMPLATE *(continued)*

Initiative—the What? Tactic—the How?	Current Performance	Target	KPI Description	Lead	Start Date	End Date	Clinical Enterprise Priority	Key Dependencies
1. Initiative: Leveraging Technology to Support Clinical Care			Expand at least two technologies initiated at a hosptial to other regional facilities Initiate two new projects (with IT) to enhance interoperability and decrease manual documentation by approximately 10 min/day Conduct two new trials on virtual interaction solutions				Care path design and adherence	

Tactic 1: Implement and Expand Specific Technologies (e.g., Vocera, IPTV, and Jive)								
Tactic 2: Enhance Interoperability Between Different Applications to Assist Daily Tasks (charting) and Transition of Care								
Tactic 3: Leverage Best Practices in Technology by Monitoring Accomplishments								
Tactic 4: Explore Venues for Virtual Interaction With Patients and Caregivers (e.g., social media for patient education)								

(continued)

TABLE 12.1 EXAMPLE OF A STRATEGIC PLAN TEMPLATE *(continued)*

Initiative—the What? Tactic—the How?	Current Performance	Target	KPI Description	Lead	Start Date	End Date	Clinical Enterprise Priority	Key Dependencies
2. Initiative: Refining Expectations/ Accountability			All nursing specific quality, patient safety, and experience metrics ***(attached)***				High reliability	
Tactic 1: Define Internal Expectation for Staff Nurses, ANMs, NMs, and NDs								
Tactic 2: Educate Patients About Their Roles, Expectations, and Experience								
Tactic 3: Monitor, Coach, Evaluate, and Celebrate Unit Specific or Individual Targets								

3. Initiative: Investing and Developing Nonlicensed Personnel to Be "Best in Class"			Number of training/develop-ment oppor-tunities provided				Caregiver roles—top of license	
Tactic 1: Extend Shared Governance to Nonlicensed								
Tactic 2: Cultivate Team-Based Culture and Support Career								
Tactic 3: Provide Training and Education								

Note: Initiatives, numeric; tactics, actions.

ANMs, assistant nurse managers; IT, internet technology; KPI, key performance indicator; NDs, nursing directors; NMs, nurse managers; YTD, year to date.

- My organization has an influential vision statement that communicates what the organization desires to achieve.
- My organization tracks its accomplishments in relation to its mission and vision.
- My organization has a strategic plan that is directly related to its mission and vision statement.
- My organization has strategic goals and objectives that are understood by employees.

Based on the results of the assessment, what are the strengths and weaknesses of your organization? What suggestions for improvement would you give?

PAYMENT MODELS

For many years, those who have been watching the U.S. healthcare system have witnessed a struggle against limited access to care, fragmented care delivery models, and a disconnect between quality and cost. These problems have resulted in a call to action requiring a transformation in healthcare. This call to action can be traced back to the IOM's 2001 report *Crossing the Quality Chasm: A New Health System for the 21st Century*. This report suggested a radical change in the way care is delivered and paid for.

In today's healthcare environment, health systems and hospitals are turning to new modes of delivery care that deliver high-quality care at a lower cost. To achieve these goals, healthcare value must increase. In all of the healthcare payment models, quality is a key component, and most arrangements tie the final payment to the achievement of key quality metrics. As value-based payment spreads, the following healthcare payment models (defined by Park, Gold, Bazemore, & Liaw, 2018) highlight its unique characteristics.

FEE-FOR-SERVICE

The most traditional of healthcare payment models, fee-for-service, requires patients or payers to reimburse the healthcare provider for each service performed. Providers are then encouraged to increase their volumes regardless of quality and financial outcomes, which places the risk for both on the insurer.

PAY-FOR-PERFORMANCE

In a pay-for-performance (P4P) or value-based reimbursement environment, healthcare providers are compensated only if they meet certain metrics for quality and efficiency. Creating quality benchmark metrics ties physicians' reimbursement directly to the quality of care they provide.

BUNDLED PAYMENT OR EPISODE-OF-CARE PAYMENT

Providers are given incentive to limit the costs for all services rendered in that episode of care.

UPSIDE SHARED SAVINGS PROGRAMS (CENTERS FOR MEDICARE AND MEDICAID SERVICES [CMS] OR COMMERCIAL)

Shared savings programs provide incentives for providers with respect to specific patient populations. A percentage of any net savings realized is given to the provider. Costs and quality of care for a defined population are the responsibility of a provider or an accountable care organization (ACO). The costs are calculated on expenditures from the prior years and supplied by the insurers.

PARTIAL OR FULL CAPITATION

In this healthcare payment model, patients are assigned a per member per month (PMPM) payment on the basis of their age, race, sex, lifestyle, medical history, and benefit design. Payment rates are tied to expected usage regardless of whether the patient visits more or less. Like bundled payment models, healthcare providers have an incentive to help patients avoid high-cost procedures and tests to maximize their compensation. Under partial- or blended-capitation models, only certain types or categories of services are paid on a basis of capitation.

SHARED GOVERNANCE

Empowering registered nurses through professional practice models includes having a strong foundation of shared governance. "Shared governance" can be defined as shared decision-making among frontline registered nurses and organizational leadership (Box 12.4). It is a model that provides direction for the professional practice of nursing. In healthcare organizations that embrace shared governance, councils are formed and are active both at the unit level and, at times, the hospital level. The characteristics of a successful shared governance council include having active participation and dedication of the frontline nurses. For shared governance to be successful, strong nursing leadership is needed that supports staff taking the time to attend the council meetings. Time needs to be given so the council can grow and develop. The framework of shared governance includes the principles of accountability, ownership, equity, and partnership. The shared governance model is often used as a strategy for healthcare organizations to ensure higher retention rates of registered nurses, increased job satisfaction, support of high reliable culture, and empowerment of frontline nurses. The essence of shared governance is to give autonomy to nursing professionals so that they can have control over their nursing practice and decisions that impact registered nurses as a means to promote quality and patient safety. The philosophy of shared governance is more than a structure; it is a way for nurses to express and manage their practice with a higher level of professional autonomy (Steckler, Rawlins, Williamson, & Suchman, 2016). In a Magnet®-designated hospital, shared governance is critical to ensure a culture of excellence, and supporting structures are critical to sustain long-term changes for a successful journey.

QUESTIONS TO CONSIDER

As you read the following case scenario, ask yourself:

- What do you think were the deciding factors for Sue to become engaged in the unit shared governance council? Do you think she would have been interested 6 months ago? Explain and provide a rationale for your answers.
- What do you think Sue and her colleagues who expressed concerns over the issues with telemetry checks should have done if others did not feel the same way about the issue?
- Think about a time during your clinical experiences when you observed an issue that may have been appropriate to bring to a shared governance council for discussion. What evidence would you need to support your concern?

QUALITY AND SAFETY EDUCATION FOR NURSES (QSEN) CONSIDERATIONS

As you read the following QSEN competencies (Box 12.5) related to understanding organizational design, ask yourself:

- Which of these competencies do I meet and which competencies do I need to develop more fully?
- What plan of action can I take to enhance those competencies in which I am weak and to develop those which I lack at this time?

BOX 12.4 THE CASE SCENARIO CONTINUES TO UNFOLD

During a recent staff meeting, the unit nurses were encouraged to join the Shared Governance Council. As a result, Sue who has been at the unit for 18 months decided to join. Sue reached out to one of the cochairs of the unit council for information about the next meeting and the topics that would be discussed. At Sue's first meeting, a fellow nurse on the unit stated that they had an issue with telemetry checks not being completed per the protocol. Sue had an interest in this topic because she shared the same concern. She volunteered to work on this issue and bring back recommendations to the next meeting. Sue and her colleagues interviewed many new and seasoned members at the unit. They discovered that the protocol had not been updated in 5 years and was not reviewed in the new-nurse orientation. Sue and her colleagues from the Shared Governance Council revised the protocol to be reflective of current workflows and created educational modules that could be used in new hire orientation and for the existing staff at the unit. They brought their work back to the Shared Governance Council, and Terri, the nurse manager, approved their work. Terri and others were then invited to the staff meeting for the unit to share the new changes to the telemetry check protocol and the new education that would be happening.

BOX 12.5 UNDERSTANDING ORGANIZATIONAL DESIGN: SELECT RELEVANT QSEN COMPETENCIES

- Recognize that nursing and other health profession students are parts of systems of care and care processes that affect outcomes for patients and families (Quality Improvement).
- Participate in structuring the work environment to facilitate integration of new evidence into standards of practice (Evidence-Based Practice).
- Appreciate that continuous quality improvement is an essential part of the daily work of all health professionals (Quality Improvement).

Source: Quality and Safety Education for Nurses Institute. (2014). QSEN competencies. Retrieved from http://qsen.org/competencies/pre-licensure-ksas

CONCLUSIONS

This chapter presented the reader with a better understanding of both organizational and system leadership. Since the release of the IOM's report on the *Future of Nursing: Leading Change, Advancing Health* (IOM, 2010), the question most leaders of healthcare organizations ask is How? The question directed to leaders in healthcare is How can they better prepare the nursing workforce for the changes in healthcare. The information discussed in this chapter provides strategies for frontline nurses to build the capabilities needed for change. Key concepts such as the organization's professional practice model, shared governance model, and participation in strategic agenda planning were discussed. There is a need for the frontline nurse leaders to be advocates for change, to drive change, and know how to be engaged members of the healthcare team. Frontline nurse leaders who are prepared, nurtured, and mentored have the potential to transform healthcare.

CRITICAL THINKING QUESTIONS AND ACTIVITIES

- Read the following article: Garcia, A. B., Rocha, F .L. R., Pissinati, P. S. C., Marziale, M. H. P., Camelo, S. H. H., & Haddad, M. D. C. F. L. (2017). The effects of organisational culture on nurses' perceptions of their work. *British Journal of Nursing, 26*(14), 806–812. doi:10.12968/bjon.2017.26.14.806
  Use the seven dimensions of organizational culture outlined in the article to assess the organizational culture in your institution. Do you feel the organizational culture influences nurses' mental health and well-being? Explain your answer.
- Using the following website, describe how you will use storytelling about experiences in your organization as it relates to culture and leadership. Steppingstones: www.lifejournal.com/articles/the-steppingstones-of-ira-progoff

REFERENCES

Evanoff, B., Potter, P., Wolf, L., Gryson, D., Dunagan, C., & Boxerman, S. (2005). Can we talk? Priorities for patient care differed among health care providers. In K. Henriksen, J. B. Battles, E. S. Marks, & D. I. Lewin (Eds.), *Advances in patient safety: From research to implementation* (Vol. 1, pp. 5–14). Rockville, MD: Agency for Healthcare Research and Quality.

Habel, M., & Sherman, R. O. (2012, September/October). Transformational leadership: A growing promise for nursing. *Heartland/Midwest*, pp. 24–29.

Heffernan, M., Quinn Griffin, M. T., McNulty, S. R., & Fitzpatrick, J. J. (2010). Self–compassion and emotional intelligence in nurses. *International Journal of Nursing Practice, 16*(4), 366–373. doi:10.1111/j.1440-172X.2010.01853.x

Institute of Medicine. (2010). *The future of nursing: Leading change, advancing health.* Washington, DC: National Academies Press. Retrieved from https://www.ncbi.nlm.nih.gov/books/NBK209880

Luzinski, C. (2011). Transformational leadership. *Journal of Nursing Administration, 41*, 501–502. doi:10.1097/NNA.0b013e3182378a71

Park, B., Gold, S., Bazemore, A., & Liaw, W. (2018). How evolving United States payment models influence primary care and its impact on the Quadruple Aim. *The Journal of the American Board of Family Medicine, 31*(4), 588–604.

Quality and Safety Education for Nurses Institute. (2014). QSEN competencies. Retrieved from http://qsen.org/competencies/pre-licensure-ksas

Steckler, N. A., Rawlins, D. B., Williamson, P. R., & Suchman, A. L. (2016). Preparing to lead change: An innovative curriculum integrating theory, group skills and authentic presence. *Healthcare, 4*(4), 247–251. doi:10.1016/j.hjdsi.2015.10.005

The Steppingstones of Ira Progoff: Bring together past, present, and future. (n.d.). Retrieved from http://www.lifejournal.com/articles/the-steppingstones-of-ira-progoff

13

INNOVATION AND CHANGE

AUDREY MARIE BEAUVAIS ● KIMBERLY SPAHN

LEARNING OBJECTIVES

After completion of this chapter, the reader will be able to

- Describe why innovation and change are needed in nursing practice.
- Assess one's own past reactions and behaviors when confronted with change.
- Describe the role of the nurse as change agent.
- Describe nursing leadership characteristics and skills that promote innovation and change.
- Distinguish planned from unplanned change.
- Apply Lewin's change theory, Kotter's eight steps to leading change, and Rogers's diffusion of innovation to innovations and changes in one's practice setting.
- Discuss effective change strategies.
- Identify factors that promote resistance to change and factors that promote change.
- Describe effective strategies to manage constant change.

Whether we like it or not, change is constant in our profession. Nursing leaders need to embrace innovation and change if we are going to help improve our nursing processes and outcomes for our patients. Innovation and change will require you to be open to new ideas, commit to continuous learning, be creative, and let go of the past (French-Bravo & Crow, 2015). In this chapter, you will find in-depth information that will be useful in creating innovations and implementing change. This chapter presents a framework for the development of skills to foster innovation and lead change.

WHY IS INNOVATION AND CHANGE NEEDED IN NURSING PRACTICE?

Before answering that question, let us define innovation and change. "Innovation" means creating something new (e.g., an idea, procedure, or device) or altering something that already exists. "Change" means implementing something new. As nurses, we want to improve our patient outcomes and our work environment and processes. However, we cannot make improvements by doing things the way they have always been done before. We have to be willing to challenge the way things have been done to make improvements. Ask yourself the following: "Why do we do things this way?" Simply pondering the question "Why?" can lead you to challenge the status quo and lead you to new ideas and innovations. Nurses new to an organization are especially valuable because they might see opportunities for improvement that have been overlooked. However, even if you have been working in an organization for a while, you should start to question why things are done in a particular way and look for ways to improve processes to obtain better results. Not only should you question, but you should also listen. Talk with others and get diverse viewpoints (Cashman, 2013). This questioning and listening can lead you to innovative ideas that in turn can be implemented to make a positive change. Change can then lead to improvements in the quality and safety of the care we provide. As a clinical leader, you will play a vital role in innovation and change!

INNOVATION

Innovation plays an essential role in nursing practice because it allows for adaptation and response in the practice environment. It helps move the nursing profession forward by optimizing patient care to improve safety and patient outcomes (Hancock, 2015). Nursing innovations can also be used to create efficiencies in our daily responsibilities (Hancock, 2015). As an associate's degree nurse, you have probably thought about your work processes and considered alternative ways of getting the job done. Nurses tend to think "outside the box" and creatively. Innovation in nursing promotes growth and progression within the nursing profession. It enhances creativity and encourages inventive problem-solving. Nursing innovations can lead to new and improved processes and/or resources that will potentially decrease cost, improve patient safety, enhance optimal patient outcomes, and advance nursing care (Hancock, 2015). As advances in healthcare technology are made and patients need greater care, nurses should be willing and able to change old practices and systems for new, innovative approaches (Kalisch & Begeny, 2010). Delivering quality care is essential as is the ability to create innovative approaches, act quickly, and take calculated risks (Kalisch & Begeny, 2010). Creativity is important to the process of innovation, but the creative idea alone cannot be sustained unless implemented in the proper environment. The feelings of patients, families,

BOX 13.1 SELF-ASSESSMENT: HOW INNOVATIVE ARE YOU?

This is not a scientific self-assessment but rather is intended to foster reflection. Please answer "yes" or "no" to the following questions:

- I have a passion for helping my patients and improving the quality and safety of patient care.
- I look for ways to solve my patients' problems.
- I am creative.
- I do not let challenges stand in my way of accomplishing my goals.
- Barriers do not stop me from achieving my patient safety goals.
- I am receptive to feedback.
- I am frequently coming up with new ideas and opportunities.
- I like to try new things.
- I like to generate new ideas.
- I have lots of ideas.
- I like possibilities.
- I take risks.
- I like the big picture.

If you answered "yes" to most of these questions, then you are most likely an innovative individual. If you answered "no" to most of these questions, then you are less likely to be innovative. Take a moment to reflect on these answers and develop three strategies to help promote your creative and innovative spirit.

employees, and other decision-makers must be considered during the innovative process (Blakeney, Carleton, McCarthy, & Coakley, 2009). Refer to Box 13.1 to assess how innovative you are.

Innovations can be simple ideas that will make a big difference to practice. The following real-life example from West Suffolk NHS Foundation Trust will help demonstrate this point. Nurse Kate Ramsey realized that the cups used for the water fountain looked exactly the same as the cups that were used for patients' soluble mediations (Ford, 2017). Patients and staff were unable to tell which cups contained medications and which contained tap water. Knowing that this could lead to medication errors, Nurse Ramsey thought of an easy innovative fix. She suggested that green cups be used to signify a cup containing a soluble medication. This simple innovation was implemented across all units in the hospital. The innovation had minimal cost and the cups were reusable and dishwasher safe. The visual difference helped to raise awareness ensuring that medications were not accidentally thrown away. Green cups were identified as a priority for patient consumption.

Another example comes from Jill Byrne, RN, a nurse at the Cleveland Clinic, who recognized a problem in the operating room (Laidman, 2017).

The problem she identified was that when the operating room doctors and nurses get hot, they get cranky. She developed a solution to the problem by creating a vest with pockets to hold ice packs. These "cool" vests are intended to be worn over the healthcare professionals' scrubs but under the plastic surgical gown that caused them to feel overheated. Nurse Byrne collaborated with Cleveland Clinic Innovations on a patent that is pending.

FACTORS AFFECTING INNOVATION

As a nursing leader, you should recognize the factors that promote and inhibit innovation among your team members. Table 13.1 highlights some of these factors.

As a clinical leader, remaining cognizant of these factors will help you to foster innovation in your healthcare setting. You should also be aware of the factors that support adopting an innovation. If your innovation has the following characteristics, the innovation is more likely to be implemented:

- Provides an improvement/advantage
- Is simple/easy to understand
- Is easy to introduce/try/use
- Is easy to measure the benefits
- Is inexpensive

In addition, the innovation is more likely to be implemented if the organization has the following characteristics:

- The organization is willing to take risks.
- The organization supports new efforts knowing that all will not succeed. It tries to learn from failure.
- The organization is not too regulated by outside agencies.

TABLE 13.1 FACTORS THAT PROMOTE AND INHIBIT INNOVATION

Factors That Can Promote Innovation	Factors That Can Inhibit Innovation
Reflection on your nursing practice individually and in team meetings	No time to reflect on your nursing practice
Willingness to take risks	Limited freedom to be creative
Having mentors and role models	Few innovative role models
Recognizing clinical heroes who make positive changes	A view that nursing does not have the status to make changes
Sharing innovative ideas at meetings	Feeling a lack of empowerment

Source: Stanley, D. J. (2012). Clinical leadership and innovation. *Journal of Nursing Education and Practice*, *2*(2), 119–126. doi:10.5430/jnep.v2n2p119

QUESTIONS TO CONSIDER BEFORE READING ON

Have you ever had (or do you have) an innovative idea? What factors promote the success of your idea? What factors inhibit the success of your idea? Does your innovation possess characteristics that would foster its implementation (provides a benefit, simple, easy, inexpensive, etc.)?

NURSES AS CHANGE AGENTS

A "change agent" refers to a person who facilitates positive transformation. A key function for nurses is to implement evidence-based practice changes (Orr & Davenport, 2014). Nurses are on the front lines of healthcare and are well aware of what works and what does not work. This keen awareness of the issues in healthcare helps to position nurses to develop innovative changes to improve the safety and quality of patient care. Nurses must have a vision and deliberately explore opportunities to be change agents (Andrews, 1993). Refer to Box 13.2 to assess how receptive you are to change.

Change often begins with you rather than with others. As a nursing leader, it will be important to use your power and influence while dealing with the logical and psychological dimensions of change (Feldman, 2008). Change should be facilitated as opposed to forced. Try to free yourself of the old processes of thinking and develop new solutions to solve problems. Remain open to feedback as well as encourage others to support the need for change. Nurses should foster certain characteristics and skills to function as change agents. Table 13.2 highlights characteristics and skills of successful nursing change agents (Feldman, 2008).

BOX 13.2 SELF-ASSESSMENT: HOW RECEPTIVE ARE YOU TO CHANGE?

There may be times when you are the innovative individual presenting ideas to others. You might then lead that innovation into a practice change. However, at other times, your superiors might be presenting innovative ideas to you and asking you to make changes. How receptive are you to new ideas? What are your reactions and behaviors when confronted with the needed change? Do you feel you are open to change or are you somewhat resistant? Take the "Change-readiness assessment" found at the following web address: http://ecfvp.org/files/uploads/2_-change_readiness_assessment_0426111.pdf. Score your attempt at the self-assessment. Reflect on the results. What about your results surprised you? What actions might you take on the basis of the results?

TABLE 13.2 CHARACTERISTICS AND SKILLS OF SUCCESSFUL CHANGE AGENTS

- Trustworthy
- Reliable
- Honest
- Competent
- Credible
- Persuasive
- Effective listening skills
- Good negotiators
- Strong work ethic
- Enthusiasm
- Respect for individual differences
- Able to think conceptually
- Able to organize thoughts logically
- Able to develop and implement plans
- Sound judgment
- Excellent communication skills
- Able to function as a coach and facilitator
- Base actions on evidence
- Have good networks

Source: Pesut, D. J., H. R. (2008). Change agents and change agent strategies. In H. R. Feldman (Ed.), *Nursing leadership: A concise encyclopedia* (pp. 103–105). New York, NY: Springer Publishing.

PLANNED AND UNPLANNED CHANGES

Healthcare organizations need to be flexible and adaptable to be successful in today's world. Many changes that are implemented in our organizations are planned as a way for the organization to reach its strategic goals. Other changes are not planned. Both are described in the following text.

PLANNED CHANGE

In an organizational setting, planned change is intentional and expected. It occurs when leaders see an opportunity for improvement and work together to organize a plan. The goal of planned change is to complete the process in a proactive, purposeful, collaborative effort with the assistance of a change agent. Planned change is necessary, but it can be resisted or challenged in nursing practice for many reasons.

Planned *internal* change refers to an organization that strategically changes some aspect of the healthcare business. This could be that it offers new services or changes the organizational structure and size (Juneja, n.d.). For example, a hospital might decide it wants to offer open heart surgery when it had never done so before. Or an organization might decide it wants to change its organizational structure by implementing service lines.

Planned *external* change refers to external factors that are introduced to an organization in a planned manner to improve the healthcare business in some way. The external factors can be technological innovations or advancements in communication and information processing (Juneja, n.d.). For example, robotics (a planned external change) can be considered a technological innovation that might be implemented in healthcare. Advancements in communication and information processing such as wireless technology and networks help make it much easier to communicate. Implementing wireless technology or an electronic medical record would qualify as a planned external change.

UNPLANNED CHANGE

Unplanned change is spontaneous and can bring about unexpected results. It typically occurs because of a surprise event, which can lead to reactive and disorganized results. Unplanned change can occur when upper management suddenly leaves an organization, or emergencies, disasters, and critical patient outcomes occur. It cannot be completely avoided, so planning for and learning from unplanned change can boost an organization's resilience (Edmonson, 2015).

Unplanned *internal* change occurs when change happens that is not strategically proposed. Rather, the change can happen as a result of such things as performance gaps (Juneja, n.d.). For example, when patients learn about poor-performing healthcare organizations, they may choose to go elsewhere for their services, thus impacting the organizations' profit margins. Unplanned *external* change can be related to modifications in governmental regulations and economic uncertainties (Juneja, n.d.). For example, the unplanned external change of alterations in governmental regulations can influence the reimbursement healthcare organizations receive.

QUESTIONS TO CONSIDER BEFORE READING ON

Think of a time you encountered unplanned change.

- How did you respond to this situation?
- What would you have done the same? What would you have done differently?

CHANGE THEORIES

Understanding change theory will help you embrace and sustain change in your work environment. Nurse leaders who use a structured change theory framework improve their chances for success (Mitchell, 2013). There are a number of change theories that leaders can use. Here, we present three of these: Lewin's change theory, Kotter's eight steps to leading change, and Rogers's diffusion of innovation.

LEWIN'S THEORY OF CHANGE

Lewin's classic change theory involves a three-step process that nurse leaders/change agents must follow before the change becomes permanent. Lewin's model provides a framework for nurse leaders to use their knowledge, skills, and attitudes to determine what needs to change, how to create the need for change through effective communication, and develop ways to sustain the new change over time (Shirey, 2013). The three-step process is as follows:

1. Unfreezing (change is needed)
2. Moving (change is initiated)
3. Refreezing (stability is obtained)

The case scenario in Box 13.3 highlights innovation and change in the clinical practice setting.

In Lewin's change theory, the **first stage**, unfreezing, involves getting ready for change, or recognizing a problem. This stage entails finding a way for people to discard an old process that was not productive in some way. The unfreezing phase helps people to overcome the status quo and get rid of the current

BOX 13.3 THE CASE SCENARIO

Read this case scenario and think about innovation and change. Can you identify an innovation that might help improve nursing practice if implemented at your place of employment as Maria has in this case scenario?

Maria has been a registered nurse (RN) for 1 year and is employed in a local community hospital on the pediatric unit. She has become more comfortable on her unit and in the hospital setting over the past year, but the transition from student nurse to RN was difficult. A few weeks after she graduated, she completed hospital orientation and received 3 months of training from experienced nurses on the unit. Once practicing on her own, she still had occasional questions about patient care, but many of the experienced nurses were not always available. She worked different shifts, on various days of the week, so the mix of RNs was always changing. During training, she was matched with different nurses every shift, and she did not have a mentor.

Maria is aware of the high attrition and burnout rate during the transition period from student nurse to RN, especially in the 2 years of practice. She has also researched the benefit of hospital mentoring programs. She knows that the RNs supported at the start of employment are more likely to develop leadership skills, increased satisfaction, and reduced first-year turnover rate (Porter & Strout, 2016). Maria has observed a high RN turnover rate on her own unit, and identified a gap between the experienced nurses and the new nurses with less than 5 years' experience. She believes that a mentoring program for new nurses could improve satisfaction and outcomes for her unit.

mindset. This phase involves creating awareness and an understanding for why the change must take place. Presenting a serious safety/quality event or problem can help get people to realize the need for change and to search for new solutions. Staff satisfaction surveys may help demonstrate that morale is low and could lead to quality and safety issues (Shirey, 2013). Educating staff regarding the need for change is an initial step. As a nurse leader, you can begin to highlight gaps between the current and desired outcomes and offer a vision of how it can change. Leaders can help staff understand what is expected of them and build their confidence that these changes are possible. Refer to Box 13.4 for the continuing case scenario and how you can apply the first stage of Lewin's change theory.

Once the problem is understood, identifying the supportive people within the organization as well as the facilitators and barriers, is essential. The **second stage**, moving or transitioning, involves a plan of action, clear communication, and shared decision-making with all team members. This is where better processes for doing things are explored. During this stage, a more productive change of thoughts, feelings, attitudes, and/or behaviors takes place. This may happen through organizational or process changes or development techniques. Often, once staff see how the change will benefit them, they will take ownership and drive the process. However, not all people will embrace the change. It may be that these individuals do not benefit from the change. People need time to adjust and lots of communication. Here are some suggestions to use as a nurse leader: communicate, get people involved in the process, immediately address any barriers of challenging people and relate them back to the need for change and better outcomes, empower people, use milestones and measures, and remain open to negotiation (Shirey, 2013). Refer to Box 13.5 for the continuing case scenario and how you can apply the second stage of Lewin's change theory.

The **third stage**, refreezing, involves stabilizing the change in practice and results in a new level of performance in the practice setting. This is where the change needs to become a new habit. If the new change is

BOX 13.4 THE CASE SCENARIO CONTINUES TO UNFOLD

Read this case scenario and describe how the information presented is related to the first stage of Lewin's change theory.

Maria identified a problem and opportunity for improvement on her unit. She completes a literature search. She considers the specific barriers and facilitators to implementing a mentoring program as well as identifies key individuals or stakeholders on her unit and within the hospital who would be involved in the decision-making process.

Maria organizes a unit meeting to discuss the problem and need for change as well as to discuss possible solutions such as a mentoring program. She provides the stakeholders and attendees with the background information and evidence on nurse-mentoring programs. She thoroughly explains why this is needed, and encourages discussion and questions.

BOX 13.5 THE CASE SCENARIO CONTINUES TO UNFOLD

Read this case scenario and describe how the information presented is related to the second stage of Lewin's change theory.

Maria's proposal for a mentoring program is approved, and the planning process begins. She does receive some negative feedback and resistance from colleagues, but takes everyone's feedback without judgment, and continues to encourage teamwork. Before implementing the program, Maria, along with the stakeholders, holds biweekly meetings to discuss the progress and provide training to the nurses.

During the initial implementation, Maria received many complaints about the original nurse orientation forms. Many of the new nurses felt that they were not realistic, and many of the experienced nurses felt that the forms took too much time to complete. Understanding that the complaint from the nurses was valid, she tried to develop a solution to address this concern. Maria thought that a secure, electronic document could potentially be attached to the electronic medical record (EMR) system so that competencies could be completed while the nurses on the unit were already documenting. This would cut down on time and improve accuracy. Maria then arranged another meeting to seek nurses' and management approval of this idea. With the help of management and information technology (IT), the improved form was created.

not made a habit, then staff will revert back to the old way of behaving or the old procedures. Some suggestions to maintain the new change involve including it in the performance appraisal system, offering rewards or incentives, celebrating successes, regularly reviewing progress with staff, and offering training when needed. Refer to Box 13.6 for the continuing case scenario and how you can apply the third stage of Lewin's change theory.

Nurses can implement change and innovation with the components of change theory to guide the process. Change is difficult if met with resistance, so teamwork and collaboration are important to function effectively during this process. Open communication, follow-up, and respect are essential.

BOX 13.6 THE CASE SCENARIO CONTINUES TO UNFOLD

Read this case scenario and describe how the information presented is related to the third stage of Lewin's change theory.

When the first 3 months of the new mentoring program were completed, adjustments and improvements were completed according to unit feedback, and the program became official on the pediatric unit. The unit celebrated its success, and, over time, this improved the satisfaction and support for new nurses on the unit.

JOHN P. KOTTER'S EIGHT STEPS IN LEADING CHANGE

John Kotter is a Harvard Business School professor who wrote about the eight-step change process in his book, *Leading Change* (1996). Box 13.7 highlights how Kotter's eight steps in leading change can be applied to the practice setting. Following these eight steps can help you embed change into your healthcare organization:

1. **Create a sense of urgency:** For a change to occur, nurses need to want that change. Creating a sense of urgency about the need for a change can help motivate nurses into action. You can help develop a sense of urgency by having discussions with nurses that provide them with convincing evidence that change is needed. Kotter explains that you need to have the majority of your staff (about 75%) on board with the change if you want to be successful.
2. **Form a strong coalition:** You need to lead change. As the leader, you should generate a sense of emotion and positive energy about being involved in this change. If you are going to convince nurses that change is needed, you need to demonstrate effective leadership skills and visible support from key stakeholders. You will need a team (coalition) of influential individuals from a variety of backgrounds.
3. **Create a vision and strategy for change:** Develop an overall vision that people can easily understand and remember. The vision should help people understand the goal. You will also need to create the strategy to help you carry out your vision.
4. **Communicate the vision:** Once you have created the vision, it should be communicated. The message about your vision needs to be delivered frequently. Do not just talk about the vision at staff meetings; rather, talk about it at every opportunity you get. Make sure your words and actions align. You need to "talk the talk" as well as "walk the walk." In other words, lead by example. During your talks, be sure to give people a chance to talk about their concerns and fears and address them as openly and honestly as you can.
5. **Enable action and remove barriers:** Support your nurses as they begin the change process. Monitor if any obstacles are prohibiting their success. Remove as many barriers as you can to empower your nurses. Check to see who might be resisting change and assist them to see what actions are needed.
6. **Make short-term wins:** Successes help motivate us. Try to give your nurses a taste of success early in the process by developing some short-term goals that are achievable. These short-term wins will not only help motivate those who are invested in the change but also help curb the critics.
7. **Build on the change:** The short-term wins are just the beginning. Make sure you do not declare victory too early or you might fail. After each short-term success, review what went well and what needs to be improved, and set additional goals.

BOX 13.7 CASE SCENARIO

As you read the following case scenario, describe how this case demonstrates the different aspects of Kotter's eight steps in leading change. Can you identify the eight steps in the scenario? Were any steps missing? If so, on the basis of the theory, what suggestions would you make?

Pam James, a chief nursing officer (CNO) at a 330-bed community teaching hospital, attended the American Nurses Credentialing Center National Magnet® Conference. She was excited and energized to learn about the benefits of becoming a Magnet-designated facility. For example, Magnet-designated facilities tend to attract and retain top talented nurses and they have improved patient care, safety, and satisfaction. On her return, she met with her leadership team to discuss the importance of this initiative at their facility. Such an initiative would help establish excellent nursing care that would most certainly positively influence patient outcomes. Pam James knew that such a designation would serve as external validation regarding the nursing care at her facility. She also knew that there was an urgency to get this designation before her competitor in the neighboring town received it. The president of the hospital was new to the facility and wanted this designation. If the CNO and leadership team could not get it, then there might be some substantial organizational changes.

Pam and her leadership team were excited to be on this journey. They recruited "Magnet champions" on each unit as a guiding coalition to help generate energy and excitement about the Magnet initiative. Pam held a Magnet retreat for the leadership team and the Magnet champions to help develop a vision and strategy to move them forward as well as to develop a timeline complete with short- and long-term goals. They created pins with a logo and vision statement on them for all the nurses to wear on their scrubs.

After the retreat, the team focused on getting the word out to all the nurses in the facility. Pam held a "town hall" meeting to tell everyone about the Magnet journey on which the facility was now embarking. The message was also shared through emails, at meetings, and with little "dog and pony" shows taken to each unit. The Magnet director was in close contact with her team and with the nurses in the hospital. If the nurses expressed that they were experiencing barriers to progressing toward their goals, then the Magnet director would work to remove those obstacles and support actions to promote positive change. As the nurses met each short-term goal, they celebrated with little events such as ice cream socials and pizza parties.

Throughout the Magnet journey, the team tried to hardwire some changes into the organization. For example, they developed a shared governance model and tied participation in such activities into the performance evaluation tools and the clinical ladder. The nursing department created an annual report and circulated it to all the nurses as well as other stakeholders to help provide a progress report and link this initiative to the success of the organization.

8. **Anchor changes in the organizational culture:** Your change needs to become part of the culture to make it lasting. The culture helps to establish what gets accomplished. As the nursing leader, you need to continue to support the change. Continue to talk about the progress with others and share success stories.

EVERETTE ROGERS'S DIFFUSION OF INNOVATIONS

Rogers's theory of diffusion of innovations helps to explain how innovations are taken up by a group (Rogers, 2003). His theory is very different than many other change theories. Rather than focusing on encouraging others to change, his framework views the change as an evolution so it becomes a fit for the needs of the person and group. In other words, with the diffusion of innovations theory, it is not about individuals who change but it is about the innovations themselves. Refer to Box 13.8, which highlights how Rogers's diffusion of innovations can be applied to the practice setting.

Each individual of the group goes through a five-step process when presented with an innovation (Rogers, 2003):

1. Knowledge: Individual is exposed to an idea and how it will function.
2. Persuasion: Individual forms a positive/negative attitude toward the innovation.
3. Decision: Individual evaluates the innovation and decides whether he or she will accept or reject the innovation.
4. Implementation: Individual puts the innovation to use at varying rates depending on the circumstances and may request other information.
5. Confirmation: Individual evaluates the results of using the innovation.

Why are some innovations accepted and implemented more readily than others? According to Rogers (2003), there are five qualities that help decide the success of an innovation:

1. Relative advantage: The extent to which the change is seen as an improvement. If the innovation is seen as an advantage, then it is more likely to be rapidly adopted.
2. Compatibility: The extent to which the innovation is seen as consistent with the values, experiences, and needs of the individual. If an idea is compatible, then it is more likely to be rapidly adopted.
3. Complexity: The extent to which the innovation is difficult to understand and use. If an idea is simple and easy to use, then it is more likely to be rapidly adopted.
4. Trialability: The extent to which an innovation can be tested. Individuals often feel that there is less risk if they can test out an innovation first.
5. Observability: The extent to which the innovation is visible to others and consequently communicated with others in either a positive or a negative light. Visible results decrease uncertainty and promote discussion.

The group can be broken down into five different categories on the basis of the probability that it will adopt a specific innovation. Each group has its own characteristics as far as attitude toward a certain innovation is concerned. As a leader, remember it is not your job to switch people to another category. That is not how this works. View these categories as fixed. An innovation will catch on when it changes to meet the needs of successive groups.

1. Innovators (2.5% of groups): They are the first people to accept an innovation. They tend to be risk takers, visionary, and imaginative. As a leader, find these people and provide them support and promote their ideas.
2. Early adopters (13.5% of groups): Once the benefits of the innovation are clear, then early adopters join in. These individuals like getting an advantage over their colleagues and like to be seen as leaders. As a leader, maintain relationship with this group by providing regular feedback. Enlist and educate some as peer coaches.
3. Early majority (34% of groups): If an innovation gets to this point, it will reach a majority audience. People in this group are often pragmatic. They are content with relatively progressive ideas, but not take action without hard evidence of the benefits. Individuals in this group tend to be followers who are cost aware and risk averse. They like easy, proven, and improved methods of doing their jobs. As a leader working with this group, make it easy and simple as well as provide strong support.
4. Late majority (34% of groups): These individuals are conservative and dislike risks and new ideas. The main reason they will follow is the fear of not fitting in because they are often influenced by the opinions of others. As a leader, emphasize the social norm as opposed to just the benefits of the innovation. Let them know that many other conservative individuals think it is a good idea. Highlight the downside of being left behind.
5. Laggards (16% of groups): These individuals are the last to change. They are adverse to change and focus on traditions. These individuals have many fears and anxieties about innovation. As a leader, you will need to address their concerns. Give them some control over the change. Help them to become familiar with the new idea. Allow them to view how other laggards have adopted the innovation.

QUESTIONS TO CONSIDER BEFORE READING ON

Think about how you can apply the change models listed in the previous section to your work environment. How could you best use these approaches in your work setting? Can you identify a needed change in your work setting that would improve safe patient care or your nursing practice?

BOX 13.8 CASE SCENARIO

As you read the following case scenario, describe how this case demonstrates the different aspects of Rogers's diffusion of innovations. Can you identify aspects of this theory? Were any concepts missing? If so, on the basis of the theory, what suggestions would you make?

Thomas Smith, a manager on a medical surgical hospital unit, attended a conference and learned about "wearable" biosensors and trackers that can be used in hospitals to detect continuous biomarkers. This technology can be placed in clothing and accessories and serves as an activity tracker, monitor, and sensor that allow the client and the clinicians to monitor health. These devices are relatively inexpensive and provide continuous physiological monitoring with little manual intervention. Thomas feels that on his busy medical surgical unit, sensors would help patient outcomes. These devices would alert nurses to sudden medical emergencies and safety issues.

Thomas speaks with the chief nursing officer, Pam James, about this new innovation. He shares with Pam the literature that he gathered at the conference. Thomas highlights key information about these wearable biosensors. He tries to help Pam see the value of the idea. Thomas knows that some of the characteristics of this innovation will help foster the adoption of the biosensors/trackers. He argues that the biosensors/trackers would help improve practice and outcomes and would be easy to incorporate into the care of the patient. The technology is simple to implement. Thomas proposes to Pam that they trial this innovation on his unit. Although Pam is in favor of the idea, the cost will be a factor that will have to be considered. Pam told Thomas that he can present the idea to his unit to get their input.

During a staff meeting, Thomas presents the idea of trialing the wearable biosensors and trackers on their unit. One young nurse was very excited about the possibility. However, the majority of the staff were concerned with how this innovation would be implemented and how it would affect their work. One older nurse was very vocal that she felt that they had enough technology on the unit and they should continue with the tradition of how things have been done because their patient outcomes are okay.

EFFECTIVE CHANGE STRATEGIES

Several different strategies can be used to implement change. When deciding what change strategy to use, keep in mind your audience and their willingness to change. Three change strategies are presented in Table 13.3 (Andrews, 1993).

It is essential to match the change strategies noted in Table 13.3 to the situation at hand. For change to be long term and attitudes/beliefs to be changed, it is most effective to use the normative re-educative approach. If immediate

TABLE 13.3 CHANGE STRATEGIES

Change Approach	Basic Assumption About What Motivates People to Change	Additional Information
Empirical-rational approach: Attempts to promote the change by providing incentives/ rewards	Assumes that individuals are rational and will change behavior if it is justified and provides some gain	Unfortunately, not all people have the capacity for rational thought
Power-coercive strategy: Involves telling others what to do rather than gaining their acceptance	Assumes that individuals will comply with plans and directions from those in power	The result is often strong resistance Used when there is high opposition and people are incapable of making their own decisions Results are unlikely to last May be effective when immediate change is needed because of an emergency situation
Normative re-educative approach: Allows individual who will experience the change to participate in problem identification, solution finding, and implementation An alteration in the person's values and perceptions helps the change to occur	Assumes that people are guided by social norms, values, and habits	Uses a democratic approach Delegates responsibilities to participants Encourages participation Openness is required Can be time-consuming

Source: Andrews, M. (1993). Importance of nursing leadership in implementing change. *British Journal of Nursing, 2*(8), 437–439. doi:10.12968/bjon.1993.2.8.437

short-term change is required, the power-coercive strategy may work. Finally if knowledge is required, then the empirical-rational strategy is useful.

FACTORS AFFECTING CHANGE

There are many factors that influence how change will be received. Nursing leaders have to provide information that is concise and understandable to those who will be affected by the change to initiate change. Multiple modes

TABLE 13.4 FACTORS AFFECTING CHANGE	
Factors That Promote Resistance to Change	**Factors That Promote Change**
If the person does not understand why the change is needed	If people understand the need
If the individual is not consulted about the change, especially if it will have a direct effect on the individual	If the need coincides with the individual's values, beliefs, and attitudes
If it will alter the person's working patterns and interpersonal relations	If the individual feels that the change's benefits outweigh the costs
If the person is not properly informed; poor communication	If the individual has a need for the change/innovation
If the person does not see the importance/value of the change	If the change is introduced gradually so people can adjust
The benefits and rewards do not outweigh the difficulty involved to make the change	
Threatens their jobs, power, or status	

of communication at numerous times will help promote successful change. Table 13.4 displays factors that affect change.

DEALING WITH CONSTANT CHANGE

The reality is that change is constant. We need to recognize and accept that change happens. As a leader, you will have to help others deal with change, which will require you to use your leadership and communication skills. The following are a few suggestions on how to help you lead and manage others through change:

- Communicate: Find out information regarding the change and how it will affect you and others. Talk to your colleagues to determine their understanding of the change. Correct misconceptions. Be transparent by sharing information as well as listening and encouraging others to speak.
- Recognize that people will resist change: Most people prefer things to remain in a constant predictable state. When change is presented, we often defend against it. As a leader, be aware and responsive to the emotional aspect of change and help people to overcome the resistance.
- Be a stabilizing force: Help others accept the change as positive by expressing how this change will help improve our profession and nursing care. Help create stability by helping others see how this change will help fulfill our purpose of providing high-quality, safe patient care.

NURSING LEADERSHIP BEHAVIORS THAT PROMOTE INNOVATION AND CHANGE

Three nursing leadership behaviors will help promote innovation and change. First, set the tone with your leadership characteristics. For example, nurse leaders who are passionate about nursing and caring for others, demonstrate a positive and enthusiastic demeanor, have a clear vision and determination, and are forward thinkers will be more apt to embrace innovation and change (Hanekom, 2016). Nurse leaders need to be bold thinkers to promote innovation and positive change.

Second, create a culture of innovation (Hancock, 2015; Hanekom, 2016). Demonstrate that you value innovation. Encourage your colleagues to think outside the box to address their concerns. This will mean that as a nurse leader, you do not micromanage your staff and colleagues, but rather give them freedom to think and pursue ideas that they feel strongly will help improve practice. Encourage colleagues to talk about their ideas and to collaborate with other disciplines if appropriate. One simple idea would be to initiate a suggestion box in your care area.

Third, build collaborative, effective teams (Hanekom, 2016). These teams can help generate ideas and solutions as well as spearhead implementing the changes. As a nurse leader, you will have to build teams that are dependable and have a clear vision. In addition, you need to foster trust among the group members. The team will need to be able to communicate openly and honestly. Team members should not fear failure because certainly not all innovations will be successful but we can learn from these failures.

Nurse leaders can help organizations through times of change through effective communication, adaptability, coordination, and the ability to remain grounded. Leaders should help develop high-functioning interdisciplinary teams that remain calm and focused. Foster your teams to be collaborative, evidence-based, respectful, and innovative. Finally, nurse leaders can prepare nurses during times of unplanned change through disaster trainings, drills, simulations, and continuous learning (Erickson, 2014).

QUALITY AND SAFETY EDUCATION for NURSES (QSEN) CONSIDERATIONS

Teamwork and collaboration are essential competencies needed for innovation and change.

Reflect on the teamwork and collaboration QSEN competencies found in Table 13.5. Conduct a self-assessment of your skills in day-to-day practice related to the competencies. Describe how you incorporate these skills into your practice. Describe one to two actions you can take to enhance your skills/practice.

TABLE 13.5 QSEN TEAMWORK AND COLLABORATION		
Definition: Function effectively within nursing and interprofessional teams, fostering open communication, mutual respect, and shared decision-making to achieve quality patient care.		
Knowledge	**Skills**	**Attitudes**
Describe own strengths, limitations, and values in functioning as a member of a team.	Demonstrate awareness of own strengths and limitations as a team member. Initiate plan for self-development as a team member. Act with integrity, consistency, and respect for differing views.	Acknowledge own potential to contribute to effective team functioning. Appreciate importance of intra- and interprofessional collaboration.
Describe scopes of practice and roles of healthcare team members. Describe strategies for identifying and managing overlaps in team member roles and accountabilities. Recognize contributions of other individuals and groups in helping patient/family achieve health goals.	Function competently within own scope of practice as a member of the healthcare team. Assume role of team member or leader on the basis of the situation. Initiate requests for help when appropriate to situation. Clarify roles and accountabilities under conditions of potential overlap in team member functioning. Integrate the contributions of others who play a role in helping patient/family achieve health goals.	Value the perspectives and expertise of all health team members. Respect the centrality of the patient/family as core members of any healthcare team. Respect the unique attributes that members bring to a team, including variations in professional orientations and accountabilities.
Analyze differences in communication-style preferences among patients and families, nurses, and other members of the health team. Describe impact of own communication style on others. Discuss effective strategies for communicating and resolving conflict.	Communicate with team members, adapting own style of communicating to needs of the team and situation. Demonstrate commitment to team goals. Solicit input from other team members to improve individual, as well as team, performance. Initiate actions to resolve conflict.	Value teamwork and the relationships on which it is based. Value different styles of communication used by patients, families, and healthcare providers. Contribute to resolution of conflict and disagreement.
Describe examples of the impact of team functioning on safety and quality of care. Explain how authority gradients influence teamwork and patient safety.	Follow communication practices that minimize risks associated with handoffs among providers and across transitions in care. Assert own position/perspective in discussions about patient care. Choose communication styles that diminish the risks associated with authority gradients among team members.	Appreciate the risks associated with handoffs among providers and across transitions in care.

(continued)

TABLE 13.5 QSEN TEAMWORK AND COLLABORATION *(continued)*

Knowledge	Skills	Attitudes
Identify system barriers and facilitators of effective team functioning. Examine strategies for improving systems to support team functioning.	Participate in designing systems that support effective teamwork.	Value the influence of system solutions in achieving effective team functioning.

Source: Quality and Safety Education for Nurses Institute. (2014). QSEN competencies. http://qsen.org/competencies/pre-licensure-ksas

CONCLUSION

Innovations involve creating something new or altering something that already exists. Innovations in healthcare can be used to make changes needed to overcome challenges and create improved outcomes in a wide variety of healthcare settings. It is important for nurse leaders to implement innovations that will address the current deficiencies. However, implementing an innovative change can be challenging. This chapter provided you with information to support why innovation is needed and ways to promote innovative thinking.

In addition, this chapter provided information on change. Change is inevitable but it is not always welcome. It is often necessary for growth. However, whether change is planned or not, it often causes anxiety and fear for those affected by it. As a result, change theories were presented in this chapter because they can provide a framework for understanding change and improving your chances of success. Nurse leaders need to use effective change strategies and help colleagues deal with constant change. Nurse leaders who support innovations and embrace positive change can help bring nursing and patient care to improved levels of performance.

CRITICAL THINKING QUESTIONS AND ACTIVITIES

- Identify a leader in your organization whom you admire who inspires innovation. What leadership skills support his or her ability to be a change agent and innovator of change? How does this leader support a creative and innovative environment? How does he or she catalyze, implement, and promote innovation? What skills does he or she use to foster creativity in successful ways? Provide a self-assessment on the extent to which you are a change agent and innovator.

(continued)

CRITICAL THINKING QUESTIONS AND ACTIVITIES *(continued)*

- Complete the following self-assessment designed to measure how innovation adept you are: http://innovationresource.com/wp-content/uploads/2012/04/Self-Ass-Innoavation-Adept.pdf
  What do the results reveal about you?
- Complete the tolerance of change scale located at the following website: https://www.mheducation.ca/college/mcshane4/student/olc/4obm_sa_15.html
  What do the results tell you? What strategies might help you increase your tolerance to change?
- Think about how change has affected you in past professional experiences. What unique leadership strengths do you possess to bring about change? How did you react to changes in the past in your nursing practice? Did you promote or hinder the changes? In what ways could you advocate for change in your current environment? How did your organization respond to change? How did your organization react to failure?

REFERENCES

Andrews, M. (1993). Importance of nursing leadership in implementing change. *British Journal of Nursing, 2*(8), 437–439. doi:10.12968/bjon.1993.2.8.437

Blakeney, B., Carleton, P., McCarthy, C., & Coakley, E. (2009). Unlocking the power of innovation. *Online Journal of Issues in Nursing, 14*(2), Manuscript 1. doi:10.3912/OJINVol14No02Man01

Cashman, K. (2013). 7 ways leaders can foster innovation. *Forbes*. Retrieved from https://www.forbes.com/sites/kevincashman/2013/08/21/7-ways-leaders-can-foster-innovation/#44dc67cd29a9

Edmonson, C. (2015). Moving forward: Lessons from unplanned change. *Journal of Nursing Administration, 45*(2), 61–62. doi:10.1097/NNA.0000000000000158

Erickson, J. (2014). Leading unplanned change. *Journal of Nursing Administration, 44*(3), 125–126. doi:10.1097/NNA.0000000000000037

Ford, S. (2017). Suffolk staff nurse's green cup innovation rolled out across hospital trust. *Nursing Times*. Retrieved from https://www.nursingtimes.net/news/hospital/nurses-green-cup-innovation-adopted-by-hospital-trust/7021249.article

French-Bravo, M., & Crow, G. (2015). Shared governance: The role of buy-in in bringing about change. *Online Journal of Issues in Nursing, 20*(2). Retrieved from http://ojin.nursingworld.org/MainMenuCategories/ANAMarketplace/ANAPeriodicals/OJIN/TableofContents/Vol-20-2015/No2-May-2015/Articles-Previous-Topics/Role-of-Buy-In-In-Change.html

Hancock, K. K. (2015). Building a culture of innovation in nursing. *Consult QD*. Retrieved from https://consultqd.clevelandclinic.org/2015/01/building-a-culture-of-innovation-in-nursing

Hanekom, J. (2016). Seven ways to foster innovation in your company. *Entrepreneur*. Retrieved from https://www.entrepreneur.com/article/282664

Juneja, P. (n.d.). Forces of organizational change: Planned vs. unplanned change and internal and external change. Retrieved from https://managementstudyguide.com/forces-of-organizational-change.htm

Kalisch, B. J., & Begeny, S. (2010). Preparation of nursing students for change and innovation. *Western Journal of Nursing Research, 32*(2), 157–167. doi:10.1177/0193945909335052

Kotter, J. P. (1996). *Leading change*. Boston, MA: Harvard Business School Press.

Laidman, J. (2017). Cool operator: Nurse creates vest with ice packs to help surgeons and others work in comfort. Retrieved from http://case.edu/think/fall2017/cool-operator.html#.W20BGzlrzcs

Mitchell, G. (2013). Selecting the best theory to implement planned change. *Nursing Management, 20*(1), 32–37. doi:10.7748/nm2013.04.20.1.32.e1013

Orr, P., & Davenport, D. (2014). Embracing change. *Nursing Clinics of North America, 50*(1), 1–18. doi:10.1016/j.cnur.2014.10.001

Pesut, D. J. (2008). Change agents and change agent strategies. In H. R. Feldman (Ed.), *Nursing leadership: A concise encyclopedia* (pp. 103–105). New York, NY: Springer Publishing.

Porter, J. S., & Strout, K. A. (2016). Developing a framework to help bedside nurses bring about change. *American Journal of Nursing, 116*(12), 61–65. doi:10.1097/01.NAJ.0000508674.23661.95

Quality and Safety Education for Nurses Institute. (2014). QSEN competencies. Retrieved from http://qsen.org/competencies/pre-licensure-ksas

Rogers, E. M. (2003). *Diffusion of innovations* (5th ed.). New York, NY: Free Press.

Shirey, M. R. (2013). Lewin's theory of planned change as a strategic resource. *Journal of Nursing Administration, 43*(2), 69–72. doi:10.1097/NNA.0b013e31827f20a9

Stanley, D. J. (2012). Clinical leadership and innovation. *Journal of Nursing Education and Practice, 2*(2), 119–126. doi:10.5430/jnep.v2n2p119

14

POWER AND POLITICS IN PROFESSIONAL NURSING PRACTICE

AUDREY MARIE BEAUVAIS

LEARNING OBJECTIVES

After completion of this chapter, the reader will be able to

- Explain the purpose of learning to use both power and politics in nursing practice.
- Describe types and sources of power used in nursing leadership.
- Examine how one can effectively use power to accomplish patient safety goals.
- Formulate strategies to enhance the development of one's personal power.
- Describe how politics can be used to improve nursing leadership skills.
- Formulate strategies to enhance the development of one's political skills.

Many nurses do not feel comfortable with the concepts of power and politics. Most likely, they feel this way because they equate the terms with dominance, coercion, and corruption. Nurses may fear that power and politics are not compatible with caring. However, the terms are compatible, and we need to get comfortable with their use in our nursing practice. We need to use both power and politics to create positive change to accomplish our healthcare goals (Beall, 2003). Nurses need to be present where the healthcare decisions are being made.

Whether you know it or not, you probably already exercise power and politics in your current position as an associate's degree nurse. For example, you have power by the fact that you are a nurse with the authority to care for clients and to delegate to nursing assistants. You also might have a role in politics as you advocate on your clients' behalf. In this chapter, we discuss the different types and sources of power exploring how to develop and use power for the improvement of client care and to further develop your knowledge about power and politics. In addition, we explore politics and how to develop your political skills to improve your nursing practice. Finally, we talk about how you can use power and politics to improve your role as a nurse leader.

QUESTIONS TO CONSIDER BEFORE READING ON

How comfortable are you with the concept of power? Do you feel that nurses by the virtue of their role hold power? Will advancing your education influence your power?

UNDERSTANDING POWER (TYPES AND SOURCES)

"Power" refers to your influence and authority over others to mobilize them to accomplish a goal (Trus, Martinkenas, & Suominen, 2017). It can be an effective tool that can lead to positive outcomes in our organizations. We all have access to power; however, that power often goes underutilized or unrecognized (Bal, Campbell, Steed, & Meddings, 2008) because we do not understand the types and sources of power and how we can use power to benefit our patients.

French and Raven (1959) conducted a study on power in leadership roles. The study identified five sources of power that are divided into two categories: formal power and personal power.

FORMAL POWER

Legitimate power (or positional power): This power is derived from a title or position in the hierarchy within the organization. For example, the nurse manager of a medical-surgical unit has authority to make requests of his or her nurses on the basis of his or her position within the organizational structure. The power comes when nurses on the unit recognize the authority of the nurse manager because of his or her title. You now have legitimate power just by the fact that you are an RN. You have the power to take care of clients and to direct others who have less education such as a nurse assistant or LPN.

Coercive power: This power arises from the capability to punish others. With coercive power, the leader penalizes or threatens to penalize others for noncompliance. For example, a nurse leader might threaten to give his or her subordinate nurse a poor performance review, not grant a requested time off, not allow attendance at an educational conference, or take a desired project away. Coercive power will likely result in resistance from the nurse if it is used in an antagonistic or manipulative way. As a nurse, you may now use coercive power by refusing to work for a coworker who did not work for you.

Reward power: This power is derived from the ability to compensate others in some way. The compensation is not always money but rather can also be any reward that is desired. For example, a nurse leader might reward a subordinate nurse with a promotion, extra time off from work, or allowing compensation time for work on a committee. As a RN, you may now reward a coworker by complimenting him or her on how he or she cared for a client with you.

PERSONAL POWER

Expert power (or skill power): This power results from one's expertise, knowledge, skills, and abilities. Nurses are experts when it comes to patient care concerns and the healthcare systems (Lanier, 2017). Unfortunately, nurses often underestimate this power. An example of expert nursing power can also be demonstrated when nurses earn specialty certifications. For example, a Wound, Ostomy, and Continence Certified nurse will have the specialized skills and experience to adequately provide expert care. Hence, this nurse's word will be powerful when making wound care recommendations to the healthcare team. As the wound care nurse gains expertise in this area and becomes a leader, the nurse can begin to gather expert power that can be used to help us meet our healthcare goals. You are an expert in that you have a nursing license and have experience in some area of nursing.

Referent power (or friendship power): This power comes from people's respect for a leader and their desire to be liked by the leader. This power is established as others trust and admire the leader. For example, a nurse leader might have referent power given his or her reputation for making sure nurses are treated fairly and coming to the defense of those who are not. The nursing profession has referent power because we have been recognized by the public as one of the most trustworthy professions for approximately 25 years (Lanier, 2017). You may have experienced this when neighbors or relatives call on you for your expertise in their time of need.

There are two other sources of power that have been mentioned in the literature. One is the *power of money*. Money is a source of power because it can impact the distribution of performance incentives (Lanier, 2017). However, money is often not a source of power for nurses and the nursing profession (Lanier, 2017). The second source is the *power in numbers*. Nurses comprise the largest percentage of the healthcare workforce because there are over 3 million nurses nationwide (Lanier, 2017). Unfortunately, nurses do not often take advantage of this source of power. Nurses can harness this power to help them to make a positive influence on our healthcare system. Power in numbers can also be used by staff nurses who feel that they are not being treated fairly with regards to their working environment. Refer to Box 14.1 and read the case scenario highlighting how the concept of power can be applied to the practice setting.

Most likely, you will use different sources of power in various situations. The skill of leadership will be to understand when to use what powers and when not to. This will require good judgment as well as practice. Refer to Box 14.2 and complete your Power Perception Profile.

BOX 14.1 CASE SCENARIO

As you read this case scenario, ask yourself the following questions:

- What type of power(s) is the nurse manager, Suzanne, exhibiting in this situation?
- What other sources of power may Suzanne find to be useful in this situation?

Suzanne works in a community hospital as a nurse manager of a medical-surgical unit. She recognizes the struggles of the staff nurse. She was once a staff nurse herself. She knows that things can go wrong and patients can get harmed. As if that is not bad enough, nurses can then be judged by others regarding these actions that unintentionally caused errors. She knows such judgment does not feel good nor does it achieve the patient safety results we strive to attain. Suzanne has developed expertise in quality improvement efforts within the hospital. Her unit is used as an exemplar throughout the hospital with its reputation of maintaining high quality standards, examining quality indicators, and taking action to improve outcomes. Suzanne has decided that she wants to pilot a program to help develop a "just culture" on her unit. A just culture will help shift its members from retrospective judgment to real-time evaluation of the actions of the healthcare team. Suzanne feels that she has an opportunity to improve patient safety by implementing a just culture. She begins by raising awareness. She does this by talking about just culture during her staff meetings. Then she decided to conduct mandatory training sessions. She is holding her staff accountable for attending these educational sessions. If nurses do not attend the mandatory sessions, then it will be noted on their performance review and scored accordingly. However, the majority of staff want to attend because they respect Suzanne's knowledge and vision as well as her ability to get results. Although Suzanne cannot pay them for attending the session, she is able to get them compensation time, which the nurses greatly appreciate.

BOX 14.2 SELF-ASSESSMENT: POWER

Reflect on what power bases you currently have as a nurse and which ones you might like to further develop to promote your growth as a nurse leader. Complete the "Power Perception Profile" created by Hersey and Natemeyer found at the following website: www.coursehero.com/file/pkiqkq/THE-POWER-PERCEPTION-PROFILE-A-measurement-devised-by-Hersey-and-Natemeyer-to. The tool will provide you with feedback on your perception of influence and power. How strong is each of your seven bases of power?

WAYS TO DEVELOP YOUR PERSONAL POWER STRATEGIES

You cannot achieve your goals without power. It is even more difficult to help others (our nursing colleagues and patients) reach their goals if you are powerless. Having power will often give you access to needed resources. Hence, it is essential as a nursing leader to learn how to build your personal power base for the benefit of yourself, your profession, and your patients. The following 11 strategies noted by Huston (2008) will help you increase your personal power base:

1. **Develop an expertise:** Try to gain unique knowledge, ability, and skills. Deliberately devote time and attention to developing your expertise. Such expertise should lead to superior performance and produce measurable outcomes. Earning a professional certification is an example of developing an expertise because it allows you to set yourself apart from your colleagues and can result in benefits to the practice environment.
2. **Find positive role models/find a mentor:** Find positive role models who are competent and well respected within your field. Although you may not know these role models personally, you can learn by studying and emulating their actions. Role models are different than mentors. Mentors are more personally involved in your career growth and development. Find a mentor who is willing to commit to a one-to-one relationship with you with the purpose of helping to promote your nursing career.
3. **Develop a network:** Your personal power can be strengthened by increasing your connectivity to members of our profession because there is power in numbers. Having a professional network helps you to influence others. Joining a professional organization is an effective way to develop your network.

4. **Develop additional skills to help you become fluid and flexible:** You can build your power base by developing skills that expand your repertoire and appeal to other employers. You obtain personal power when you have options. You decrease personal power when an employer knows that you cannot afford to change your job or that you do not possess the skills to do so.
5. **Be reflective and self-aware:** Reflect on your values and beliefs so that you can demonstrate consistency in action. You will increase your power by maintaining your values and principles despite pressures to act to the contrary.
6. **Focus on your goals:** People do not want to follow someone who does not have goals. Hence, make sure you have well-written, meaningful goals. The goals will help you to use your time sensibly.
7. **Select your battles wisely:** Battles often result in hard feelings. Do not enter battles lightly. However, when the issues are significant, you must be willing to stand up for what is right. When an issue is important enough to fight for, it helps to be transparent regarding what is negotiable, and anticipate what the damages of the battle may be.
8. **Take risks:** Examine the costs and benefits of your choices. Be willing to take risks because thoughtful risk takers often increase their power. Take risks by being innovative and self-assured when presenting your ideas. Challenge the existing state of affairs.
9. **Let go of your ego:** If you want to increase your personal power, it helps to be relatable. People want leaders who are humble, genuine, and human. Make sure you can laugh at your mistakes and allow others to laugh with you.
10. **Be a hardworking team player:** Earn respect by paying your dues through hard work and dedication. Likewise, be a team player who is genuinely interested in the members, demonstrates strong interpersonal skills, and offers support to help the team reach its goals.
11. **Practice self-care:** Make sure you take time to relax, reflect, and have fun. These activities are vital so that you have other reserves available when professional activities drain your energy.

Additional strategies for increasing your power base can be found in Table 14.1. These strategies were based on the findings of a study from the Center for Creative Leadership (Bal et al., 2008).

Using the strategies in Table 14.1 can help you increase your personal power base. Developing your power base will take time and effort, but will be worthwhile when it helps you to reach your goals. Refer to Box 14.3 to complete a self-assessment of your power.

TABLE 14.1 POWER STRATEGIES	
Establish and maintain healthy relationships	Develop trusting relationships. Establish a positive identity in your community. Identify people who can help you reach your goals and establish meaningful relationships with them.
Downplay your personal agenda	Focusing on your personal agenda may lead others to perceive you as self-serving or deceitful.
Communicate	Explore ways to improve your communication network. Locate people who might help you find other sources of information.
Share information	With integrity, be generous in sharing information with others. Withholding information from others can make you appear as though you are doing so for personal gain. Naturally, do not reveal confidential information and do not gossip.
Find ways to communicate your authority	Make the most of your position by communicating your formal leadership role. For example, you can include your title on your email signature, speak up in meetings, and dress the part.
Develop authentic charisma	Increase your ability to connect with people by developing your own charisma. For example, you can convey a sense of energy, make eye contact, and smile.
Establish your expertise	Obtain expertise such as advancing your education or obtaining a specialty certification. Put your credentials on your email signature to help make your credibility visible.
Reward others	Incentivize people through rewards that are appealing to the recipient. For example, not all people would like to be rewarded with an ice cream social at work. Others might find it more rewarding to have recognition in the monthly newsletter.
Verbally recognize others	Praise people often and praise them in front of others.
Provide feedback	Hold people accountable. Privately offer constructive feedback to those who are not meeting expectations. Enforce the standards while providing support. Be clear regarding the consequences for not meeting expectations and follow up accordingly.
Teach	Empower others by teaching them.

Source: Bal, V., Campbell, M., Steed, J., & Meddings, K. (2008). The role of power in effective leadership [White paper]. *Center for Creative Leadership.* Retrieved from https://www.ccl.org/articles/white-papers/the-role-of-power-in-effective-leadership

BOX 14.3 SELF-ASSESSMENT: POWER

Do you feel you are powerful at work? List behaviors that you use to exert power. What type of power do you use? Do you use your power effectively? Consider how you could improve your use of power. Can you identify organization barriers that prevent you from being as powerful as you could be? How can you help others gain power? Develop a specific plan as to how you can take action in each of the strategies described in this section and in Table 14.1 to enhance your power base. Set a time line as to when you plan to implement these strategies.

QUESTIONS TO CONSIDER BEFORE READING ON

What is politics? What sources of power are helpful in politics? How can nurses increase their political skills to help benefit patients, the nursing profession, and the healthcare system?

UNDERSTANDING POLITICS

Nurses have the unique opportunity to take on the advocacy role and to promote positive patient outcomes, and improve both nursing practice and our healthcare system (Hahn, 2009). The key will be for us to translate our clinical concerns into policy issues (Hahn, 2009). Nurses have knowledge, expertise, insights, and problem-solving abilities that make them ideal for helping to advocate for change. Not only do nurses have expert power that can influence politics, but, as mentioned earlier, nurses also have power in numbers. Think about what could happen if we collectively use our voices to stand behind key healthcare issues. Your professional nursing practice includes an obligation to work in advocacy roles in politics. Refer to Box 14.4 for a case scenario that highlights how politics can be applied to the practice setting.

What exactly is politics? "Politics" can be defined as the process by which people generate decisions that have the capacity to impact events (Hahn, 2009). Take some time to view the following websites that can help promote your understanding of politics:

- Legislative action in Congress: www.congress.gov (search nursing, healthcare, bill numbers as keywords)
- Academy of Medical Surgical Nurses: www.amsn.org
- American Nurses Association: www.nursingworld.org
- Contact the president and vice president: www.whitehouse.gov/CONTACT
- White House press releases: www.whitehouse.gov
- U.S. House of Representatives: www.house.gov
- U.S. Department of Health and Human Services: www.hhs.gov
- National Academy of Medicine: https://nam.edu

BOX 14.4 CASE SCENARIO

As you read this case scenario, ask yourself the following questions:

- What political skills did Lauren use?
- What sources of power will be useful to Lauren?
- How can Lauren leverage her power?
- What other political strategies can Lauren use to help positively change the healthcare system to address the opioid crisis in our nation?

Lauren is an emergency room nurse at a local hospital. She has become concerned because the number of individuals in her community coming to the emergency department with opioid overdoses has increased substantially. The problem really hit home when she recently lost a cousin to a heroin overdose. This promoted her to take political action. She started to educate herself and others by raising awareness. She went to the dean of her alma mater and asked about the possibility of hosting an opioid panel event open to the public. The dean embraced the idea and helped to organize and host the event with key influential experts on the topic serving on the panel. The dean suggested that they also invite legislators and include the media to get more widespread attention to the issue. At the opioid panel event, Lauren made a point of introducing herself to the legislators and sharing her stories because she knew that they would have a powerful impact. She offered to serve as a resource to the legislators when it came to this topic.

Nurse leaders should take time to understand politics and to develop their political skills. Nurses should read the news daily to stay abreast of issues that influence the nursing profession and patients (Dailey, 2008). They should be familiar with the views of the different political parties and individual candidates to determine which group/individuals best align with their views (Dailey, 2008). The following website is useful to help familiarize you with the political parties: www.politics1.com/parties.htm. If you are not already registered to vote, please do so and then exercise that right! Table 14.2 has some additional steps you can take to develop your political skills.

USING POWER AND POLITICS AS A NURSE LEADER OR MANAGER

Nurse leaders must harness their power and political skills to help move healthcare forward. Nurses should use their legitimate power along with their strong decision-making and assertiveness skills. Furthermore, our nurse leaders have to gain confidence and feel comfortable to speak up and express their views (Montalvo, 2015). Political skills are a critical competency for

TABLE 14.2 STEPS TO DEVELOP YOUR POLITICAL SKILLS	
Network	Share your ideas and concerns with your colleagues. Join your state and national nurses associations, which will provide you with the opportunity to learn about the political concerns affecting nursing and give you an opportunity to participate in the political process. Consider joining the nursing legislation coalition in your state (Dailey, 2008; Hahn, 2009).
Educate yourself	Earlier in the chapter, we talked about educating yourself by reading the news and joining your professional organization. Also, consider reading your professional organization's journals and newsletters because they will help you understand the key issues influencing your practice. Educate yourself on our political system (i.e., how a bill becomes a law). Review bills that are introduced in the U.S. Congress and in your state legislature (Dailey, 2008). The following websites may be useful to you: • www.congress.gov/resources/display/content/How+Our+Laws+Are+Made+-+Learn+About+the+Legislative+Process • www.house.gov/the-house-explained/the-legislative-process • www.llsdc.org/state-legislation
Develop political relationships	Make an effort to get to know your federal and state legislators. Introduce yourself as a nurse and offer to serve as a resource on healthcare issues. Share your stories because they have powerful influence. Contact legislators by email or phone when you encounter issues that are important to healthcare and the profession of nursing (Dailey, 2008; Hahn, 2008).

leaders in healthcare (Montalvo, 2015). They require social astuteness, interpersonal influence, networking ability, and sincerity as nurse leaders pursue goal-directed behavior to achieve outcomes (Montalvo, 2015). Developing power and political skills as a nurse leader will help with professional development, career advancement, and the ability to positively influence healthcare. Refer to Box 14.5 to complete a self-assessment of your political skills.

BOX 14.5 SELF-ASSESSMENT: POLITICAL SKILLS

This is not a scientific-based self-assessment tool but includes questions that are intended to foster reflection on ways to increase your political involvement. Answer "yes" or "no" to the following statements to assess your political skills:

- I share ideas and concerns about patient care, the nursing profession, and the healthcare system with my colleagues.
- I belong to my state nurses association.
- I belong to a national nurses association.
- I stay appraised of healthcare issues by reading the news and/or my professional nursing organization's journals/newsletters.

BOX 14.5 SELF-ASSESSMENT: POLITICAL SKILLS (*continued*)

- I know who my federal and state legislators are.
- I have contacted my federal or state legislator about issues that are important to me as a nurse.
- I have offered expert testimony on healthcare issues at legislative committee hearings.
- I have helped a legislator with campaign activity.
- I have sought a position on a political committee of a nursing organization.

If you answered "yes" to the majority of these statements, then you have demonstrated that you have already taken steps to develop your political skills. If you answered "no" to the majority of these statements, then you have opportunities to strengthen your political skills through the strategies we discussed in this chapter. On the basis of this information, describe the way you plan to enhance your political involvement.

QUALITY AND SAFETY EDUCATION for NURSES (QSEN) CONSIDERATIONS

The following QSEN competencies (Box 14.6) can be related to power and politics. As you read the following QSEN competencies related to leadership, ask yourself:

- Which of these competencies do I meet and which competencies do I need to develop more fully?
- What plan of action can I take to enhance those competencies in which I am weak and to develop those that I lack at this time?

BOX 14.6 SELECTED QSEN COMPETENCIES RELATED TO POWER AND POLITICS

- Describe own strengths, limitations, and values in functioning as a member of a team.
- Demonstrate awareness of own strengths and limitations as a team member.
- Initiate plan for self-development as a team member.
- Acknowledge own potential to contribute to effective team functioning.
- Recognize that nursing and other health profession students are parts of systems of care and care processes that affect outcomes for patients and families.
- Give examples of the tension between professional autonomy and system functioning.
- Value own and others' contributions to outcomes of care in local care settings.

Source: Quality and Safety Education for Nurses Institute. (2014). QSEN competencies. Retrieved from http://qsen.org/competencies/pre-licensure-ksas

CONCLUSIONS

Nurse leaders should take a vested interest in influencing the decision-making process when those decisions will influence nursing and healthcare (Katriina et al., 2012). They can do this by exerting their power and political skills and ensuring that they are present where those decisions are being made. Nurse leaders need to harness their power and take political action to improve patient care. Nurses tend to focus on individual patient care without looking at the larger context of healthcare. We cannot continue as we have in the past and assume others will fix our healthcare problems. We have to start to take command and steer healthcare in the right direction.

CRITICAL THINKING QUESTIONS AND ACTIVITIES

- Identify a nurse leader who you feel is powerful. List the specific actions the leader uses in exerting that power. What type of power is the leader using? How effective is the leader? Could you envision yourself using power in a similar way?
- Consider completing the Political Skills Inventory at the following website: www.d.umn.edu/~scastleb/Political%20Skills%20survey.pdf. On the basis of your results, develop a personal plan to increase your political skills.
- Review the political websites noted throughout this chapter. Specifically, look for any healthcare legislation that has been proposed in your state. Analyze how that legislation will impact your nursing practice.

REFERENCES

Bal, V., Campbell, M., Steed, J., & Meddings, K. (2008). The role of power in effective leadership [White paper]. *Center for Creative Leadership.* Retrieved from https://www.ccl.org/articles/white-papers/the-role-of-power-in-effective-leadership

Beall, F. (2003). Nurses, power and politics. *Georgia Nursing, 62*(4), 3–11.

Dailey, M. A. (2008). Mastering the art of politics. *Pennsylvania Nurse, 63*(3), 4–7.

French, J., & Raven, B. (1959). The bases of social power. In D. Cartwright & A. Zander (Eds.), *Group dynamics* (pp. 259–269). New York, NY: Harper & Row.

Hahn, J. (2009). Power dynamics, health policy, and politics. *MEDSURG Nursing, 18*(3), 197–199.

Huston, C. J. (2008). Eleven strategies for building a personal power base. *Nursing Management, 39*(4), 58–61. doi:10.1097/01.NUMA.0000316063.50564.57

Katriina, P., Sari, V., Anja, R., Christina, S., Paula, A., & Tarja, S. (2013). Nursing power as viewed by nursing professionals. *Scandinavian Journal of Caring Sciences, 27*, 580–588. doi:10.1111/j.1471-6712.2012.01069.x

Lanier, J. (2017, March/April). Feel the power. *Ohio Nurses Review*, 6–7.

Montalvo, W. (2015). Political skill and its relevance to nursing: An integrative review. *Journal of Nursing Administration, 45*(7-8), 377–383. doi:10.1097/NNA.0000000000000218

Quality and Safety Education for Nurses Institute. (2014). QSEN competencies. Retrieved from http://qsen.org/competencies/pre-licensure-ksas

Trus, M., Martinkenas, A., & Suominen, T. (2017). International nursing: How much power do nurse managers have? *Nursing Administration Quarterly, 41*(4), 337–345. doi:10.1097/NAQ.0000000000000247

15

MANAGING QUALITY AND SAFETY

DAVID M. DEPUKAT

LEARNING OBJECTIVES

After completion of this chapter, the reader will be able to

- Define quality improvement and safety in healthcare.
- Describe approaches that nurses can take to evaluate the quality of care through measurement and benchmarking.
- Explain the influence of variation on the quality of care and apply a framework to improve reliability.
- Differentiate prepatient events, safety events, and serious safety events.
- Describe how human factors contribute to events of harm.
- Define the culture of safety and its elements, including event reporting, event disclosure, and accountability in a just culture.
- Explain the process for determining actual and potential failures in processes.
- Describe the characteristics needed to maintain a high-reliability organization.

Providing the highest quality of care to clients, and keeping them safe, is a priority for all nurses. You have probably heard the terms "quality" and "safety" used in clinical practice, sometimes interchangeably. While closely related, these two concepts differ. A deeper understanding of these concepts will provide you with the knowledge and skills needed to improve the quality of care being provided and expand the culture of safety in your practice setting. The American Nurses Association's (ANA's, 2015) *Scope and Standards of Practice* calls on all nurses to use nursing practice to assess and to improve both the quality and the safety of care. This imperative encompasses essential Quality and Safety Education for Nurses (QSEN) competencies for nurses, as displayed in Table 15.1. Shift to shift and day to day, nurses perform a variety of interventions, use critical thinking, and use

TABLE 15.1 MANAGING QUALITY AND SAFETY: RELEVANT QSEN COMPETENCIES
Appreciate that continuous quality improvement is an essential part of the daily work of all health professionals. (Attitude)
Describe the benefits and limitations of quality improvement data sources, and measurement and data analysis strategies. (Knowledge)
Select and use relevant benchmarks. (Knowledge)
Explain common causes of variation in outcomes of care in the practice specialty. (Knowledge)
Describe common quality measures in the practice specialty. (Knowledge)
Select and use quality measures to understand performance. (Skill)
Describe human factors and other basic safety design principles as well as commonly used unsafe practices (e.g., workarounds and dangerous abbreviations). (Skill)
Describe the benefits and limitations of selected safety-enhancing technologies (e.g., barcodes, computer provider order entry, and electronic prescribing). (Skill)
Delineate general categories of errors and hazards in care. (Knowledge)
Describe factors that create a just culture and culture of safety. (Knowledge)
Describe processes used to analyze causes of error and allocation of responsibility and accountability (e.g., root cause analysis and failure mode effects analysis). (Knowledge)
Use national patient safety resources: (Skill) • For own professional development • To focus attention on safety in care settings • To design and implement improvements in practice

Source: American Association of Colleges of Nursing. (2012). *Graduate level QSEN competencies: Knowledge, skills, and attitudes*. Washington, DC: Author.

decision-making to ensure patient safety. As organizations move toward becoming high-reliability organizations, month-to-month and quarter-to-quarter trends become important in viewing the overall effectiveness of maintaining safety and quality. This chapter outlines the key concepts related to quality and safety in nursing practice on the journey to becoming highly reliable.

In this chapter, an evolving case scenario will follow a nurse's exploration of quality and safety on her patient care unit, which is introduced in Box 15.1.

QUALITY

QUALITY IMPROVEMENT

Quality improvement is the responsibility of all healthcare professionals. Batalden and Davidoff (2007) defined "quality improvement" as "the combined and unceasing efforts of everyone—healthcare professionals, patients and their families, researchers, payers, planners and educators—to make

BOX 15.1 CASE SCENARIO

Madelyn is a bachelor of science in nursing (BSN)-prepared clinical nurse on a medical unit in a large, urban academic medical center. She has been practicing for 7 years, and she recently became certified in her specialty. Recently, Madelyn has become interested in how the quality of care on her unit has been measured as well as its performance. After a discussion of these interests with her manager, Madelyn was appointed the safety and quality leader for the unit. She was asked to review quality data for falls with injury in the previous quarter.

the changes that will be to better patient outcomes (health), better system performance (care), in better professional development (learning)" (p. 6). No single healthcare discipline is responsible for the improvement of quality. In addition, improvement requires strong partnerships between the providers and the consumers of healthcare. Nurses at all levels of practice are poised to both participate in and lead quality improvement activities. This level of engagement requires a thorough understanding of measurement of quality and tools to support its improvement.

QUESTIONS TO CONSIDER BEFORE READING ON

Think about the nursing care in your practice area. How is the quality of nursing care measured?

What quality indicators are important to your practice area?

MEASURING QUALITY

Types of Measures

Donabedian (1988) seminally proposed the methods for measuring the quality of care. Structures, or structural elements, are aspects of the care environment. These structures may include policies, pieces of equipment, or workflows. Structures are designed or developed to achieve an outcome of care to improve the quality of care. Processes of care measure adherence or compliance to a structural element, often in a percentage. Outcomes are directly related to the health of the client and best quantify the quality of care. Table 15.2 provides examples of structures, processes, and outcomes. Balancing measures have been introduced as a complement to outcome measures. These measures aim to capture unintended changes in other

TABLE 15.2 STRUCTURES, PROCESSES, AND OUTCOMES

Structure	Process Measures	Outcome Measures
Barcode medication administration technology	Patient-scanning and medication-scanning rates (adherence to policy)	Rate of medication errors (number of medication errors per 1,000 medications administered)
Nurse-driven urinary catheter removal protocol	Percent of urinary catheters with provider-ordered nurse-driven removal protocol	Catheter-associated urinary tract infection (CAUTI) rate (incidences of CAUTI per 1,000 catheter days)

measures during the quality improvement process. Balancing measures may also improve as outcome measures improve, but these measures may also deteriorate over time. For example, a behavioral health nurse may lead a quality improvement team to reduce the use of mechanical restraints. In doing so, this nurse suggests tracking physical assaults and chemical restraints as balancing measures. Although a reduction in restraints may be beneficial, an unanticipated increase in physical assaults because of the restraint reduction would require further attention.

Basic Statistics

The most elementary form of measuring quality is through incidences of events in a specific time frame. For example, a patient care area may have four falls with injury in a month. This time frame—a month—allows for comparison. In the month prior, this patient care area had five falls with injury. The incidences of falls with injury decreased from the first month to the next month. Similarly, this approach can be taken to compare two or more patient care areas. Perhaps in a month's time, a medical intensive care unit had two falls, a cardiac surgery unit had three falls, and an oncology unit had one fall. A nurse may conclude that the cardiac surgery unit had the most falls. However, these approaches fail to account for volume. Was the number of patients the same between the months? Are the units the same size? The calculation of incidences divided by volume is called a "rate." The inclusion of a denominator decreases the bias of an incidence or prevalence measure (Pronovost et al., 2006). Most quality data are reported using rates.

The use of rates becomes very important in quality improvement. Unlike incidences, rates correct for volume. Most often, patient volume accounts for the denominator. For example, the falls with injury rate is reported in events for every 1,000 patient days. This volume may not always be patient volume; other volumes may be more appropriate. For example, the rate of medication errors may best be volume-corrected by the number of medication administrations in a period of time. In tracking catheter-associated urinary tract infections, the incidences of these infections are often volume-corrected by the numbers of days that patients had urinary catheters in place, which is calculated similarly to the patient days. With the implementation of the electronic health record (EHR), these denominators are usually easily calculated.

Benchmarking

Basic statistical principles allow patient care areas and organizations to view quality over time. However, these approaches do not allow for comparison with other organizations. Benchmarking is the process that allows organizations to do so. Organizations submit quality and safety data to an agency for benchmarking. The National Database of Nursing Quality Indicators (NDNQI) provides benchmarking for nursing-specific quality indicators such as falls with injury, hospital-acquired pressure ulcers, and hospital-acquired infections. The Centers for Disease Control and Prevention's National Healthcare Safety Network (NHSN) provides benchmarking for many infections such as catheter-associated urinary tract infections and central line–associated bloodstream infections.

An organization cannot compare itself with a single organization through benchmarking. Rather, organizations are benchmarked using the benchmarking agency's database mean or median. These data are calculated from all data submitted by organizations. Data are benchmarked in one of the following two ways: the mean or median. The use of the database mean, or average, reveals how far above or below the mean (or average) the organization's quality indicator is. Albeit dependent on the indicator, being below the mean with a smaller number is desired. This result would imply a lower rate of an event, such as falls with injury. The mean, however, is affected by extreme values or skewed results. The median, or the middle value, of the data submitted is less affected by these types of values. Therefore, organizations will often view their performance against the database mean and median to evaluate performance. Another approach to viewing an organization's performance is percentile rank. Depending on the measure, a higher percentile rank implies a better performance. The median performance is the 50th percentile. In addition, most agencies provide organizations with the ability to adjust the databases used to calculate the mean or median. This adjustment occurs based on the organization's characteristics. For example, a rural community hospital could modify the calculation to include other rural hospitals with similar bed size. Organizations can compare internal quality measures with similar organizations on the basis of its characteristics, making the comparison more valuable.

In Box 15.2, Madelyn will explore her unit's benchmarked falls with injury rate.

BOX 15.2 THE CASE SCENARIO CONTINUES TO UNFOLD

In reviewing her unit's fall rates from the previous quarter, Madelyn found that the falls with injury rate was 4.2 per 1,000 patient days. She looked to benchmarking data for comparison to better understand her unit's quality. In the previous quarter, the unit ranked at the 47th percentile and above the database mean (which was 4.8 per 1,000 patient days). By both accounts, Madelyn understood that her unit was not in the better performing 50% of reporting units. However, she wondered what organizational characteristics were used in the benchmarking process. After asking her manager, Madelyn discovered that her unit's performance was benchmarked using other large (more than 500 beds), academic medical centers.

PERFORMANCE MEASURES

Nursing-Sensitive Indicators

Nursing-sensitive indicators are structural, process, and outcome measures on which nurses have primary influence (Montalvo, 2007). Hospital-based nursing divisions have focused much attention on these outcomes, such as falls with injury and physical/sexual assaults in behavioral health settings. Although the ANA (2015) and others stress the role of nursing in these measures, all healthcare professionals are responsible for the quality of care, as evidenced by aligning the definition of quality improvement. Nursing-sensitive outcomes measured by NDNQI are shown in Table 15.3. The American Academy of Ambulatory Care Nursing expanded nursing's interest in ambulatory-based outcomes of care, which become important as nursing's role expands in these settings (Martinez, Battaglia, Start, Mastal, & Matlock, 2015; Mastal, Matlock, & Start, 2016).

Core Measures

Although nursing-sensitive indicators are performance measures primarily influenced by nurses, core measures provide performance measures for the entire team of healthcare professions. The Joint Commission (TJC) collaborated with the Centers for Medicare & Medicaid Services (CMS) and others to develop a standardized set of measures for organizations. These organizations aimed to reduce the burden of healthcare organizations by determining which outcomes of care to measure as well as develop a structure for reporting and benchmarking. This approach focuses all of healthcare's attention on core quality measures. Many core measures are publically available at the following website: https://www.medicare.gov/hospitalcompare/search.html. The core measure sets are shown in Table 15.3.

TABLE 15.3 NURSING-SENSITIVE INDICATORS AND CORE MEASURES

Nursing-Sensitive Indicators	Core Measure Sets
• Patient falls with injury • Central-line–associated bloodstream infections (CLABSI) • Catheter-associated urinary tract infection (CAUTI) • Ventilator-associated pneumonia • Pressure ulcer prevalence • Psychiatric physical/sexual assault rate • Restraint prevalence • Pediatric peripheral intravenous infiltration rate	• Acute myocardial infarction • Children's asthma care • Emergency department • Hospital outpatient department • Hospital-based inpatient psychiatric services • Immunization • Perinatal care • Stroke • Substance use • Tobacco treatment • Venous thromboembolism

Sources: The Joint Commission. (2017). Core measure sets—measures. Retrieved from https://www.jointcommission.org/core_measure_sets.aspx; Montalvo, I. (2007). The national database of nursing quality indicators (NDNQI). *Online Journal of Issues in Nursing, 12*(3), Manuscript 2. doi:10.3912/OJIN.Vol12No03Man02

QUESTIONS TO CONSIDER BEFORE READING ON

In your organization, find two nursing-sensitive indicators or core measures:

- What is the rate of the measure?
- What processes measures do you use to support the outcome measure? For example, what compliance measures are important for that outcome?
- How does your organization's performance compare with that of other organizations when benchmarked? What characteristics of your organization are important to modify the database for benchmarking?

THE EFFECT OF VARIATION IN THE QUALITY OF CARE

Variation in processes and practices affects the quality of care and its outcomes; variations are highly affected by the culture within an organization down to its patient care areas (Pronovost et al., 2006). Nursing in high-reliability organizations may approach variation in different ways. Processes and practices become standardized using best practices from other organizations and evidence-based practice. In this way, nursing provides consistent, high-quality interventions. The development of any process must also consider reliability. Process reliability implies that a process is done consistently each time. Organizations accomplish this concept through the simplification of processes and the removal of inefficiencies and redundancies. In doing so, organizations create processes that are easier to complete without deviation or using a workaround.

Pronovost et al. (2006) described a framework for improving reliability in organizations, which included the following steps:

- Identify evidence-based practices that have been demonstrated to improve an outcome.
- Select those practices with the greatest influence on the outcome and convert to behaviors.
- Develop measures to ensure reliability and reduce variation.
- Measure performance over time.
- Ensure healthcare professionals are using, and patients are receiving, the evidence-based practices through professional accountability.

MODELS AND TOOLS FOR IMPROVEMENT

Plan–Do–Study–Act

The Institute for Healthcare Improvement (IHI) and other quality organizations have adopted the Plan–Do–Study–Act (PDSA) model for improvement in healthcare (Langley et al., 2009; Ogrinc et al., 2012). Sometimes, this model is referred to as the Plan–Do–Check–Act (PDCA). This model structures rapid cycles of change, or PDSA cycles, with four phases in each cycle. The **Plan** phase defines the purpose of the cycle of change; develops a measurable, objective, and time-limited goal; and details an implementation plan for the cycle of change. This goal should support the outcome measure, or a process measure to support that outcome, aimed for improvement. The **Do** phase carries out the plan. The **Study** phase reviews the progress toward the goal of the PDSA cycle including effects on outcome measures and balancing measures. The **Act** phase considers the cycle of change's effectiveness and begins planning the next cycle of change. Each four-step cycle repeats until the outcome of the quality improvement activity improves to the desirable rate. However, healthcare professionals often misunderstand the purpose of the PDSA cycles. Usually, each cycle results in the continuous addition of new practices without evaluation of their effectiveness. Within the PDSA model for improvement, each cycle of change is a *test* of that change rather than a full implementation. After a cycle of change, the practice is adopted, adapted, or abandoned, which depends on the evaluation of the cycle's effectiveness.

Common Cause Analysis

The common cause analysis (CCA) is a tool used in the initial steps of quality improvement, which is used by Madelyn in the case scenario (Box 15.3). Prior to the first cycle of change, quality improvement teams must better understand the outcome of interest. The CCA seeks to discover recurrent themes or characteristics of many events. For example, a quality improvement team seeking to improve a patient care area's falls with injury rate may perform a

BOX 15.3 THE CASE SCENARIO CONTINUES TO UNFOLD

In preparing for a CCA of all falls with injury occurring in the previous 6 months, Madelyn considered possible data to assess for trends, including the following:

- Day of the week and time of day when the fall occurred
- Staffing mix at the time of the fall
- Patient's fall risk assessment
- Medications administered within 2 hours of the fall
- Fall risk precautions in place at the time of the fall

CCA of all fall events in the previous 6 months. These data can be analyzed for trends and recurring themes. Those characteristics and themes revealed by the CCA can be used in the planning of the PDSA cycles of change.

QUESTIONS TO CONSIDER BEFORE READING ON

- In preparing for the CCA on falls with injury, what data would be important to assess for trends and themes aside from those mentioned by Madelyn?
- Madelyn is hesitant to include too much data, which can be overwhelming and difficult to manage. What data would not be important? Why?

SAFETY

The Institute of Medicine (IOM) published *To Err Is Human* (1999) and *Crossing the Quality Chasm* (2001), which invigorated the emphasis for patient safety in the United States. In this report, the IOM estimated that approximately 44,000 to 98,000 patients died each year from *preventable* medical mistakes and errors. These death rates are equivalent to a Boeing 737 (at least) or a Boeing 747 (at most) crashing each day. In 2010, the *New England Journal of Medicine* estimated that as many as 18% of patients are harmed by these medical errors (Landrigan et al., 2010). Through the lens of safety, these events leading to harm and death are preventable. Although clients in healthcare settings die from their disease processes despite medical and nursing care, deviations in standards of practice may contribute to these events. These standards of practice come from many sources include the ANA's *Scope and Standards of Practice*, professional nursing organization's standards of practice, organization-specific policies and procedures, and regulatory agencies (e.g., the CMS) and accrediting agencies (e.g., TJC). Decreased variation, adherence to standards of care, and highly reliable human behaviors contribute to improvements in safety.

Many organizations, perhaps even yours, are on the journey to becoming a high-reliability organization (Reason, 1997; Weick & Sutcliffe, 2007). These organizations have taken a critical approach to improving safety through the elimination of preventable events of harm. This preoccupation with safety considers all possible failures in processes and practices to make them more reliable. Commercial air travel and nuclear power industries, for example, have taken this approach to safety to eliminate preventable events that cause harm (Frankel, Leonard, & Denham, 2006). Who would travel on a commercial airline if an airplane crashed each day? High-reliability organizations in healthcare take characteristics from these industries to eliminate events of harm. After all, safety is an essential right of all patients.

In Box 15.4, you will see how Madelyn reviews a safety event a bit differently than quality measures.

GENERAL CATEGORIES OF ERRORS AND HAZARDS IN CARE

Many organizations defined safety event classification systems; the American Society for Healthcare Risk Management's (ASHRM, 2014) system is offered here. These events are considered preventable errors resulting from a deviation from standards of practice. The ASHRM defined the three types of events. Prepatient events are considered unsafe situations where an error is caught by a barrier designed to prevent it. These errors do not reach the patient. An example of a prepatient event is an incorrect medication found during the barcode medication administration (BCMA) process. A safety event reaches the patient with minimal or no detectable harm. For example, a patient who received 800 mg of ibuprofen instead of 400 mg (as ordered) likely caused no detectable harm. A serious safety event causes moderate to severe harm or death. An unfortunately common serious safety event is the overdose of a child when dose-based calculations are done incorrectly. Serious safety events are often traumatic for both

BOX 15.4 CASE STUDY

After reviewing the rate of falls with injury on her unit, Madelyn was asked by her nurse manager to review a medication event. A patient was admitted from the emergency department with a diagnosis of atrial fibrillation. Prior to hospitalization, the patient took 8 mg of warfarin daily to prevent blood clots associated with the atrial fibrillation. Five days into the admission, the patient developed a pulmonary embolism that required admission to the intensive care unit. On investigation by the manager, the patient had been receiving only 5 mg of warfarin daily since admission. Madelyn was asked to assist in finding the cause of this error.

clinicians and families. The understanding of all types of events and the causes of all events are important for an organization on its journey to becoming a high-reliability organization.

BASIC SAFETY DESIGN PRINCIPLES AND HUMAN FACTORS

As organizations attempt to prevent errors, various structures are developed to be barriers to prevent the occurrence of an error. Barriers include the implementation of technology, policies, procedures, and workflows. These structures are placed into practice to prevent the events of harm. However, latent weaknesses exist in each barrier. No single barrier will prevent all errors each time from reaching a patient. Deviations from policies or errors in human behavior contribute to barriers not being successful. Reason (1997) introduced the "Swiss cheese model," which describes how events of harm occur despite multiple barriers. As each barrier is represented by a "slice" of Swiss cheese, the "slices" of the cheese line up, and the event of harm occurs bypassing the barriers through the "holes" (which are their latent weaknesses). Safety improvements occur by finding and correcting the latent weaknesses in barriers and preventing human errors.

Human behavior can be unreliable. Failure to pay attention to details, ineffective communication, nonadherence to policies and procedures, and other human behaviors contribute to events of harm. Organizations have evaluated structures and processes to improve the reliability of human behavior. These organizations have approached human behavior in generally three ways: simplification of processes, implementation of safe behaviors for all staff members, and tools to decrease reliance on memory. Complicated processes become error-prone as the required time and complexity are met with healthcare professionals using workarounds or being noncompliant with the practice. Because processes are built as barriers to prevent events of harm, these behaviors can contribute to the safety events.

Safe behaviors by all healthcare professionals—including both clinical and nonclinical—improve the reliability of behavior. So much of healthcare is communicated, hence tools such as phonetic clarification ("T as in Tom, A as in Apple") and numeric clarification (150 spoken as "One-Five-Zero" because one fifty [150] and one fifteen [115] can be easily confused) contribute to a safe environment. Succinct communication using the situation, background, assessment, and recommendation (SBAR) format focuses the attention of the sender and the receiver of the communication. Key phrases such as "I have a clarifying question" signal the need for clarity to the team.

Because human memory can contribute to skills-based, rule-based, and knowledge-based errors, organizations implement strategies to alleviate the reliance on memory. For example, organizations seeking to reduce the rate of central line–associated bloodstream infections may implement procedural checklists for the maintenance of the central line. Clinical informatics solutions, such as EHR and computerized physician order entry (CPOE), can provide reminders and advisories on the basis of documentation. For example, an advanced practice registered nurse may get notified of a potential interaction between two medications being ordered, or the EHR may recommend a constant companion for a patient endorsing suicidal ideation after a nurse documents this finding. In all, organizations use a variety of approaches to make human behavior more reliable. However, instances may exist where human behavior is purposefully unreliable, for example, noncompliance with a policy or standard of practice. Insufficient time, lack of technical resources, or burdensome priorities may contribute to noncompliance. Normalized deviance also contributes to human factors associated with events of harm. Consider traveling a few miles per hour above the speed limit to "keep up with traffic." The notion of deviating from a practice standard or policy, or in this case a law, because others are doing the same defines normalized deviance. This behavior can contribute to a culture that is inherently unsafe.

QUESTIONS TO CONSIDER BEFORE READING ON

Think about your practice setting and different safety events that have occurred.

- Would the event be classified as a prepatient event, safety event, or a serious safety event?
- What was the deviation from the policy or practice standard?
- Did human behavior impact the safety event? How?

BENEFITS AND LIMITATIONS OF COMMONLY USED SAFETY TECHNOLOGY

As technology emerged to support the work of healthcare professionals, the meaningful use of technology to improve care coordination, safety, and quality becomes important (CMS, 2015). Examples of these technologies include the EHR, CPOE, and BCMA technologies. These technologies aim to improve safety by decreasing the variation and increasing the reliability of human behavior. For example, CPOE eliminates handwritten orders that potentially were difficult to read or transcribe. BCMA technologies connect the orders in CPOE to the patient identification band to confirm the correct medication is to be administered. The EHR provides advisories when medications have interactions or contraindicate with an allergy. These technologies provide benefits by adding barriers of protection for patients (Powell-Cope, Nelson, & Patterson, 2008).

However, safety technology has its limitations. As technology becomes widespread, healthcare professionals may become overly focused on technology. Organizational factors such as training, policies, procedures, and the culture of safety contribute to its implementation. Social factors also impact the benefits of technology. Ideally, processes and workflows are designed to support the technology as a barrier to prevent harm. Technological limitations, in regards to design and implementation, may cause workarounds by healthcare providers if the processes are time-consuming, burdensome, or not perceived as effective. These workarounds remove the barriers that the technology was designed to address. For example, patient identification bands used for BCMA may become unusable after 2 or 3 hospital days, causing nurses to preprint duplicate bands. If these duplicate bands are used for the BCMA process, the purpose is defeated. Technologies are the most meaningful and appropriately used when healthcare professionals are involved in their design and implementation (Powell-Cope et al., 2014).

Box 15.5 depicts a conversation in the case scenario that Madelyn has with colleagues about the role of BCMA and safety, as well as how complex measurement of safety is.

CULTURE OF SAFETY

Organizations have many priorities including targets for patient volume, finances, and patient satisfaction scores. However, high-reliability organizations adopt a culture of safety that prioritizes safety above other operational and financial performance targets. Maintaining a focus on safety is difficult in an age of increased patient complexities and decreasing reimbursements for care. However, improving safety requires a dedication to the culture of safety at the levels of the patient care area, the clinical specialty division, and the organization. Hofmann, Jacobs, and Landy (1995) found that common visions pertaining to safety between management, leadership, and frontline employees were necessary for the organization to value safety.

BOX 15.5 THE CASE SCENARIO CONTINUES TO UNFOLD

Each month, the manager of Madelyn's unit shares the BCMA scanning compliances rates with the nursing team. After these rates were posted, Madelyn discussed the importance of the BCMA processes with two of her colleagues. Sal shared his support of the technology to improve the safety of the unit, and he maintained a compliance of 97% for all medication administrations for the past 3 months. Brandon expressed frustrations with the technology and has been compliant with 89% of administrations. In the discussion, Sal shared two events where an incorrect medication was administered. In both instances, he did not follow the BCMA process. Having had no medication errors since starting this process, Brandon asked Madelyn the value of BCMA. In response, Madelyn explained the necessity of safety barriers, such as the BCMA process, to improve the reliability of human behavior. Although technology helps with that improvement, errors can still exist with deviations in human behavior.

The ANA (2016), among other organizations, defined the elements of this culture. Within the culture of safety, nurse leaders must understand the causes of individual errors and ensure that appropriate action is taken based on the findings. The culture of safety supports an open discussion about safety and events of harm without individual blame. Without openness and trust, clinical staff and leaders may not be truthful in reporting unsafe conditions or behaviors. These concepts directly impact the reporting of errors and events of harm. In alignment with the ANA's (2012) *Principles for Nurse Staffing*, the culture of safety ensures that staffing and other resources meet the needs of the patients served in both volume and acuity. The culture of safety calls for accountability of all individuals to support safety as a principal priority. However, it is imperative for leadership to enculturate safety, for an ineffective culture of safety has been associated with many adverse events (Smetzer, Baker, Byrne, & Cohen, 2010). This enculturation can be measured using a validated survey, such as the Agency for Healthcare Research and Quality Surveys on Patient Safety Culture. These surveys are specific to patient care settings, including hospitals, long-term care facilities, and others.

Reporting Errors to the Organization and Those Affected

The culture of safety views errors as learning experiences to find weaknesses in those barriers aimed to prevent events of harm. Every healthcare professional possesses the responsibility to be transparent and communicate openly about safety and events of harm (Frankel et al., 2006). Organizations encourage healthcare professionals to use event reporting to capture all events of harm and unsafe situations. Many organizations adopted electronic formats. Many event-reporting systems allow the submitter to remain anonymous; although this may seem in contradiction to the culture of safety, disallowing these submissions may decrease overall reporting. Organizations build these systems with data fields to allow for further data analyses through common cause and other analyses. However, event-reporting systems may capture only a portion of actual events and unsafe situations, be perceived as burdensome, and may not be trusted by healthcare professionals working in a culture of blame (Wolf & Hughes, 2008). Despite these limitations, electronic event-reporting systems provide organizations with the tools and the data to respond to safety events and analyze trends over time.

Communicating errors to patients and families is often difficult, particularly when the error caused harm. Fear of litigation and professional liability, as well as feelings of guilt and shame, increase the difficulty. However, the culture of safety promotes transparency with those individuals affected by the event as much as with healthcare professionals (National Patient Safety Foundation's Lucian Leape Institute, 2015). Maintaining trust between the patient and the healthcare team provides the core imperative. Although healthcare professionals may be hesitant, patients desire full error disclosure and clarity; the lack of understanding may contribute to increased litigation, decreased trust, and nonadherence to treatment recommendations (Wolf & Hughes, 2014). Therefore, the clear and timely disclosure of events in accordance with organizational policy, which may require consultation with risk management or use of a structured process, aligns with the culture of safety and best practices for the patient's care.

UNDERSTANDING CAUSES OF ERRORS AND ACCOUNTABILITY

Root Cause Analysis

Unlike the CCA, the root cause analysis (RCA) investigates a single event or situation. High-reliability organizations use the RCA in all serious safety events (Wolf & Hughes, 2008). The purpose of the RCA is to determine the causation or the relationship among the deviations from normal processes in the event of harm. A healthcare professional conducting an RCA starts at the event of harm and maps every contributing action to that event. The RCA has limited generalizability of its findings regarding human behavior trends and environment of care causes. These limitations arise from the single-event nature of the RCA. However, these analyses are powerful tools to determine causes of the events of harm, particularly when the causes are practices or processes (Wolf & Hughes, 2008). Unfortunately, the RCA can be used only after an event has occurred.

In Box 15.6, Madelyn uses the RCA process to review the safety event.

Failure Mode and Effect Analysis

Although RCA is a method for evaluation of causes and effects in a specific event, the failure mode and effect analysis (FMEA) evaluate processes to identify steps that can go wrong (failure modes) and the impacts of these steps going wrong (effect; Reiling, Knutzen, & Stoecklein, 2003). The RCA aims to reconstruct processes and actions as they occurred in relation to an event of harm (to discover what went wrong); the FMEA maps processes and actions using policies, procedures, and standards of practice (to discover what could go wrong). The FMEA, then, aims to detect and fix weak processes before events of harm. Teams consider three aspects to prioritize the impact of a failure mode:

- Probability (*P*): What is the probability this failure mode will happen?
- Severity (*S*): If the failure mode were to happen, what is the likely severity or its contribution to an event of harm?
- Detection (*D*): What is the unlikelihood that other barriers would detect the failure mode?

Failure modes with a high probability of occurrence, potentially high severity in patient harm, and the high unlikelihood of detection would be considered unacceptable in a high-reliability organization. The FMEA may use ratings of 1 to 10 for each aspect; the product of these aspects ($P \times S \times D$)

is used to rank the failure modes. By using a FMEA for processes either in development or in use, organizations can study and prevent events of harm before their occurrence.

Just Culture

Punitive cultures in healthcare cause the underreporting of safety events, for healthcare providers carry a fear of personal risk for reported safety events. Within the culture of safety, organizations must take a nonpunitive approach to managing errors (National Patient Safety Foundation's Lucian Leape Institute, 2015; Sammer, Lykens, Singh, Mains, & Lackan, 2010). However, instances may exist where disciplinary action is appropriate. These concepts compose the "just culture." The AHRQ (2008) noted clearly: "A just culture is one where people can report mistakes, errors, or waste without reprisal or personal risk. This does not mean that individuals are not held accountable for their actions, but it does mean that people are not held responsible for flawed systems in which dedicated and trained people can still make mistakes" (p. 47). The ANA (2010) and many other organizations support the full adoption of the just culture through position statements on the matter. However, the implementation of the just culture may give healthcare managers and leaders challenges. Marx (2008) created a methodological algorithm to support managers and leaders in addressing deviations of human behavior that cause events of harm. For example, human behavior errors done without a conscious decision ("by mistake" or "accidentally") are managed differently than those behaviors when one consciously decides to deviate from a standard of practice or a policy. In this manner, healthcare professionals are held accountable for their actions while promoting the culture of safety. Chassin and Loeb (2013) recommend that organizations formalize ways to separate human error and system design errors from purposeful actions that result in harm.

SUSTAINING A HIGH-RELIABILITY ORGANIZATION

The journey to becoming a high-reliability organization requires changing the essential culture of an organization. Implementing the culture of safety and the just culture begins the journey to eliminating preventable events of harm. The sustainment of this culture requires specific actions to maintain initial successes and further improve the safety of healthcare consumers. Five characteristics define how a high-reliability organization sustains its commitment to safety (AHRQ, 2008):

1. Preoccupation with failure: High-reliability organizations persistently investigate ways that systems and processes may fail and lead to harm. This characteristic includes an evaluation of all near-miss safety events for failure modes and recommendations to remedy weaknesses in systems and processes.

BOX 15.6 THE CASE SCENARIO CONTINUES TO UNFOLD

Madelyn assisted her manager in conducting an RCA of the warfarin medication error. Madelyn was surprised to see that the weaknesses of the barriers "line up" for an event of harm to occur. The RCA showed the following, from admission:

- In the emergency department, the patient reported being unsure of his medications and doses; the emergency department physician entered "To Be Determined" in the medication reconciliation process. On arrival to the patient care area, a nurse reviewed the patient's home medication list with his wife and found that warfarin was missing. The nurse approached the resident physician and asked for the medication to be ordered.
- The resident physician asked the nurse to write the dose down. Running late to rounds, the physician called the pharmacy to enter a telephone order. However, the handwritten 8 was mistaken for a 5. When the order was entered, the nurse reviewed the order. The nurse was confused when seeing 5 mg ordered but assumed that there was a reason.
- The primary team ordered blood work on the second hospital day for the patient. However, the phlebotomist had not correctly labeled the tube for the prothrombin time and international normalized ratio. The laboratory technologist used a new function in the EHR to notify the nurse and physician, but these providers did not review the message because the functionality was not fully adopted.

During this patient's hospital stay, Madelyn realized the many system and process failures that contributed to the event of harm. A barrier would have likely detected one of the failures, but in accordance with the "Swiss cheese model," the weaknesses "lined up." In the just culture, no healthcare professional would likely be held personally accountable. Rather, a breakdown of processes and unintended human behaviors contributed to the event of harm.

2. Sensitivity to operations (situational awareness): High-reliability organizations seek a detailed understanding of all clinical and nonclinical operations with attention to any effect on patient care delivery.
3. Resilience: High-reliability organizations develop systems with multiple barriers such that one or more barrier failures would be detected by another barrier.
4. Deference to expertise: High-reliability organizations value the recommendations of all healthcare professionals regardless of rank, tenure, or profession.
5. Reluctance to simplify: High-reliability organizations develop and simplify systems to improve their reliability; however, these organizations are reluctant to simplify the understanding of failures and events of harm. This understanding is developed through rigorous processes such as RCA.

PATIENT SAFETY AND QUALITY RESOURCES, INITIATIVES, AND REGULATIONS

After *To Err Is Human* (IOM, 1999) highlighted the state of healthcare in the United States, various organizations provided direction to the quality and safety of care. In 2005, the Patient Safety and Quality Improvement Act of 2005 (PSQIA) created legislation to further understand safety trends. The PSQIA established a reporting system for participating patient safety organizations to trend and analyze patient safety data. This legislation provides organizations with confidentiality protection when transmitting patient safety information, which aimed to improve the reporting of events of harm. These legislations also limit the use of patient safety information derived from internal investigations in litigation. The PSQIA, through its protections, encourages individuals and organizations to report events of harm.

Both federal and private agencies provide direction and resources for the improvement of quality and safety. The AHRQ, as an agency of the U.S. Department of Health and Human Services, directs the quality and safety of organizations throughout the country. The CMS provides federal regulatory oversight for organizations participating in these programs, and state departments of public health act on the behalf of the CMS in assessing organizations' safety. The CMS sets standards for safe practice through its Conditions of Participations. TJC, through its accreditation process and National Patient Safety Goals (NPSGs), sets quality and safety expectations (called "elements of performance") and surveys organizations for adherence to these expectations. NPSGs are used by many organizations to guide their safety and quality improvement trajectory (TJC, 2018). The IHI develops tools, resources, and strategies to improve the quality of care in addition to providing free education to healthcare professionals through its Open School. Many organizations—private and public—are dedicated to the improvement of safety and quality.

SELF-ASSESSMENT

Visit the following website: https://members.rmpsi.com/MembersOnly/RM_ToolChest_HCF/Risk%20Management/RMPSSelfAssessment.pdf, and complete the Risk Management and Patient Safety Self-Assessment Questionnaire. What strengths do you identify? What improvements can be made?

CONCLUSION

Dedication to quality and safety is the responsibility of all healthcare professions in partnership with the consumers of care and their families. This chapter outlined essential concepts in quality improvement and patient safety. Quality improvement aims to improve the outcomes of care—rather than processes of care—through measurement over time. Performance measures such as nursing-sensitive indicators and core measures demonstrate the impact of healthcare professionals on the health of its consumers. Models and tools for improvement were discussed. Safety was described as an approach to minimize, and then eliminate, preventable events of harm by increasing the reliability of human behavior and systems. The culture of safety and the concepts of high-reliability organizations were used as the lens to view safety. Human factors affecting safety and strategies to improve these factors were identified. Tools for determining the causes and effects of these events were identified. Finally, additional resources for patient safety were presented. All healthcare professionals, including you, are called to improve the safety and quality of care provided. As a nurse, you are well positioned to provide the leadership to unit-based and organization-wide quality improvement and safety initiatives.

CRITICAL THINKING ACTIVITIES

- Using the website www.ihi.org/education/IHIOpenSchool/resources/Pages/Activities/Mutiny.aspx, review the case of a physician escalating safety concerns. Reflect on challenges of escalating concerns in the culture of safety. How would you feel if this involved you and a senior nurse? You and a physician? You and your manager?
- Review TJC NPSGs, available using the website www.jointcommission.org/standards_information/npsgs.aspx. What are some activities your organization is doing to address these goals? What outcome measures match these goals?
- The death of Josie King made national news and demonstrated failures contributing to an event of harm. Watch the video using the website www.ihi.org/education/ihiopenschool/resources/Pages/CourseraVideo1.aspx. Describe the failures in human behavior that led to the event of harm.
- If your organization has participated in a culture of safety survey—for example, the Agency for Healthcare Research and Quality Surveys on Patient Safety Culture—review your organization's results. What is one element that surprised you? Did you expect to see the results that you did?

REFERENCES

American Association of Colleges of Nursing. (2012). *Graduate level QSEN competencies: Knowledge, skills, and attitudes*. Washington, DC: Author.

American Nurses Association. (2010). Position statement: Just culture. Retrieved from https://www.nursingworld.org/~4afe07/globalassets/practiceandpolicy/health-and-safety/just_culture.pdf

American Nurses Association. (2012). *ANA's principles for nurse staffing*. Silver Spring, MD: Author.

American Nurses Association. (2015). *Code of ethics for nurses with interpretive statements*. Silver Spring, MD: Author.

American Nurses Association. (2016). Creating a culture of safety. *The American Nurse*. Retrieved from http://www.theamericannurse.org/2016/02/05/creating-a-culture-of-safety

American Society for Healthcare Risk Management. (2014). Serious safety events: A focus on harm classification: Deviation in care as link. Retrieved from http://www.ashrm.org/pubs/files/white_papers/SSE-2_getting_to_zero-9-30-14.pdf

Batalden, P. B., & Davidoff, F. (2007). What is "quality improvement?" and how can it transform healthcare? *Quality and Safety Health Care, 16*(1), 2–3. doi:10.1136/qshc.2006.022046

Centers for Medicare & Medicaid Services. (2015). Meaningful use definition and objectives. Retrieved from https://www.healthit.gov/providers-professionals/meaningful-use-definition-objectives

Chassin, M. R., & Loeb, J. M. (2013). High-reliability health care: Getting there from here. *Milbank Quarterly, 91*(3), 459–490. doi:10.1111/1468-0009.12023

Donabedian, A. (1988). The quality of care: How can it be assessed? *Journal of the American Medical Association, 260*, 1743–1748. doi:10.1001/jama.1988.03410120089033

Frankel, A. S., Leonard, M. W., & Denham, C. R. (2006). Fair and just culture, team behavior, and leadership engagement: The tools to achieve high reliability. *Health Services Research, 41*(4 Pt 2), 1690–1709. doi:10.1111/j.1475-6773.2006.00572.x

Hofmann, D. A., Jacobs, R., & Landy, F. (1995). High reliability process industries: Individual, micro, and macro organizational influences on safety performance. *Journal of Safety Research, 26*(3), 131–149. doi:10.1016/0022-4375(95)00011-E

Institute of Medicine. (1999). *To err is human: Building a safer health system*. Washington, DC: National Academies Press.

Institute of Medicine. (2001). *Crossing the quality chasm*. Washington, DC: National Academies Press.

The Joint Commission. (2018). 2018 National patient safety goals. Retrieved from https://www.jointcommission.org/standards_information/npsgs.aspx

The Joint Commission. (2017). Core measure sets–measures. Retrieved from https://www.jointcommission.org/core_measure_sets.aspx

Landrigan, C. P., Parry, G. J., Bones, C. B., Hackbarth, A. D., Goldmann, D. A., & Sharek, P. J. (2010). Temporal trends in rates of patient harm resulting from medical care. *New England Journal of Medicine, 363*, 2124–2134. doi:10.1056/NEJMsa1004404

Langley, G. J., Moen, R. D., Nolan, K. M., Nolan, T. W., Norman, C. L., & Provost, L. P. (2009). *The improvement guide: A practical approach to enhancing organizational performance*. San Francisco, CA: Jossey-Bass.

Martinez, K., Battaglia, R., Start, R., Mastal, M. F., & Matlock, A. M. (2015). Nursing sensitive indicators in ambulatory care. *Nursing Economic$, 33*(1), 59–66.

Marx, D. (2008). *The just culture algorithm*. Plano, TX: Outcome Engineering.

Mastal, M. F., Matlock, A. M., & Start, R. (2016). Ambulatory care nurse-sensitive indicators series: Capturing the role of nursing in ambulatory care. *Nursing Economic$, 34*(2), 92–97.

Montalvo, I. (2007). The national database of nursing quality indicators (NDNQI). *Online Journal of Issues in Nursing, 12*(3), Manuscript 2. doi:10.3912/OJIN.Vol12No03Man02

National Patient Safety Foundation's Lucian Leape Institute. (2015). *Shining a light: Safer health care through transparency*. Boston, MA: National Patient Safety Foundation.

Ogrinc, G. S., Headrick, L. A., Moore, S. M., Barton, A. J., Dolansky, M. A., & Madigosky, W. S. (2012). *Fundamentals of health care improvement: A guide to improving your patients' care* (2nd ed.). Chicago, IL: The Joint Commission.

Powell-Cope, G., Nelson, A., & Patterson, E. (2008). Patient care technology and safety. In R. G. Hughes (Ed.), *Patient safety and quality: An evidence-based handbook for nurses*. Rockville, MD: Agency for Healthcare Research and Quality.

Pronovost, P. J., Berenholtz, S. M., Goeschel, C. A., Needham, D. M., Sexton, J. B., Thompson, D. A., … Hunt, E. (2006). Creating high reliability in health care organizations. *Health Services Research, 41*(4 Pt 2), 1599–1617. doi:10.1111/j.1475-6773.2006.00567.x

Pronovost, P. J., Needham, D., Berenholtz, S., Sinopoli, D., Chu, H., Cosgrove, S., … Goeschel, C. (2006). An intervention to decrease catheter-related bloodstream infections in the ICU. *New England Journal of Medicine, 355*(26), 2725–2732. doi:10.1056/NEJMoa061115

Reason, J. T. (1997). *Managing the risks of organizational accidents*. London, UK: Ashgate.

Reiling, G. J., Knutzen, B. L., & Stoecklein, M. (2003). FMEA: The cure for medical errors. *Quality Progress, 36*, 67–71.

Sammer, C. E., Lykens, K., Singh, K. P., Mains, D. A., & Lackan, N. A. (2010). What is patient safety culture? A review of the literature. *Journal of Nursing Scholarship, 42*(2), 156–165. doi:10.1111/j.1547-5069.2009.01330.x

Smetzer, J., Baker, C., Byrne, F. D., & Cohen, M. R. (2010). Shaping systems for better behavioral choices: Lessons learned from a fatal medication error. *Joint Commission Journal on Quality and Patient Safety, 36*, 152–163. doi:10.1016/S1553-7250(10)36027-2

Weick, K. E., & Sutcliffe, K. M. (2007). *Managing the unexpected* (2nd ed.). San Francisco, CA: Jossey-Bass.

Wolf, Z. R., & Hughes, R. G. (2008). Error reporting and disclosure. In R. G. Hughes (Ed.), *Patient safety and quality: An evidence-based handbook for nurses.* Rockville, MD: Agency for Healthcare Research and Quality.

IV

MANAGING HUMAN AND FISCAL RESOURCES

16

MANAGEMENT AND LEADERSHIP ROLES IN PROFESSIONAL NURSING

KRISTY DIXON STINGER

LEARNING OBJECTIVES

After completion of this chapter, the reader will be able to

- Define management.
- Explain the relevance of managing human and fiscal resources.
- Analyze different theories of management.
- Explain the management process describing nursing skills needed in each phase.
- Identify management skills and qualities needed to be an effective nurse leader.
- Perform a self-assessment of one's own management skills.

We are living in a new era of healthcare that is constantly changing and evolving. Healthcare policy is impacting the way we provide care to our patients. It dictates who receives care, where one receives care, what types of services are reimbursed, and how care is delivered. It is a constant struggle to reduce costs while trying to improve processes and enhance patient care. Leadership and management skills are vital to navigate through these ever-changing times. The nurse can use different management theories with which to work and implement ongoing changes to improve the quality of patient care and increase organizational productivity. Management theories help us understand why people practice certain behaviors and provide insight into how individuals work together. Managers and nurses can use management theories when implementing new programs, practices, and policies in the workplace. An effective manager will understand which theory best fits his or her style and is best suited for his or her coworkers and situation. This means using different theories in different situations or combining components from various theories. Nurses can use a variety of strategies to lead quality initiatives in their workplace.

As a practicing registered nurse (RN), you work daily with interprofessional teams to care for a variety of patients in all settings. The management and leadership information presented during your associate's degree program has helped to prepare you with the latest knowledge and skills to be an effective nurse advancing the care and health of the patients for whom you care. It is well known that education has a significant impact on the knowledge and competencies of a nurse clinician (American Association of Colleges of Nursing [AACN], 2008). Nurses need to be able to meet the increasing complexity of the healthcare system and effectively lead and manage practice. This chapter reinforces what you have learned in your associate's degree program regarding management theory and technique and you have applied within your own clinical experience as an RN. It challenges you to think of the management styles of those with whom you have worked and the management style that you aspire to implement in your own practice. It adds to your current knowledge and experience as a RN and as a leader in healthcare today so you can successfully integrate the knowledge and experience you have to effectively lead those with whom you work.

WHAT IS MANAGEMENT?

In Chapter 3, we defined and discussed the difference between leadership and management in addition to describing a variety of leadership theories. As you will remember, leadership requires skills to lead and influence others, whereas management requires skills to effectively use resources to accomplish tasks. You already do some of both at some level in your current role as an RN. For example, you use an extensive set of skills from planning and delegating to communicating and motivating. As an RN, you have also now had the experience of working with a manager in your place of work. In this chapter, we explore nursing management roles in more depth, focusing on the management of human and fiscal resources. We also discuss management theories, the management process, and management skills. Finally, you also assess your own current personal management skills and identify areas in which you may enhance these skills.

QUESTIONS TO CONSIDER BEFORE READING ON

- Recalling the information presented in Chapter 3, do you think that leadership and management skills are distinct?
- Do you believe there is some overlap? Explain.

THE IMPORTANCE OF MANAGING HUMAN AND FISCAL RESOURCES

Most likely, you entered the nursing profession because you wanted to provide compassionate care to those in need. Why then would we tell you that it is important to manage the human and fiscal resources associated with care? The answer is relatively simple. Healthcare is a business. If that business is not managed appropriately, we will not be in business any longer. As a nurse, you have a unique perspective and the ability to examine the resources we use. You know what is necessary to care for your patients and what is wasteful. The following case scenario helps illustrate how nurses might be called upon to manage resources and control costs.

The case scenario given in Box 16.1 highlights how nurses can be called upon to manage fiscal resources such as equipment and supplies. For example, you might learn that your unit tends to use butterfly needles because the staff believe that they are easier to draw blood on the first try as well as are less painful for the patient given the smaller needle size. However, you are also well aware that they are more costly. Nurses at the bedside know what is necessary (and not necessary) to care for their patients. The goal is to reduce expenses without impairing the service to our patients.

QUESTIONS TO CONSIDER BEFORE READING ON

Within your area of practice:

- What fiscal resources are essential for you to perform your nursing role?
- What fiscal resources do you feel could be managed better?

BOX 16.1 CASE SCENARIO

James Hernandez is the nurse manager of the medical surgical unit at Springfield Hospital. He holds a meeting to share difficult news with his staff. He tells the staff that the hospital is losing money despite the fact that its patient volume is up. He has been asked by senior management to control their resources. This means that their request for new IV pumps will be placed on hold. It also means that they will need to carefully watch their staffing, overtime, and use of supplies. James asked the staff for their input to help control costs while maintaining the high-quality healthcare for their patients.

The case scenario given in Box 16.1 also highlights the need to manage human resources. Staffing overages, overtime, and staff turnover can have large negative repercussions on the budget. Nurse leaders know what staffing is necessary to provide safe quality care as well as what may be excessive. It is our job as nurse leaders to be mindful of this. Another cost associated with human resources is burnout and staff turnover. Unfortunately, the turnover rate for RNs continues to rise. The 2016 National Healthcare Retention & RN Staffing Report states that turnover statistics for bedside RNs in 2014 were 16.4%, and they rose to 17.2% in 2015.

Having a high turnover rate can have devastating consequences on a hospital's budget and impact its profit margin. According to the 2016 National Healthcare Retention & RN Staffing Report, the average cost of turnover for a nurse ranges from $37,700 to $58,400. Hospitals can lose $5.2 million to $8.1 million annually. The costs and consequences of burnout and turnover are significant. The good news is that there are ways for both nurses and hospital administrations to combat nurse burnout. Nurses play a vital role in maintaining the quality care that hospitals provide. However, we need nurse leaders who will work closely with the leadership team to avoid nurse burnout. We need to support nurses at the bedside, give them the resources they need, and provide them with emotional support and positive recognition. Healthcare organizations are taking steps to reduce nurse burnout by allowing self-scheduling, decreasing overtime, and providing support and mentorship programs. Strong management skills are vital to accomplish this.

Managing resources is a continuing challenge in today's healthcare environment while focusing on both cost containment and quality. It requires specific skills that you may have observed being performed by nurse mangers in your practice area. As you read about the following theories, think about those in your practice setting.

From the time that nurses and healthcare professionals began forming organizations with goals and objectives, managing has been essential to ensure the coordination of efforts. As we have progressed and organized groups have grown, the job of nurse managers has become more and more complex. Management of human and fiscal resources is the process of designing and maintaining an environment in which individuals, working together in groups, efficiently accomplish selected aims in a cost-effective manner (Koontz & Weihrich, 1990, p. 4). Nursing management is the process of directing or administering nursing practice. A nurse manager is one who administers, initiates, organizes, maintains, and monitors results in practice. Nurse managers focus on resources and are objective with goals and outcomes. A manager focuses on the organization and coordination of resources to achieve specific initiatives and objectives. Formal nurse managers are individuals who are officially appointed to a position of authority within an organization. However, nurse managers are not the only individuals who can rely on management principles and theory to help guide them in the workplace. Informal clinical leaders can also use management theories. The words "leader" and "manager" are often confused and used interchangeably. Although a manager is someone who has an assigned role and title within an organization, a leader excels at interpersonal relationships and inspires those with whom he or she works. Leaders use their own influence and skills to empower others. They, too, can use management theories in their practice and create change.

MANAGEMENT THEORIES

It is important to look at the past to see how today's leadership theories and management theories have evolved to understand from where they evolved (Hill, Jones, & Schilling, 2014). Management theories came into development in the mid to late 1800s during the Industrial Revolution because it was during the Industrial Revolution that organizations were growing from small, home-grown companies to mass-production facilities. These theories focused more on control of both resources and people. Beginning in the 1930s through the 1950s, the human relations movement began and recognized the importance of examining employee behaviors. From there, leadership theories developed, recognizing the importance of the leaders' role in leading others (refer to Chapter 3 for a review of leadership theories). The following is a description of classical theories (late 1800s—scientific, bureaucratic, administrative) and newer theories (contingency, systems, chaos, and theories X and Y).

SCIENTIFIC MANAGEMENT THEORY

The scientific management theory was developed by Frederick Taylor and looks for the specification and measurement of all organizational tasks (Waring, 2016). It came about at the turn of the century and represents the start of modern management. During that time, large organizations were created to manufacture a variety of products all of which were done with careful measurement and specification of activities and results. On the basis of a systematic study of people, tasks, and work behavior, the theory broke the work process down into the smallest possible units in an effort to determine the most efficient method possible for completing a particular job. This theory asserts that organizations should identify the best way to train workers to handle each element in a predetermined manner and set up a system of rewards for improved productivity (Gladwin, Kennelly, & Krause, 1995). The goal of this theory is to improve economic efficiency. It was one of the earliest attempts to apply science to the engineering of processes and to management and introduced the concept of breaking a complex task into a number of subtasks, thus optimizing performance. Taylor believed that employees were economically motivated and that was what drove their work ethic and drive.

BUREAUCRATIC MANAGEMENT THEORY

The bureaucratic management theory developed by Max Weber is a theory that contains two essential elements. First, it encourages structuring an organization into a hierarchy and establishing strong lines of control and authority. Second, it identifies the importance of having clearly identified rules to help govern an organization and its members (Cole, 2004). Similar to the scientific management theory, Weber advocated for a system on the basis of standardized procedures and a clear chain of command. Weber suggested that organizations develop comprehensive and detailed standard operating procedures for all routine tasks. Max Weber focused on dividing organizations into strong lines of authority and control. He believed in a hierarchy of authority, standardized procedures, and hiring employees only if they met the specific qualifications for the job and had clearly defined job roles (Bush, 2007). He wanted to eliminate favoritism in organizations. His theory has been critiqued as being very impersonal with little human-level interaction between its members.

ADMINISTRATIVE THEORY

The administrative theory developed by Henri Fayol is a theory that is focused at the management level. Henri Fayol believed that management is a science that can be learned. Fayol believed that management had five principal roles: to forecast and plan, to organize, to command, to coordinate, and to control (Kiggundu, Jørgensen, & Hafsi, 1983). He developed 14 principles of administration to go along with the five principal roles. The principles are as follows: specialization/division of labor, authority with responsibility, discipline, unit of command, unity of direction, subordination of individual interest to the general interest, remuneration of staff, centralization, scalar chain/line of authority, order, equity, stability of tenure, initiative, and esprit de corps. He believed that an ideal organization was based on team dynamics and personal effort.

CONTINGENCY THEORY

The contingency theory asserts that managers make decisions not on the basis of a "one-size-fits-all" method but rather on the basis of the situation at hand. Management effectiveness is contingent or dependent on circumstances (Otley, 2016). The way one manages should change depending on the circumstance at hand. Managers need to look at the current situation and take appropriate action. There is no best way to run a business, organization, or company. Internal and external situations need to be evaluated and considered when making management decisions.

SYSTEMS THEORY

The systems theory is a theory that encourages managers to examine patterns and events within the workplace. It considers a system as a set of distinct parts that form a complex whole (Schneider, Wickert, & Marti, 2017). It treats an organization as either an open or a closed system. A closed system is not affected by its environment; however, an open system is affected by its environment (Shafritz, Ott, & Jang, 2015). The theory is based on the premise that managers need to recognize and understand how different systems affect a worker and how a worker affects the system around him or her. Managers need to coordinate programs to work as a collective whole for the overall goal or mission of the organization rather than for individual or for isolated departments.

CHAOS THEORY

The chaos theory is a branch of mathematics focused on the behavior of dynamical systems (Burke, 2017). It is based on the concept that change is constant and inevitable. It looks at certain systems that are very sensitive and unpredictable. These systems may be organizations, weather patterns, ecosystems, or anatomical functions. Within this theory, the term "butterfly effect" became popular, meaning that a small change in one state can result in large differences in a later state, for example, a butterfly flapping its wings in Brazil can cause a tornado in Texas (Boeing, 2016). Although certain circumstances and events can be controlled in an organization, others simply cannot be controlled. This theory recognized that systems can be unpredictable. Organizations are encouraged to see the organizational shape that emerges from a distance (Bums, 2016). In other words, managers need to look for patterns that lead to certain types of behaviors within the organization.

THEORY X AND THEORY Y

Theory X and theory Y are two contrasting theories that explain how managers' beliefs about what motivates their employees can affect their own management style (Mohamed & Nor, 2013). Managers who believe that workers naturally lack ambition and need incentives to increase their productivity within the workplace lean toward the theory X management style. These managers tend to use an authoritarian style of leadership. Theory X managers tend to micromanage their employees' work to make sure that it is accomplished properly. Theory Y managers believe that workers are naturally driven and take responsibility for their work and actions. Theory Y managers are not authoritarian; they encourage participation from their workers. Managers who fall into the theory Y category trust their staff to take ownership for their work and do it effectively by themselves.

QUESTIONS TO CONSIDER BEFORE READING ON

After reading the management theories noted earlier, can you relate your own management functioning to any of those theories?

- Describe the management style of a manager you have had in the past that would bring out the best in your work.
- Think of a time that the area in which you work has been reorganized or changed. How was the task approached? How did the affected employees respond to the reorganization and change?

As you read the continued case scenario that follows, reflect on the aforementioned management theories and determine which theory best fits the nurse manager.

The case scenario given in Box 16.2 continues to highlight how nurses can be called upon to manage fiscal resources. As a nurse, you can play an important role in helping to reduce costs by reducing expenses without impairing the service provided to patients. Meeting this challenge takes innovative thinking and involvement of all staff.

BOX 16.2 THE CASE SCENARIO CONTINUES TO UNFOLD

James Hernandez takes time at his monthly departmental meeting with his medical surgical staff to brainstorm with staff as to how they can control staffing and overtime. He provides education on how the department budget is developed and monitored and demonstrates to the staff how a small amount of overtime can have significant effects on the departmental budget. James and his staff brainstorm about how they as a unit can decrease overtime. All agree that any staff overtime must be approved by James or his assistant nurse manager on an individual, daily basis. Staff can no longer stay over their shift and not tell anyone about it. Another idea that the group came up with was to develop a small unit-based subcommittee to review staffing schedules to minimize overtime and assure proper nurse-to-patient ratios are followed. James explains to his staff that staffing may be adjusted pending the unit census. The staff are engaged and agree to work as a team to improve the unit's fiscal performance. James promised to give his department monthly updates on their performance and celebrate any success they have.

THE MANAGEMENT PROCESS

Nurses are expected to perform basic managerial functions in their day-to-day role. The AACN (2008) recognizes that nursing has the potential to make the biggest impact on transformation of healthcare delivery to a safer, higher quality, and more cost-effective system. Leadership and management skills are needed that emphasize ethical and critical decision-making, delegation, and conflict resolution strategies. This is critical to promoting high-quality care. It is vital for nurses to demonstrate leadership and communication skills. The management process can be followed to productively manage staff and resources to achieve goals. It is a systematic way of doing things. The process can be applied universally to all professions. The management process stemmed from Henry Fayol's management theory (Fayol, 1949) and includes five managerial steps or functions: planning, organizing, commanding, coordinating, and controlling. Although Chapter 3 introduced these concepts, in the following text we provide a little more detail:

1. **Planning:** Planning is a crucial first step as it creates the blueprint and path one must follow to see a project or activity through from beginning to end. Strategic planning involves looking ahead into the future and determining the course of action one will follow to achieve one's desired goals and objectives. It involves decision-making. Planning involves four elements (Barnat, 2014):
   a. Evaluating environmental forces and organizational resources
   b. Establishing a set of organizational goals
   c. Developing strategies and plans to achieve those goals
   d. Formulating a decision-making process

   For example, when rolling out a new clinical initiative such as a safe patient-handling program on a clinical unit, the planning of how this will be accomplished is vital. In the planning phase, a strong manager will assess his or her unit by recognizing the goals of the organization and looking at resources he or she has and resources he or she needs. He or she will set specific goals for his or her unit/staff. For example, all patients who meet the requirements for safe patient-handling equipment will be moved or mobilized using specific equipment. The expectation is that all staff will be trained on how to use the equipment and will use the equipment when providing patient care. A desired outcome from implementing a process such as this is that patient falls will decrease and employee injuries from patient handling will decrease. Both of these outcomes can be measured and results shared with staff.
2. **Organizing:** Once a plan has been made, the next step is to organize and gather the resources that are necessary to complete the project

at hand. Organizing involves creating an intentional structure for individuals to fill. Three elements are essential to organizing (Barnat, 2014):

a. Developing the structure of the organization
b. Acquiring and training human resources
c. Establishing communication patterns and networks

Continuing with our earlier example, when initiating a safe patient-handling program, the manager will identify the resources he or she will need to complete this initiative. The initiative will be led by the manager of the clinical unit and the assistant nurse manager. Key staff members will be designated as superusers and will attend an in-depth specialty-training session to learn how to use the equipment and, in turn, help teach their fellow colleagues and be a resource on the unit. Education will be provided on the unit and at designated times before and after shifts begin. This initiative will be discussed at monthly departmental meetings and through daily muster sessions on the unit.

3. **Commanding:** Managers must supervise their employees daily. It is the responsibility of managers to share with staff the vision and goals of the organization for which they work. They need to inspire their staff to work as a team to attain those goals. Commanding a subordinate must be consistent with company policies and all subordinates must be treated fairly and consistently.

   The nurse manager leading the safe patient-handling initiative has the overall authority and responsibility for implanting this initiative on his or her unit. He or she must supervise the employees and make sure that they are following the policies and procedures of the organization. All employees must be treated fairly and consistently.

4. **Coordinating:** In the management process, leading involves influencing individuals to work together to achieve a common goal. Many believe that management and leading should go hand in hand. A good, effective manager should be a good, effective leader. However, not all managers can lead effectively and not all leaders are good, effective managers. Leading takes skill. Managers must harmonize the procedures and activities performed by the company and coordinate processes among departments and employees. Three components make up the leading function that allows a manager to coordinate an initiative (Barnat, 2014):

   a. Influencing employees
   b. Motivating employees
   c. Forming effective groups

   The nurse manager leading the safe patient-handling initiative will discuss the initiative and goals of the initiative with all staff—nurses and nursing aides, physical therapy, and transportation—and explain the importance of this initiative. It is his or her job to motivate employees and get them engaged and involved in this patient-safety initiative. Staff will need to hold each other accountable and help each other.

5. **Controlling:** Controlling is comparing, measuring, and correcting the activities that are performed to achieve the goal or objective at hand. It involves monitoring and evaluating activities. By controlling what individuals are working on, organizational outcomes can be controlled. All activities must be in line with the company's organizational policies and objectives.
   Three basic components constitute the control function (Barnat, 2014):
   a. Elements of a control system
   b. Evaluating and rewarding employee performance
   c. Controlling financial, informational, and physical resources
      Daily, the nurse leader will work with staff and round on patients to assure that the safe patient-handling program is in place and that equipment is being used when transferring, moving, and ambulating patients. The manager will share and post employee injury rates and patient fall rates and share the results with staff, celebrating any success stories they have and also sharing any challenges. Staff will be engaged in solving any issues and challenges that may arise. The manager will have oversight for the financial impact this initiative has on his or her unit. This includes the following: monitoring the costs of education and potential overtime for staff to attend the education and the costs involved with ordering necessary equipment and supplies. The manager will also need to have oversight of the physical allocation of equipment on his or her unit. This may involve coordinating with facilities and materials management to move items around or order new equipment. The manager will also need to review how the implementation of this program will affect documentation in the electronic medical record. Policies and procedures for patient handling will also need to be updated to include this new initiative.

QUESTIONS TO CONSIDER BEFORE READING ON

- How can the steps of the management process be used in healthcare? Can you think of an example of a time when you have used these steps to successfully complete a project? What worked well? What did not?

MANAGEMENT SKILLS

What are the essential management skills that help make one an effective nurse leader?

- **Strategic planning/objective setting**
  It is vital that a manager establishes and communicates a clear direction to his or her team to reach the desired outcome. Strategic planning with clear objectives is vital.
- **Communication**
  Managers need to have excellent communication skills, written and verbal. This is a vital skill that enables them to build positive relationships with their colleagues and peers and motivate them to achieve their potential.
- **Emotional intelligence**
  As discussed in detail in Chapter 2, emotional intelligence is an important skill a good manager should possess. Emotional intelligence is the ability to identify and manage one's own emotions and the emotions of others. It is the ability to harness emotions and apply them to tasks such as thinking and problem-solving.
- **Decision-making ability**
  One must be able to view the various options at hand, make effective decisions, and take the appropriate action to be an effective manager.
- **People development**
  A good manager must have the ability to coach and mentor his or her staff to maximize performance. The ability to manage people and provide constructive feedback is vital to maximize performance and achieve objectives and goals.

MANAGEMENT ROLES IN PROFESSIONAL NURSING: RELEVANT QUALITY AND SAFETY EDUCATION for NURSES (QSEN) COMPETENCIES

As nurses work with various leaders and managers in the healthcare setting, certain values and competencies are vital and essential to practice for both graduate and undergraduate nurses. QSEN in collaboration with the Institute of Medicine (IOM, 2003) developed specific competencies to prepare nurses to have the knowledge, skills, and attitudes (KSAs) necessary to continuously improve the quality and safety of the organizations in which they work (Cronenwett et al., 2007). Patient-centered care, teamwork and collaboration, evidence-based practice, quality improvement, safety, and informatics are all vital competencies for nursing leadership and management. Table 16.1 highlights those QSEN competencies that are relevant to management roles in professional nursing.

Assess your own management skills in relation to the QSEN competencies. What skills, knowledge, and attitudes do you still need to develop (Box 16.3)?

TABLE 16.1 QSEN COMPETENCIES RELEVANT TO MANAGEMENT ROLES
Evidence-based practice **Integrate best current evidence with clinical expertise and patient/family preferences and values for delivery of optimal healthcare**
• Participate in structuring the work environment to facilitate the integration of new evidence into standards of practice (evidence-based practice: Skills) • Value the need for continuous improvement in clinical practice on the basis of new knowledge (evidence-based practice: Attitudes)
Quality improvement **Use data to monitor the outcomes of care process and use improvement methods to design and test changes to continuously improve the quality and safety of healthcare systems**
• Practice aligning the aims, measures, and changes involved in improving care and use measures to evaluate the effect of change (quality improvement: Skills) • Appreciate that continuous quality improvement is an essential part of the daily work of all health professionals (quality improvement: Attitudes)
Safety **Minimize risk of harm to patients and providers through both system effectiveness and individual performance**
• Describe processes used in understanding causes of error and allocation of responsibility and accountability (e.g., root cause analysis and failure mode effects analysis; safety: Knowledge) • Use national patient safety resources for own professional development and to focus attention on safety in care settings (safety: Skills) • Apply technology and information management tools to support safe processes of care (informatics: Skills)
Informatics **Use information and technology to communicate, manage knowledge, mitigate error, and support decision-making**
• Recognize the time, effort, and skill required for computers, databases, and other technologies to become reliable and effective tools for patient care (informatics: Knowledge) • Use information management tools to monitor outcomes of care processes (informatics: Skills) • Appreciate the necessity for all health professionals to seek lifelong, continuous learning or information technology skills (informatics: Attitudes) • Value nurses' involvement in design, selection, implementation, and evaluation of information technologies to support patient care (informatics: Attitudes)

BOX 16.3 SELF-ASSESSMENT OF MANAGEMENT SKILLS

Think of how you manage in various situations. How would you rate your personal management skills?

Skill	Unsatisfactory	Weak	Average	Good	Excellent
Organization					
Strategic planning/ objective setting					
Time management					
Interpersonal and relationship building					
Communication					
Problem-solving					
Leading					
Delegation					
Emotional intelligence					
Decision-making ability					
Controlling costs					
People development					
Discipline					
Conflict resolution					

CONCLUSION

This chapter reviewed the concept of management and provided a general description of each of the management theories. The importance of managing human and fiscal resources was highlighted. The steps of the management process were reviewed and key management skills that are beneficial for a manager or leader to possess were discussed. Analyzing one's personal management was explored and related to QSEN.

CRITICAL THINKING QUESTIONS AND EXERCISES

- Assess your management skills using the quiz on the following website: www.mindtools.com/pages/article/newTMM_28.htm. Review your quiz results. With what skills are you comfortable? What skills could use further development? What surprised you? How will you use these results to make improvements in how you manage as a nurse?
- Ask your supervisor whether it is possible to review the budget. What are the biggest expenses for your practice area? Is it the staffing, equipment, supplies, or some other line item? Are costs increasing or decreasing? What actions can be taken to reduce costs while still maintaining the quality of care? How much of the budget is spent on staffing? Is there overtime? If so, how much is overtime affecting the bottom line?
- Work with your supervisor to determine the turnover rate in your practice area. Determine what it costs to hire and orient a new nurse to your practice area.

REFERENCES

American Association of Colleges of Nursing. (2008). *The essentials of baccalaureate education for professional nursing practice*. Washington, DC: Author.

Barnat, R. (2014). Strategic management: Formulation and implementation. Retrieved from http://www.introduction-to-management.24xls.com/en107

Boeing, G. (2016). Visual analysis of nonlinear dynamical systems: Chaos, fractals, self-similarity and the limits of prediction. *Systems, 4*(4), 37. doi:10.3390/systems4040037

Bums, J. S. (2016). Chaos theory and leadership studies: Exploring uncharted seas. *Journal of Leadership and Organizational Studies, 9*(2), 42–56. doi:10.1177/107179190200900204

Burke, W. W. (2017). *Organization change: Theory and practice*. Thousand Oaks, CA: Sage.

Bush, T. (2007). Educational leadership and management: Theory, policy and practice. *South African Journal of Education, 27*(3), 391–406.

Cole, G. A. (2004). *Management theory and practice* (6th ed.). Boston, MA: Cengage Learning EMEA.

Cronenwett, L., Sherwood, G., Barnsteiner, J., Disch, J., Johnson, J., Mitchell, P., ... Warren, J. (2007). Quality and safety education for nurses. *Nursing Outlook, 55*(33), 122–131. doi:10.1016/j.outlook.2007.02.006

Fayol, H. (1949). *General and industrial management*. London, UK: Pitman & Sons.

Gladwin, T. N., Kennelly, J. J., & Krause, T. S. (1995). Shifting paradigms for sustainable development: Implications for management theory and research. *Academy of Management Review, 20*(4), 874–907. doi:10.2307/258959

Hill, C. W., Jones, G. R., & Schilling, M. A. (2014). *Strategic management: Theory and integrated approach*. Boston, MA: Cengage.

Institute of Medicine. (2003). *Health professions education: A bridge to quality*. Washington, DC: National Academies Press.

Kiggundu, M. N., Jørgensen, J. J., & Hafsi, T. (1983). Administrative theory and practice in developing countries: A synthesis. *Administrative Science Quarterly, 28*(1), 66–84. doi:10.2307/2392387

Koontz, H., & Weihrich, H. (1990). *Essentials of management*. New York, NY: McGraw-Hill.

Mohamed, R. K. M. H., & Nor, C. S. M. (2013). The relationship between McGregors X-Y theory management style and fulfillment of psychological contract: A literature review. *International Journal of Academic Research in Business and Social Sciences*, 3(5), 715.

Otley, D. T. (2016). The contingency theory of management accounting and control: 1980-2014. *Management and Accounting Research*, 31, 45–62. doi:10.1016/j.mar.2016.02.001

Schneider, A., Wickert, C., & Marti, E. (2017). Reducing complexity by creating complexity: A systems theory perspective on how organizations respond to their environments. *Journal of Management Studies*, 54(2), 182–208. doi:10.1111/joms.12206

Shafritz, J. M., Ott, J. S., & Jang, Y. S. (2015). *Classics of organization theory*. Boston, MA: Cengage Learning.

Waring, S. P. (2016). *Taylorism transformed: Scientific management theory since 1945*. Chapel Hill: University of North Carolina Press.

17

CARE DELIVERY MODELS, STAFFING, AND SCHEDULING

KAREN BURROWS

LEARNING OBJECTIVES

After completion of this chapter, the reader will be able to

- Describe patient and nursing care delivery models for staffing.
- Analyze the strengths and weaknesses of patient classification systems and nursing workload measurement systems.
- Compare and contrast nurse staffing and scheduling methods and models.
- Discuss leader and manager responsibilities to meet staffing needs.

Nurses understand the importance of having the correct number of nursing staff to provide safe, quality care to patients. Currently, 17 states have legislation that addresses staffing levels in hospitals (Tevington, 2011), with California remaining as the only state mandating staffing ratios. The other states have legislation that surrounds staffing plans with staff input or chief nursing officer (CNO)-driven staffing plans. The American Nurses Association (ANA) supports the development of unit-specific staffing plans that can account for changes occurring on a nursing unit and are flexible to ensure patient safety and provision of quality care (ANA, 2017). As nurses, we know that ratios require knowledge of patient acuity to make sound staffing decisions. One size does not fit all. Budgets often dictate the number of staff we can have based on a historical average of nursing hours needed per patient day (NHPPD). Yet the budget does not account for the amount of nursing time needed by the patient.

Appropriate scheduling can help to decrease nursing overtime, thus providing better management of fiscal resources. Unfortunately, even the best schedule is subject to unexpected changes. An unforeseen nursing absence on a unit with an inexperienced charge nurse may lead to a unit shortage requiring a manager "borrowing" a nurse from another unit or adjusting the schedule and having someone come in on a different day. This shifting of employees will buy time to fix the staffing shortage but may lead to issues further in the week.

Safe, appropriate staffing is a challenge for hospitals to manage. This chapter reviews patient and nursing care models, patient classification systems (PCSs), staffing and scheduling models, leader and manager staffing and scheduling responsibilities, and ways to make self-scheduling a positive experience for nurses. As part of our accountability to our patients and the profession, nurses need knowledge of the process of staffing and scheduling and to be actively involved in the process.

The case scenario given in Box 17.1 highlights concerns around safe/ appropriate staffing.

QUESTIONS TO CONSIDER BEFORE READING ON

- What type of nursing care or patient delivery model is used at your place of employment?
- What are the benefits and disadvantages of the model used?

NURSING AND PATIENT CARE DELIVERY MODELS

A nursing care delivery model describes how nursing care is delivered to the patient in a specific health system (Davidson, Halcomb, Hickman, Phillips, & Graham, 2006). It often takes into account the skill mix and number and type of staff and available resources on a given unit or at a specific facility and serves as the "infrastructure" for how care should

BOX 17.1 CASE SCENARIO

As you read the following case scenario, reflect on the situation. What could be done to help alleviate the staffing issue? How did staffing influence the quality and safety of care provided?

Tom is the night charge registered nurse (RN) on a 36-bed geriatric medical surgical floor that is filled to capacity. It is Friday night and the unit experienced two sick calls leaving four of the required nurses. By 4 a.m., neither Tom nor the other three RNs have had the ability to take a break or ensure that all patients have been toileted every 2 hours. It is then that they hear a loud crash and find Mrs. Jones, admitted with dehydration and a urinary tract infection (UTI), unconscious on the floor on her side. The roommate states that Mrs. Jones was getting up to use the bathroom. Mrs. Jones suffered an epidural hematoma, and likely will never regain consciousness.

be provided (Jost, Bonnell, Chacko, & Parkinson, 2010). Some of the more traditional nursing models are task driven, whereas others look to understand the patient and needs for timely discharge (Rhéaume et al., 2015). Some models are more innovative and look at how the nurse will be used in a virtual patient care environment (Klingensmith & Knodel, 2016). Despite the variety of models available, research has shown that nurses adapt and change their roles regardless of model to meet the needs of the current patients for whom they care (Rhéaume et al., 2015). Some of the more traditional nursing care delivery models are explained in the subsequent text and in Table 17.1.

The **patient-focused care (PFC) model** originated in the United States in the 1980s with the goal of cost containment combined with the provision of more direct nursing care. Nurses achieved this goal providing

TABLE 17.1 NURSING CARE DELIVERY MODELS

Care Model	Advantages	Disadvantages
Primary nursing: The same nurse cares for the same patients when he or she works (Seago, 2001)	• Consistency with plan of care • Better patient outcomes	• All-RN model, no UAP • Does not take acuity into consideration
Team/functional nursing: Team members are assigned care duties on the basis of their skill set and scope of care. Examples: RN as IV medication nurse, CNA completing vital signs and baths, LPN as the PO medication nurse (Seago, 2001)	• Allows for coordination of a greater number of patients with fewer staff • Can be used with LPN and UAP	• All are working under the scope of the RN's license • Trust must exist between team members that tasks are completed and all changes are communicated to the team
Modular nursing: Care provided in pods. Each pod is made up of licensed staff and may contain unlicensed workers. Staff always care for patients in one geographic location on the unit (Mensik, 2014)	• Uses the primary care model • Reduces RN fatigue from time spent in a search or find • Everything needed is located in the pod • Workers have > autonomy in the pod	• Less familiar with other pods if census requires a pod shift • Could miss trends more easily identified when looking at the unit as a whole (e.g., side effects of new medications)
Float nursing: One nurse is left without an assignment to be assigned to help out where needed (e.g., doing the admissions for a nurse completing discharges; Mensik, 2014)	• Can help in high-volume-turnover units	• Hard to quantify work done during the shift to provide evidence of necessity • Perceived inequities in who gets the help can occur

CNA, certified nursing assistant; IV, intravenous; LPN, licensed practical nurse; PO, oral; RN, registered nurse; UAP, unlicensed assistive personnel.

more individualized care in the role of care managers, with unlicensed assistive personnel (UAP) completing task-oriented care roles such as performing electrocardiograms (ECGs) and drawing blood. The advantages of the model are continuity of care, better understanding of individualized needs of the patient as a whole making it holistic in nature, and improved nurse satisfaction. The disadvantages are perceived increased in workload left to the bedside nurse and assistive personnel (Kjörnsberg, Karlsson, Babra, & Wadensten, 2010).

The **primary/total patient care delivery model** is the oldest model with its origins coming from the work of Florence Nightingale, and echoed in patient care provided by nursing students in the 1930s; it made a resurgence in the 1980s. In this model, the RN delivers total nursing care to the patient and cares for the same patient during the patient's stay (Tiedeman & Lookinland, 2004). This model aligns the most to professional nursing practice. Advantages include the nurse has fewer patients and cares for the same patients, improving continuity of care even when not present via the care plan. The length of stay is usually decreased. Disadvantages include the lack of UAP to provide patient care, requiring the nurse to complete all the administrative patient care tasks as well as physical care tasks, and an all-RN staff is used, which is more costly than use of UAPs and LPNs (Jost et al., 2010).

In the 1950s, the **team-based nursing model** was developed with the premise that improved care could be given using a team of individuals versus a single individual. In team nursing, the entire team provides care for all patients under the direction of a nurse who functions as team leader. Care is assigned by the leader on the basis of skills, knowledge, and the complexity of the patient (Jost et al., 2010). The advantage of this model is that it requires collaborative care and communication, both of which are needed for quality patient care (IOM, 2003). The disadvantages are that it requires a team leader who has strong leadership skills along with hands-on care experience to ensure effective communication, and it remains one of the most expensive models of care (Jost et al., 2010).

In **modular nursing**, patients are cared for in care pods. Care provided is location based where one nurse and UAP might care for four to six patients. The nurse is assigned mostly to the same pod. The advantages of this model are continuity of care and reduced length of stay. The disadvantage is that assignment workload is not taken into consideration, which could result in heavy assignments, poor staff satisfaction, reduced quality, and poor patient outcomes (Mensik, 2014).

Functional nursing had its debut in the 1940s. In functional nursing, each member of the nursing team completed a function for the patient on the basis of an individual's skill and knowledge. Tasks were delegated in a top-down, hierarchical approach. Functional nursing was dependent on following policies and procedures. Some of the tasks assigned were to the dressing nurse and to the medication nurse. The nurse manager was responsible to ensure the completion of all skills, whereas the charge nurse made all care decisions. The advantage is cost-effectiveness with the ability to complete tasks in a timely manner similar to an assembly line. Disadvantages include fragmentation of care (only the manager knew the entire patient picture), and bedside nurses never had opportunities for professional nursing growth through clinical decision-making (Tiedeman & Lookinland, 2004).

Float nursing is when there is a nurse without an assignment who helps out on the unit where needed. This can occur using any of the aforementioned models. The advantage of this model is that it can help to decompress heavy workloads such as high-volume admissions and discharges. The disadvantages are the cost of always having one extra person around without an assignment and lack of measurable productivity for unit budgeting. Depending on a unit's staffing mix of licensed and unlicensed staff, one model may be better than another and it may mean that one model cannot be consistently used (Mensik, 2014).

The final model whose popularity is increasing on the horizon is the **innovative care delivery model.** This model uses technology to expand the area to which nursing care is provided through the use of telehealth and videoconferencing equipment. The advantage of this model is that it allows for cost-effective quality outcomes for patients in areas where they would not have had access to care earlier. It also allows nurses to develop critical thinking skills and advanced nursing knowledge. The disadvantages include the cost of high-resolution equipment and the inability of the nurse to provide a complete hands-on assessment (Klingensmith & Knodel, 2016).

Patient care delivery models are broader than nursing care delivery models and describe how all members of the health team operate, not just nurses. They depict how the team (nurse, physician, administration) operates to provide quality patient care. A couple of examples of patient care delivery models are highlighted as follows (Mensik, 2014):

- **Planetree patient-centered care:** All staff members (nurses, unit clerks, physicians, etc.) are caregivers whose role is to meet the patients' needs. Patients are viewed as unique individuals with diverse needs who are partners in their care.
- **Transitional care model:** In this model, care is provided and coordinated by the same master's-prepared advanced practice RN in partnership with the patient, the family caregivers, the physician, and other health team members (Naylor, 2012). The transitional care model focuses on the identification of patients' health goals, the design and implementation of the plan of care, and continuity of care across settings and across providers throughout episodes of illness.
- **Magnet® hospital environment/shared governance:** Magnet organizations are distinguished by a high degree of nursing autonomy, physician–nurse collaboration, and nurse control of practice. This model allows for shared decision-making by the nurses and managers.

QUESTIONS TO CONSIDER BEFORE READING ON

- Does your healthcare agency in which you are employed use a patient classification system (PCS) or nursing workload measurement?
- If yes, what measures does it use and why?
- If not, explain why a PCS or nursing workload measurement is not used.

PATIENT CLASSIFICATION SYSTEMS

Patient classification systems (PCSs) are used to provide a quantitative measure of workload for the determination of staffing needs by measuring the amount of care a patient requires using objective measures such as vital signs, treatments, and number of medications (Daraiseh, Vidonish, Kiessling, & Lin, 2016). Initially, PCSs were used to analyze physician practice patterns and resource utilization of hospitalized patients (Arbitman, 1986; Swan & Griffin, 2005). Some examples of these PCSs include diagnosis-related groups (DRGs) and medical illness severity grouping systems (MEDIS-GRPS).

NURSING WORKLOAD MEASUREMENT SYSTEMS

Historically, when nurses left private duty and joined to provide care in hospitals after World War II, the cost for nursing care was made part of the room and board charges. Ever since, nurses have been trying to separate out what they provide for care to quantifiably measure it (Welton, 2007). This has now been termed "nursing workload."

The case scenario given in Box 17.2 highlights nursing workload measurement systems and how they influence patient care.

BOX 17.2 CASE SCENARIO

As you read this case scenario, reflect on how the lack of a nursing workload measurement system may have influenced patient care. What are the benefits of patient ratios?

Joan is working nights on a medical surgical nursing unit. The nurse-to-patient ratio for her floor is one nurse to six patients. The hospital does not have a nursing workload measurement system and assigns patients on the basis of pods. Joan's assignment consists of three patients on precautions for hospital-acquired infections, a patient with pneumonia requiring frequent suctioning, a day 2 knee replacement, and fresh postoperative thyroidectomy. Joan is concerned about her assignment because the patient with pneumonia has been evaluated six times by the Rapid Evaluation Team today.

Nursing workload measurement system measures the intensity with which nurses care for patients and is inclusive of direct and indirect care provided (Myny et al., 2011). It also takes into account the time for provision of direct patient care (Shullanberger, 2000). To clarify, many terms are used when referring to nursing workload measures such as workload management systems, nursing workload, PCSs/instruments, and timed activity classification systems (Swan & Griffin, 2005). No matter what term is used, these systems were developed to quantify nursing practice.

Considering that nurses play a vital role in the well-being of our patients and provide the greatest number of care hours for patients, it is essential that we understand the work nurses perform. That is where patient classification and workload measurement systems come in for nursing. These systems grew from our need to be able to forecast the number of nurses needed to care for patients in the hospital on a daily basis. Initially, these systems looked at nursing tasks.

The original measure of nursing workload, the PCS, was developed in the 1960s. The PCS uses indicators and characteristics to categorize patients requiring different levels of care and has undergone several revisions over the years resulting in several systems on the basis of patient type (Siew & Ghani, 2006). An example of a workload system specific to a patient population is the therapeutic intervention scoring system (TISS) for critically ill children. The TISS looks at patient acuity as well as nursing care interventions on the basis of the latest evidence to determine workload and appropriate unit staffing for the pediatric ICU (Trope, Vaz, Zinger, & Sagy, 2015).

Over time, the workload systems have advanced, allowing us to incorporate elements such as risk, complexity of services, and skill level. Typically, these systems look at discriminating indicators intended to place a patient into the correct patient type so we can measure the nursing workload for that patient. Data from the system in conjunction with other measures can be used for staffing decisions, trending, tracking, and budgeting. Although these systems initially were used in hospital settings, they are now also used in other settings such as ambulatory care (Swan & Griffin, 2005). It is important to note that not all organizations chose to use patient classification and nursing workload measurement systems. Strengths and weaknesses of these systems are noted in a paper published by the Registered Nurses Association of Ontario (2005) and some are highlighted as follows:

Strengths of workload measurement systems:

- They can be used to make decisions regarding the allocation of resources.
- They can be integrated with electronic health record to link workload with patient characteristics and clinical outcomes.
- They can be integrated with electronic health record to link standards with financial data to ascertain costs.

- They can potentially contribute to the quality of care by providing justification for appropriate resource distribution.

Weaknesses of workload measurement systems:

- Not all systems have been integrated into the electronic health record.
- The success of systems that are integrated into the electronic health record has not been consistent.
- Not all workload measurement systems have been validated and thus may not accurately reflect the work of nursing.
- Some have unrealistic expectations about the application of the measurement systems.
- Workload measurement systems may be used to control costs, which is not their intended purpose. This in turn will lead to staff not endorsing or participating in the systems.

QUESTIONS TO CONSIDER BEFORE READING ON

Does your institution have policies and procedures developed for nursing staffing and scheduling models? If yes, what do they say? Have the policies and procedures been developed collaboratively? Were needs assessment data incorporated into the nursing staffing and scheduling model?

STAFFING AND SCHEDULING

One of the most important decisions to be made in hospitals has to do with nurse staffing and scheduling as these decisions are directly related to quality of patient care (Aiken, Clarke, Cheung, Sloane, & Silber, 2003; Person et al., 2004). Such decisions are not easy because they are influenced by the need for round-the-clock staffing on hospital units, delivery of quality patient care, and cost containment. Often times, patients are kept in the hospital only if they need highly skilled nursing care. The case scenario in Box 17.3 highlights a staffing and scheduling concern in nursing.

Given the variability on patient care units, nursing leaders can spend an incredible amount of time dealing with scheduling and staffing issues. Although scheduling is done weeks in advance, the management of staffing levels is handled on a daily basis. Staffing and scheduling are typically grouped together but they are not interchangeable terms.

STAFFING

"Staffing" refers to having sufficient nurses with the right mix of expertise to care for the patient workload (Rose, 2016). Although unit schedules are created months in advance, the actual required unit staffing is often projected

BOX 17.3 CASE SCENARIO

Consider the following questions as you read this case scenario:

- In this scenario, the charge nurse will be working with the manager to fill the shift vacancy created by the "sick call-in." What is the manager's role in this scenario?
- Is it the manager's responsibility that the next shift is now short a nurse?
- What should Suzy do first to fix the staffing vacancy?

Suzy is the day shift charge nurse for the second time today. It is 10 a.m. and she is looking at the staffing for the next shift with the knowledge that the unit will be receiving eight postoperative orthopedic patients between 2 p.m. and 4 p.m. She also has six planned patient discharges that have been staggered from 11 a.m. to 2 p.m. Between discharges and admissions, the unit will be full at 26 patients. The nursing staffing matrix for her unit indicates that for 26 patients, she is allowed six nurses and no certified nursing assistants (CNAs). She currently has five registered nurses (RNs) for evenings because of one "sick call-in" from an RN. There is no availability from the staffing office or sister unit.

no further than 24 hours in advance of a weekday shift and 48 hours for weekends or holidays.

The full-time equivalents (FTEs) are usually calculated from the average daily census (ADC) and average NHPPD from the prior year (Kirby, 2015) to determine the required number of staff for a given unit. The total number of required staff for a unit takes into account vacation/holiday/sick (VHS) days and paid time off (PTO). An FTE is equal to one person working 40 hours per week (Marquis & Huston, 2015).

SCHEDULING

"Scheduling," as opposed to staffing, refers to determining a set number and skill mix of staff for a future time period on the basis of factors such as census, acuity, and anticipated volumes (Rose, 2016). Each unit/hospital will have a set time frame for which they schedule. For example, a unit may have 4-week schedules, whereas others book as far out as 3 months.

Scheduling for a unit requires that there be the correct skill mix of licensed and unlicensed care providers to meet the needs of the unit. Schedules are made to ensure that there is sufficient staff to operationalize the unit's care delivery model. The schedule should have the correct mix of full-time and part-time employees to ensure adequate staffing with coverage for sick days, leaves, and vacations. This can be seen in the partial schedule in Table 17.2. The task of staff scheduling is either centralized or decentralized.

TABLE 17.2 SAMPLE SCHEDULE

Name	FTE	Saturday	Sunday	Monday	Tuesday	Wednesday	Thursday	Friday	Saturday	Sunday
RN1	1.0	7	7	7	3	3	Off	7	Off	Off
RN2	.8	Off	Off	7	7	Off	Off	7	7	7
RN3	1.0	7	7	Off	Off	7	7	3	Off	Off
RN4	1.0	Off	Off	7	7	3	Off	7	7	7
RN5	1.0	7	7	3	Off	Off	7	3	Off	Off
RN6	1.0	Off	Off	3	3	3	3	Off	7	7
RN7	1.0	7	7	Off	7	7	3	3	Off	Off
RN8	.6	Off	Off	Off	3	3	Off	Off	7	7
RN9	1.0	7	7	7	Off	7	7	3	Off	Off
RN10	.6	Off	Off	7	7	Off	Off	Off	7	7
RN11	.6	7	7	Off	3	3	Off	7	Off	Off
RN12	.6	Off	Off	3-SC	3	Off	Off	Off	7	7
RN13	.8	3	3	Off	Off	7	3	3	Off	Off
RN14	.8	Off	Off	3	V	V	Off	Off	3	3
RN15	.6	3	3	Off	Off	3 sick	3	3	Off	Off
RN16	.6	Off	Off	3	3	Off	Off	Off	3	3

RN17	PD	3	3	Off	Off	7-SC	3	Off	Off	Off
RN18	.6	Off	Off	3	3-SC	Off	Off	Off	3	3
RN19	.8	3	3	Off	Off	7	7	7	Off	Off
RN20	.8	Off	Off	3	3	Off	3	Off	3	3
RN21	.8	3	3	Off	7	7	Off	7	Off	Off
RN22	.8	Off	Off	7-SC	7	Off	7	Off	3	3
RN23	PD	3	3	V	V	V	V	V	Off	Off
RN24	.8	Off	Off	7	7	Off	7	Off	3	3
RN25	PD	M	M	M	M	M	M	M	M	M
Day total		6	6	7	7	7	6	6	6	6
Eve total		6	6	7	7	6-5	6	6	6	6

3, 3 p.m. to 11.30 p.m.; 7, 7 a.m. to 3.30 p.m.; FTE, full-time equivalent; M, maternity leave; PD, personal day; RN, registered nurse; SC, shift cancelled; V, vacation.

Centralized Staffing

Centralized staffing means that one department handles the staffing for all units in the hospital. This includes all call-ins, call-outs, and floats. With centralized staffing, the burden of finding staff is left to someone outside the unit who may or may not be a nurse (Marquis & Huston, 2015). With centralized staffing, it is imperative that the charge nurse communicate the unit's needs with regards to admissions, transfers, and patient acuity to the centralized staffing personnel. The centralized team will make all staffing decisions (vacations, time off, etc.) on the basis of the needs of the facility in a cost-efficient manner while ensuring that staffing policies are followed (Marquis & Huston, 2015).

The centralized staffing model has both advantages and disadvantages. An advantage of the centralized system is that it takes the nurse manager out of handling the last-minute call-outs and scheduling errors so his or her time can be used more effectively. In addition, it looks at the staffing needs of the entire organization so resources are deployed on an as-needed basis. For example, a nurse leader/manager might be overstaffed on one unit and would send the extra nurse home; with centralized staffing, that nurse would be sent to assist another unit lacking staff required for that shift so resources are more efficiently used. A disadvantage of the centralized system is that the centralized staffing employee(s) may not know the appropriate skill mix needed to maintain safe, quality patient care (Crist-Grundman & Mulrooney, 2011). Therefore, it is important that unit nurse managers/leaders clearly communicate staffing needs to the centralized staffing team.

QUESTION TO CONSIDER BEFORE READING ON

Using the prior case scenario, if the centralized office told Suzy it does not have a nurse but can give her two nurses' aides, would this be appropriate given the number of admissions and discharges?

Decentralized Staffing

Decentralized staffing means that the nursing manager or designee decides on the level of staffing required prior to and during the shift (Marquis & Huston, 2015). According to the ANA, it is the manager's role to ensure that staff have the resources to do their job with the highest level of quality (ANA, 2016). An advantage of decentralized staffing is that it ensures that the correct staffing mix is used based on census (Mensik, 2014). All staffing decisions to increase and decrease numbers of staff are at the discretion of the manager, allowing control over the unit's staffing budget.

A disadvantage is that there is no way to get emergency staffing relief from outside the unit unless a sister unit (a like or similar unit) is part of the decentralized staffing plan. Hospitals have found this model to be more costly, despite increased staff satisfaction, because it frequently results in an increase in hours per patient day without a change in the flat rate payment system (Shullanberger, 2000).

Decentralized staffing allows for the deployment of self-scheduling. Self-scheduling is known to improve staff work satisfaction as well as improve quality patient outcomes (Shullanberger, 2000). Units must have a clear knowledge of the unit as well as hospital staffing policies and they must be consistently enforced for self-scheduling to be effective. Some staffing software systems allow for staffing guidelines to be built in for building an electronic self-schedule taking into consideration nursing skill sets, required weekends, and holidays.

QUESTIONS TO CONSIDER BEFORE READING ON

- Using Table 17.3 as a guide, how many FTEs will be needed to cover nights? The staffing matrix maximum number of RNs needed is six, and each RN must work every other weekend.
- What care model have you used in your practice? Do you think another model would be more efficient in providing care and why?
- Does your current unit use LPNs and CNAs? If so, what is the skill mix you have to have if the unit is full?

As nurses become increasingly involved in making staffing and scheduling decisions for their unit, it is important for them to engage in effective communication and understand unit quality metrics that represent sufficient staffing, as well as technology used for scheduling and quality metric management as part of their nursing practice. Quality and Safety Education for Nurses (QSEN) has developed such competencies for the baccalaureate-prepared nurse, and the ones pertaining to staffing and scheduling have been outlined in Table 17.3.

CRITICAL THINKING EXERCISE

Given the aforementioned schedule, help Suzy plan her next steps. Who can Suzy call to assist her with coverage for Wednesday evenings?

TABLE 17.3 DEVELOPING STAFFING AND SCHEDULING SKILLS: RELEVANT QUALITY AND SAFETY EDUCATION FOR NURSES (QSEN) COMPETENCIES
• Examine how the safety, quality, and cost-effectiveness of healthcare can be improved through the active involvement of patients and families (patient-centered care, Knowledge)
• Participate in building consensus or resolving conflict in the context of patient care (patient-centered care, Skills)
• Value continuous improvement of own communication and conflict resolution skills (patient-centered skills, Attitudes)
• Explain how authority gradients influence teamwork and patient safety (teamwork and collaboration, Knowledge)
• Value the need for continuous improvement in clinical practice on the basis of new knowledge (evidence-based practice, Knowledge)
• Describe strategies for learning about the outcomes of care in the setting in which one is engaged in clinical practice (quality improvement, Knowledge)
• Use measures to evaluate the effect of change (quality improvement, Skills)
• Value the contributions of standardization/reliability to safety (safety, Skills)
• Describe examples of how technology and information management are related to the quality and safety of patient care (informatics, Knowledge)
• Value nurses' involvement in design, selection, implementation, and evaluation of information technologies to support patient care (informatics, Skills)

Source: Cronenwett, L., Sherwood, G., Barnsteiner, J., Disch, J., Johnson, J., Mitchell, P., ... Warren, J. (2007). Quality and safety education for nurses. *Nursing Outlook, 55*(3), 122–131. doi:10.1016/j.outlook.2007.02.006; Quality and Safety Education for Nurses Institute. (2014). QSEN competencies. Retrieved from http://qsen.org/competencies/pre-licensure-ksas

QUESTIONS TO CONSIDER BEFORE READING ON

What staffing model(s) are used at your organization? Explain the advantages and disadvantages of this model(s).

STAFFING MODELS

There are three main staffing models (budget based, nurse–patient ratio, and patient acuity). However, no one model is suitable for all settings and all situations. Many hospitals will use several methods to modify the staffing approach to meet their particular needs. Staffing models are highlighted in Table 17.4.

TABLE 17.4 STAFFING MODELS

Staffing Models	How Calculated/ Determined	When to Use/When Not to Use
Budget based, NHPPD	Number of nursing hours worked in 24 hours/ADC	• Used to determine the budgeted FTE for a care unit using the following: • NHPPD × volume annually/2,080 (hours in one FTE per year) • Budgeted NHPPD should not be used to develop static staffing tables (Kirby, 2015)
Patient care ratios	Set by unions, legislation, and organizations Unit-specific RN to patient limits	• Good when trying to achieve minimal staffing measures • Does not take into account the acuity of the patients (Welton, 2007)
Acuities	Uses patient characteristics (vital signs, number of IVs, and invasive equipment, etc.) to determine direct care hours required. Calculated usually by a software program	• Used for leveling assignments and justifying excess staff • Does not take into account user entry discrepancies for nonconcrete measures such as independence (Sherman et al., 2010)
Care workload	Computer generated from existing databases	• Yet to be determined in development (Miller, 2016)

ADC, average daily census; FTE, full-time equivalent; NHPPD, nursing hours per patient day; RN, registered nurse.

BUDGET-BASED STAFFING MODELS

Budget-based staffing models allocate nursing staff on the basis of the NHPPD. Typically, the number of hours per patient day is divided by the total number of patient days to determine the staffing levels on the basis of regional or national benchmarks.

When discussing RN-only staffing, NHPPD is most commonly used to look at nursing workload and is a reportable quality metric to the National Database of Nursing Quality Indicators (NDNQI), where data have demonstrated that higher NHPPD resulted in improved quality outcomes (Montalvo, 2007). The trending of NHPPD and patient outcomes by NDNQI is closely monitored by the ANA to determine when workforce policy will need to be developed (ANA, 2016).

NHPPD is easily calculated and allows institutions to compare staffing levels with quality outcome measures. It is based on the average historical care hours needed for a particular unit. This type of model is driven by the ADC, where the number of hours worked in 24 hours is divided by the census, essentially assigning every patient the same number of care hours (Kirby, 2015). This methodology works when patients are of varying levels of acuity, and does not work when the census exceeds the ADC. This particular model requires managers to constantly track changes in patient volume to ensure that staffing is adjusted (Sherman, Martinez-Soto, Peters, Mathew, & Pischke-Winn, 2010).

NURSE–PATIENT RATIO

Nurse–patient ratio staffing models use the number of patients on the unit to determine the number of nurses. This model often does not factor in the patient needs, acuity levels, or nursing judgment. It indicates exactly how many nurses are allowed per shift per number of patients. Some states mandate the nurse–patient ratios. Each patient is allowed the same number of hours from the RN per shift. When using ratios, once a unit hits its maximum allotted patients per nurse, it can refuse future admissions until more staff are obtained. In hospital-driven ratios, minimal and maximal staffing can be adjusted to meet the needs of the patient, so ratios are what hospitals strive to achieve (Mensik, 2014). It is important to note that Buerhaus (2009, 2010) reviewed outcomes from the mandated ratios in California and found that set ratios did not reduce pressure ulcer prevalence or falls. As a result, perhaps set ratios are not the best methodology to improve care quality.

STAFFING MATRIX

Staffing matrices are similar to ratios in that they allow a set number of care providers of varied skill levels on the basis of the census from the prior shift. Unit staffing matrices are commonly built based on ADC and NHPPD data that are either historical or projected. The goal is to control the staffing budget by keeping NHPPD neutral. This model differs from ratios as it allows for assignment adjustments on the basis of acuity. For example, if the preferred unit ratio is one nurse to six patients and one patient requires more intensive nursing care, then one RN may have seven patients so the RN caring for this patient can spend the additional time (Loden, 2011). The case scenario in Box 17.4 highlights a staffing issue in a hospital that uses a staffing matrix.

PATIENT ACUITY

Patient acuity staffing models use the patient's level of care complexity to determine the staffing needs. Acuities use specific patient characteristics from nursing assessment to determine their complexity and direct care hours required (Sherman et al., 2010). The problem with acuity-based systems is the variability in measures collected as well as the variability in the individual completing the assessment. It is also not a measure that can be compared nationally with access quality care outcomes.

BOX 17.4 THE CASE SCENARIO CONTINUES TO UNFOLD

As you read this case scenario, try to answer the following question:

What type of nursing staffing model should Suzy consider because she no longer has an all-RN team to care for the 26 patients on the night shift? What other solutions would you suggest to Suzy?

Suzy does not work in a state with mandated nurse–patient ratios. Her hospital uses a staffing matrix to determine the number of staff required for her floor. Suzy has been alerted to a sick call by the centralized staffing office. If she is unable to persuade someone to come in, she will have to increase the number of patients for each nurse, not following the prescribed matrix. Suzy understands that this could affect the quality of patient care so she opts to accept the two nurses' aides from the centralized staffing office to ease the burden on the remaining RNs.

CARE WORKLOAD

A future staffing model called "care workload" is currently in development. Software engineers are developing and testing products that will take into account census, acuity on the basis of the number of direct and indirect care interventions, as well as skill mix required for clinicians. This computer program will generate the needed staffing for a given unit taking into consideration the factors discussed earlier. This calculation is referred to as a care workload because it encompasses the nursing process, patient teaching, emotional support, administrative work done to care for patients, as well as an element of unpredictability, or as we nurses call it the "what if" factor, making this new measure the closest thing to quantify what a nurse truly does on a daily basis (Miller, 2016).

THE AMERICAN NURSES ASSOCIATION'S VIEW ON STAFFING

The ANA (2012) staffing principles state that staffing needs to take into account the number and skill mix of individuals needed to provide safe quality care. They state that the RN must be a part of the staffing decision process, as well as a collaborator with other healthcare officials. In 2015, the Registered Nurse Safe Staffing Act was introduced, requiring all hospitals that receive Medicare funds to develop staffing plans and levels that ensure safe patient care. This act also required that hospitals form staffing committees and have in place whistleblower protections for those who report unsafe staffing levels (Senate Bill 1132, 2015). This was supported by the ANA and allowed states to develop flexible nurse staffing plans (ANA, 2016).

According to Becker's Hospital Review, the American Hospital Association (AHA), direct care providers are responsible for over 50% of a hospital's costs. The AHA is in agreement that correct levels of staffing are required for patient safety/quality care. It also knows that staffing overages are fiscally irresponsible, and could financially ruin healthcare institutions. Given that the fiscal health of the facility is at stake, they believe that acceptable staffing levels should be determined by the hospital rather than by legislative mandated ratios or union-based staffing minimums (Schouten, 2013).

The ANA has called for the transparent reporting of staffing and skill mix data to the National Quality Forum (NQF) to improve patient outcomes. The retrospective study of Aiken et al. (2014) looked at patient outcomes on the basis of increased workload and nursing education level. In this study, she identified that for every one patient increase in a nurse's workload, there was a resultant 7% increase in an inpatient dying within 30 days of admission to the hospital. She also found that she could decrease that 7% by 7% for every 10% of nurses who held their BSN. These results support that the nursing skill mix must be rich with BSN-prepared nurses to reduce hospital mortality.

THE NURSE MANAGER'S RESPONSIBILITY FOR STAFFING AND SCHEDULING

According to the American Organization of Nurse Executives (AONE) competencies for nurse managers, the responsibilities of the manager include the following: staff selection, evaluation of staffing patterns, matching staff competencies to assignments, defining the role of the staff members within their scope of practice, and completing and evaluating the orientation process (AONE, 2015). In this era of cost reduction in healthcare, nurse managers need to take responsibility of their staffing budget and ensure that safe staffing levels are met in a fiscally responsible manner (Schouten, 2013). Part of this is trending unit data to determine where staffing levels fall short. For example, consider if all nurses start at 7 a.m. and the staffing takes into account admissions and discharges taking place at 11 a.m. or later. Would it be better to have a nurse start later in the shift and overlap the next until patients are settled and documentation completed? Staggered starts are a way managers can make a fiscally responsible improvement to staffing.

When decentralized staffing methods are used, the unit staffing requires 24/7 manager accountability. Because the manager is not present 24/7, this means that the manager must provide staff with the necessary resources and guidelines so they can provide safe quality care in a fiscally responsible manner. The manager should engage staff in the scheduling process so members feel ownership and control over the schedule, while at the same time using hospital policy to guide the schedule, such as every nurse works every other weekend.

The manager's role in staffing will vary in centralized staffing on the basis of the organizational requirements of the manager (Marquis & Huston, 2015). In a centralized staffing model, the manager will have to ask the central office to find staff to fill vacancies. That said, most managers will work to ensure that safe staffing occurs for all shifts regardless of the way staffing is determined for their organizations.

CONCLUSION

This chapter reviewed the different nursing care and patient delivery models used in healthcare organizations, how patient classifications are used, how workload is measured, how staffing levels and schedules are determined based on unit staffing models, as well as the ANA's view on staffing and manager accountability. New terminology such as FTE and NHPPD should start and look like calculations, and you may already be answering that question of "why didn't they let us have that extra nurse last night?" with "I need to talk about a float nurse role to our manager." Remember, regardless of the staffing model used, the end goal is safe, cost-effective, quality care being provided to patients.

CRITICAL THINKING QUESTIONS AND EXERCISES

- You are a member of the self-scheduling committee on your floor and you are preparing to release the Thanksgiving to New Year's schedule for staff self-schedule. In preparation, you marked in everyone's weekend requirement, made a list of what everyone worked the past year, as well as noted the hospital policy on working holidays. Once the schedule is posted for sign up, you noticed that no one has scheduled himself or herself to work the holidays, and several senior staff have stated that the unit policy always said that after 20 years, you need to work only one major holiday a year. This policy is opposite of the hospital nursing policy, which says every other holiday. What action should you take as a leader of the self-scheduling team? What could you have done prior to posting the schedule?
- You are making assignments for the next shift and identify that the staffing matrix on the basis of ADC and NHPPD says that you can keep five of your seven nurses. Hospital policy allows you to float and cancel staff in 4-hour increments. These decisions must be decided within 2 hours of the start of shift. You cancel one RN for 4 hours and commit a second RN to float to your sister unit in the opposite wing. This unit is short three nurses for the coming shift. One hour prior to change of shift, you get two unexpected admissions from the emergency department, changing the number of nurses you need to six. What do you do? Discuss the pros and cons for your choice.
- Make a mock schedule for a newly proposed unit with an anticipated ADC of 20 patients. This unit will use patient ratio–based staffing, five patients to one nurse. The calculated NHPPD for a census of 20 is (96/20 = 4.8) is 4.8. The approved budgeted FTEs for your unit is 16.85. Have you been given enough FTEs to staff your unit 24/7 working 8-hour shifts? How many full-time and part-time persons will you need? Can anyone take a day off?

REFERENCES

Aiken, L. H., Clarke, S. P., Cheung, R. B., Sloane, D. M., & Silber, J. H. (2003). Educational levels of hospital nurses and surgical patient mortality. *Journal of the American Medical Association, 290*(12), 1617–1623. doi:10.1001/jama.290.12.1617

Aiken, L. H., Sloane, D. M., Bruyneel, L., Van den Heede, K., Griffiths, P., Busse, R., Diomidous, M., ... RN4CAST consortium. (2014). Nurse staffing and education and hospital mortality in nine European countries: A retrospective observational study. *Lancet, 383*(9931), 1824–1830. doi:10.1016/S0140-6736(13)62631-8

American Nurses Association. (2012). *ANA's principles for nurse staffing* (2nd ed.). Silver Spring, MD: Author. Retrieved from https://www.nursingworld.org/nurses-books/anas-principles-for-nurse-staffing

American Nurses Association. (2016). Nurse staffing. Retrieved from https://www.nursingworld.org/practice-policy/advocacy/state/nurse-staffing/

American Nurses Association. (2017). Nurse staffing. Retrieved from http://www.nursingworld.org/MainMenuCategories/Policy-Advocacy/State/Legislative-Agenda-Reports/State-StaffingPlansRatios

American Organization of Nurse Executives. (2015). *AONE Nurse manager competencies*. Chicago, IL: Author. Retrieved from http://www.aone.org/resources/nurse-manager-competencies.pdf

Arbitman, D. B. (1986). A primer on patient classification systems and their relevance to ambulatory care. *Journal of Ambulatory Care Management, 9*(1), 58–81. doi:10.1097/00004479-198602000-00007

Buerhaus, P. I. (2009). Avoiding mandatory hospital nurse staffing ratios: An economic commentary. *Nursing Outlook, 57*, 107–112. doi:10.1016/j.outlook.2008.09.009

Buerhaus, P. I. (2010). What is the harm in imposing mandatory hospital nurse staffing regulations? *Nursing Economic$, 28*(2), 87–93. Retrieved from http://libdb.fairfield.edu/login?url=http://search.ebscohost.com/login.aspx?direct=true&db=rzh&AN=105174958&site=ehost-live&scope=site

Crist-Grundman, D., & Mulrooney, G. (2011). Effective workforce management starts with leveraging technology, while staffing optimization requires true collaboration. *Nursing Economic$, 29*(4), 195–200.

Cronenwett, L., Sherwood, G., Barnsteiner, J., Disch, J., Johnson, J., Mitchell, P., ... Warren, J. (2007). Quality and safety education for nurses. *Nursing Outlook, 55*(3), 122–131. doi:10.1016/j.outlook.2007.02.006

Daraiseh, N. M., Vidonish, W. P., Kiessling, P., & Lin, L. (2016). Developing a patient classification system for a neonatal ICU. *Journal of Nursing Administration, 46*(12), 636–641. doi:10.1097/NNA.0000000000000419

Davidson, P., Halcomb, E., Hickman, L., Phillips, J., & Graham, B. (2006). Beyond the rhetoric: What do we mean by a model of care? *Australian Journal of Advanced Nursing, 23*(3), 47–55. Retrieved from http://libdb.fairfield.edu/login?url=http://search.ebscohost.com/login.aspx?direct=true&db=rzh&AN=106440795&site=ehost-live&scope=site

Institute of Medicine. (2003). *Health profession education: A bridge to quality*. Washington, DC: National Academies Press. Retrieved from https://www.nap.edu/read/10681/chapter/1

Jost, S. G., Bonnell, M., Chacko, S. J., & Parkinson, D. L. (2010). Integrated primary nursing: A care delivery model for the 21st-century knowledge worker. *Nursing Administration Quarterly, 34*(3), 208–216. doi:10.1097/NAQ.0b013e3181e7032c

Kirby, K. K. (2015). Hours per patient day: Not the problem, nor the solution. *Nursing Economic$, 33*(1), 64–66.

Kjörnsberg, A., Karlsson, L., Babra, A., & Wadensten, B. (2010). Registered nurses' opinions about patient focused care. *Australian Journal of Advanced Nursing, 28*(1), 35–44. Retrieved from http://libdb.fairfield.edu/login?url=http://search.ebscohost.com/login.aspx?direct=true&db=rzh&AN=104964616&site=ehost-live&scope=site

Klingensmith, L., & Knodel, L. (2016). Mercy virtual nursing: An innovative care delivery model. *Nurse Leader, 14*(4), 275–279. doi:10.1016/j.mnl.2016.05.011

Loden, K. C. (2011). Need to improve patient satisfaction? Consider a staffing matrix. *Nursing Management, 42*(7), 46–48. doi:10.1097/01.NUMA.0000398916.71011.ad

Marquis, B. L., & Huston, C. J. (2015). *Leadership roles and management functions in nursing: Theory and application* (8th ed.). Philadelphia, PA: Wolters Kluwer Health/Lippincott Williams & Wilkins.

Mensik, J. (2014). What every nurse should know about staffing. *American NurseToday, 9*(2), 1–7. Retrieved from https://www.americannursetoday.com/what-every-nurse-should-know-about staffing

Miller, D. (2016). Moving away from HPPD to optimize nurse staffing resources. Retrieved from http://blogs.Infor.com/healthcare/2016/01/moving-away-from-hppd-tooptimize-nurse-staffing-resources.html

Montalvo, I. (2007). The National Database of Nursing Quality Indicators™ (NDNQI®). *Online Journal of Issues Nursing, 12*(3), Manuscript 2. doi:10.3912/OJIN.Vol12No03Man02

Myny, D., Van Goubergen, D., Gobert, M., Vanderwee, K., Van Hecke, A., & Defloor, T. (2011). Non-direct patient care factors influencing nursing workload: A review of the literature. *Journal of Advanced Nursing, 67*(10), 2109–2129. doi:10.1111/j.1365-2648.2011.05689.x

Naylor, M. D. (2012). Advancing high value transitional care: The central role of nursing and its leadership. *Nursing Administration Quarterly, 36*(2), 115–126. doi:10.1097/NAQ.0b013e31824a040b

Person, S. D., Allison, J. J., Kiefe, C. I., Weaver, M. T., Williams, O. D., Centor, R. M., & Weissman, N. W. (2004). Nursing staffing and mortality for Medicare patients with acute myocardial infarction. *Medical Care, 42*(1), 4–12. doi:10.1097/01.mlr.0000102369.67404.b0

Quality and Safety Education for Nurses Institute. (2014). QSEN Competencies. Retrieved from http://qsen.org/competencies/pre-licensure-ksas

Registered Nurses Association of Ontario. (2005). Reporting on…Nursing workload measurement systems: A discussion of the issues. Retrieved from http://rnao.ca/sites/rnao-ca/files/storage/related/1554_RNAO_Workload_Measurement.pdf

Rhéaume, A., Dionne, S., Gaudet, D., Allain, M., Belliveau, E., Boudreau, L., & Brown, L. (2015). The changing boundaries of nursing: A qualitative study of the transition to a new nursing care delivery model. *Journal of Clinical Nursing, 24*(17-18), 2529–2537. doi:10.1111/jocn.12846

Rose, V. L. (2016). Staffing and quality. *Long-Term Living: For The Continuing Care Professional, 65*(5), 28–31.

Schouten, P. (2013). Better patient forecasts and schedule optimization improve patient care and curb staffing costs. Retrieved from https://www.beckershospitalreview.com/hospital-management-administration/better-patient-forecasts-and-schedule-optimization-improve-patient-care-and-curb-staffing-costs.html

Seago, J. A. (2001). Nurse staffing, models of care delivery, and interventions. In A. J. Markowitz (Ed.), *Making Health care safer: A critical analysis of patient safety practices* (pp. 423–446). Rockville, MD: Agency for Healthcare Research and Quality. Retrieved from https://archive.ahrq.gov/clinic/ptsafety/chap39.htm

Senate Bill 1132. (2015). S.1132 - Registered nurse safe staffing act of 2015. Retrieved from https://www.congress.gov/bill/114th-congress/senate-bill/1132

Sherman, L., Martinez-Soto, E., Peters, B., Mathew, B., & Pischke-Winn, K. (2010). Nursing research: Implementation of acuity based staffing. *CHART Journal of Illinois Nursing, 107*(1), 11–12.

Shullanberger, G. (2000). Nurse staffing decisions: An integrative review of the literature. *Nursing Economic$, 18*(3), 124–148.

Siew, C. T., & Ghani, N. D. (2006). An overview of nurses workload measurement systems and workload balance. Retrieved from http://www.academia.edu/3055752/An_Overview_of_Nurses_Workload_Measurement_Systems_and_Workload_Balance

Swan, B. A., & Griffin, K. F. (2005). Measuring nursing workload in ambulatory care. *Nursing Economic$, 23*(5), 253–260.

Tevington, P. (2011). Mandatory nurse-patient ratios. *Medsurg Nursing, 20*(5), 265–268. Retrieved from http://libdb.fairfield.edu/login?url=http://search.ebscohost.com/login.aspx?direct=true&db=rzh&AN=104699212&site=ehost-live&scope=sit

Tiedeman, M. E., & Lookinland, S. (2004). Traditional models of care delivery: What have we learned? *Journal of Nursing Administration, 34*(6), 291–297. doi:10.1097/00005110-200406000-00008

Trope, R., Vaz, S., Zinger, M., & Sagy, M. (2015). An updated therapeutic intervention scoring system for critically Ill children enables nursing workload assessment with insight into potential untoward events. *Journal of Intensive Care Medicine, 30*(6), 344–350. doi:10.1177/0885066613519938

Welton, J. M. (2007, September 30). Mandatory hospital nurse to patient staffing ratios: Time to take a different approach. *Online Journal of issues in Nursing, 12*(3), Manuscript 1. doi:10.3912/OJIN.Vol12No03Man01

18

BUDGETING AND MANAGING FISCAL RESOURCES

DEIRDRE O'FLAHERTY ● JEAN MARIE DINAPOLI

LEARNING OBJECTIVES

After completion of this chapter, the reader will be able to

- Evaluate objectives, programs, and activities of the nursing services and the fiscal resources needed to accomplish them.
- Define basic budget terminology.
- Discuss the role of nursing leadership in preparing a budget and increasing the awareness of nursing costs.

As a registered nurse, your main priority is patient care. When identifying resources or supplies that would benefit the patient and the nurse experience, it is often frustrating to be denied what you perceive is needed because of budgetary reasons. The financial aspect of patient care is not often taught to nurses in school but it is the foundation of today's healthcare delivery system. Although budgets are not a top priority for registered nurses (as they should be), it is important to have a basic understanding of what a budget is and how it will affect your ability to care for your patients.

The information in this chapter helps you expand your current knowledge of a healthcare agency's budgetary process. It provides you with an overview of techniques and tools used to design a unit budget and to create staffing plans. Definitions for terms often used in developing budgets are discussed. A budget can be described as a written plan defining allocation of resources to serve as a guide to ensure that expenses are met and comply with organizational needs. A good budget is based on objectives and standards. It is simple, flexible, and balanced and uses available resources first to avoid increasing costs (Finkler & Jones, 2013). Typically, budgets are

BOX 18.1 CASE SCENARIO

As you read this case scenario, reflect on your current practice setting and think about what you would change in the patient care environment. These are a few questions that you may want to consider. Is there enough space allocated for patient care and for staff to complete tasks? Have you ever had the opportunity to participate in the plans to design a patient room? If so, what would your ideal exam room look like? How about redesigning the space in your work station? Is there a budget to cover the expenses? If not, do you know from where these funds come?

You are a registered nurse working in an outpatient primary care practice. The practice is open Monday to Friday from 8:30 a.m. to 5 p.m. Tensions have been high lately because another primary care practice merged into the same floor a year ago. This caused space constraints because there are not enough exam rooms for the 12 doctors to see their patients. This has become increasingly frustrating for you as room assignments have been your primary responsibility since you started in the practice 5 years ago. In addition to the lack of space for patients, the waiting area is often crowded causing frustration to staff and patients because of the inability to move patients through their visit.

Your nurse manager approaches you with the exciting news that the clinic may be expanding to another floor in the building. She has asked you to join her and to represent the nursing staff on the planning committee. The purpose of this committee will be to discuss staffing and to determine space needs and proposed patient flow on the new floor. This will be a major expense for the hospital and a detailed budget will need to be approved before the expansion can proceed. Your nurse manager gives you a brief overview of what to expect and what will be discussed in the meetings to prepare you for the first meeting.

associated with revenues and expenses but they are also used to monitor nonfinancial aspects such as supplies and equipment. Budgets are used to help coordinate the efforts of an organization by determining what resources will be used by whom, when, and for what purpose (Tomey, 2009).

The case scenario in Box 18.1 highlights how budgeting and managing fiscal resources can be applied to the practice setting.

QUESTIONS TO CONSIDER BEFORE READING ON

- Have you ever attended a budget meeting?
- What is the role of the nurse manager at budget meetings and typically who attends these meetings?
- Are there minutes or agendas from previous meetings that are available for you to review?

BUDGET OVERVIEW

In large organizations such as hospitals, it is imperative that costs of each unit/department are distinct to allow for financial accountability. Hospitals are unique organizations with many competing priorities. The healthcare team's main concern is the patient. They want to ensure that patients in their care are exposed to the latest technology, the newest equipment, and the most up-to-date treatments without concern for cost. However, what the healthcare team can forget is the fact that healthcare agencies are a business with competition from other healthcare facilities. "The complexity of the healthcare system today challenges hospitals to provide safe, patient-centered and cost effective care. Economic constraints, changes in payment structures, the shift to value-based care, and increased emphasis on prevention are important forces in healthcare delivery" (DiNapoli, O'Flaherty, Musil, Clavelle, Fitzpatrick, 2016). With this in mind, it is important for all members of the healthcare team to be fiscally responsible.

The success of the organization requires that an operational and financial balance exist so that there are enough capital funds to be able to meet expenses. Maintaining a balance between quality and cost is a challenge in today's healthcare arena. Funds are not unlimited; reimbursement rates and value-based care all impact the bottom line. This poses a challenge as funds might be restricted and often are allocated or designated for special purposes. Operational expenses such as purchasing new and innovative equipment, repairs, and staffing all potentially impact quality. The decision makers are typically the chief financial officer, finance committee, nursing in collaboration with other departments, and key stakeholders. Data collection and technological advances are reviewed and evaluated and taken into consideration before approval of items to be purchased.

Expenses are categorized as either capital or operational. Budgets are developed in both categories. Therefore, there is a "capital" budget and an "operational" budget. A capital budget is the money allocated for the acquisition or maintenance of fixed assets such as the building and equipment. Hence, money that is designated to cover the expense of purchasing new beds and stretchers for inpatients is considered a capital expense, as is, for example, the purchase of new telemetry monitors and equipment; either of these items has the potential to impact quality and safety. This is discussed again later in the chapter. An operational budget is money allocated to the functioning of the organization such as labor costs. Successful budgeting with positive outcomes requires collaboration among many stakeholders with conflicting agendas. The overall mission and responsibility of the organization is to ensure that patients receive compassionate and comprehensive care in the most effective and efficient manner.

The nurse manager and the leadership team are charged with managing cost to maximize revenue, eliminate redundancy, and improve quality. Managing cost to maximize revenue sources in today's turbulent economic arena, all while trying to keep employees engaged and motivated to minimize turnover, is daunting. Communicating budgeting decisions and including and empowering the staff in the decision-making process is instrumental to achieving unit goals. The "theory of structural empowerment" has been widely applied in nursing research and practice and is defined as the ability to get things done in an organization by having access to information, resources, opportunity, and support. Kanter, the founding theorist, acknowledged that management plays a significant role in the provision of these structural factors and posits that empowered leaders are more effective in empowering their employees, resulting in an increased commitment to ensure that the organizational goals are achieved (DiNapoli, Garcia-Dia, & O'Flaherty, 2014). Communication is the key driver in successful leadership and collaboration.

The budgeting process usually starts during the second half of each fiscal year. The yearly budgets become effective on the first day of each fiscal year. The fiscal year is the 12-month period over which the organization budgets its spending. The fiscal year is not always January 1 to December 31. It can occur over any 12-month period. Other common time frames for the fiscal year are July 1 to June 30 as well as October 1 to September 30. In most institutions, nursing administration partners with the finance department to review current budgets and forecast for the future to allow for expansion of equipment, staffing, and technology to meet the changing needs of patient care.

QUESTIONS TO CONSIDER BEFORE READING ON

This is an opportunity to reflect on the current practice at your institution, and review the current literature, economic forecasts, and reimbursement rates to be prepared to lead your team.

- Have you ever thought about how your unit budget affects your day-to-day ability to render care?
- How aware are you of your unit's/agency's budget? Does your nurse manager ever mention the budget and what it entails?
- Do you understand the impact your unit's/agency's budget has on the financial stability of the institution for which you work?

BUDGET COMPONENTS

BUDGET

A budget is an agreed-upon financial plan in which your manager and the organization have determined that specific funds are allocated for the purpose of meeting costs to manage the unit or cost center. The nurse manager's role is to ensure that this plan is met and that the unit stays within budgetary goals and provides safe and cost-effective care. The case scenario in Box 18.2 describes a planning meeting in which budgeting terminology is encountered.

BOX 18.2 THE CASE SCENARIO CONTINUES TO UNFOLD

As you continue with this case scenario, reflect on your work experience and situations where staffing was ideal. Think of the role of nurse leaders with whom you have interacted and what made them successful in negotiating staffing or other unit needs such as new equipment. Did their communication style contribute to interacting with the team?

You have attended the first planning committee meeting and were joined by members of the interdisciplinary team. You and the nurse manager of your unit have been asked to review your current staffing and patient volume to determine whether additional staff will be needed when the new unit is opened. Terms such as full-time equivalent (FTE), projected growth, cost center, and direct care worker were all discussed during the meeting. You recognized a few of these terms but a lot of this information is new to you, because your leadership class in school was very basic. Let us review some of the budget terminology to prepare for the next meeting.

Operating budget provides an overview of an organization's functions by projecting the planned operations, usually for 1 year. Line items often included on operating budgets are employee salaries and benefits (also known as "fringe"), medical–surgical supplies, office supplies, laundry services, drugs and pharmaceuticals, and repairs/maintenance for equipment. If a clinical area is off-site, line items would also include rent, housekeeping, and utilities to the operating budget. In determining a budget, the manager often relies on current expenses to forecast what will be needed next year. There are often unforeseen expenses that need to be projected into the budget for overhead such as electricity, depreciation of equipment, and unexpected projects or repairs. Because of this, operating budgets need to have some cushion funds added to provide for changes and expenses outside the control of the unit. Table 18.1 is an example to provide you with a better understanding of what an operating budget entails.

Capital budget provides funds for the cost of major purchases, maintenance, renovations, remodeling, and expansion, and often requires a justification for expenses or expenditures over a certain dollar figure decided by your institution. As reimbursement structures have changed to a value-based payment structure, capital planning for health systems has evolved to becoming a more strategic investment across the healthcare system (Hegwer, 2016). Capital budgets differ from operating budgets because the expenses are for large purchases or remodeling and need to be justified and approved often by not only finance but sometimes even the hospital's board of directors. Capital budget items are usually major investments because it takes a long time to recover the costs of the purchases.

(Text continued on page 350)

TABLE 18.1 BUDGET FOR 2017: SUPPLIES AND EXPENSES

Description	Account	Total	January	February	March	April	May
Uniforms	2,130	2,000	167	167	167	167	167
Dressing and bandages	2,180	154	13	13	13	13	13
Sutures	2,220	444	37	37	37	37	37
Medical/surgical disposable	2,260	25,231	2,103	2,103	2,103	2,103	2,103
Needles and syringes	2,300	5,022	419	419	419	419	419
Lab supplies	2365	18,300	1,525	1,525	1,525	1,525	1,525
Office supplies	2,399	10,224	852	852	852	852	852
Duplicating services	2,450	96	8	8	8	8	8
Minor equipment	2,465	164	14	14	14	14	14
Electrical supplies	2,480	500	42	42	42	42	42
Building maintenance	2,500	130,328	10,861	10,861	10,861	10,861	10,861
Nonmedical equipment	2,530	450	38	38	38	38	38
Janitorial supplies	2,555	654	55	55	55	55	55
Electricity	2,590	50,672	4,223	4,223	4,223	4,223	4,223
Water and sewer	2,610	13,200	1,100	1,100	1,100	1,100	1,100
Telephone	2,650	610	51	51	51	51	51
Wireless/cell phones	2,680	5,864	489	489	489	489	489
Answering services	2,700	50,498	4,208	4,208	4,208	4,208	4,208
Tel. move, add, change (MAC)	2,720	625	52	52	52	52	52
Pagers	2,740	860	72	72	72	72	72
Off-site telecom/ data services	2,760	2,309	192	192	192	192	192

	June	July	August	September	October	November	December	Spread
	167	167	167	167	167	167	163	MO
	13	13	13	13	13	13	11	MO
	37	37	37	37	37	37	37	MO
	2,103	2,103	2,103	2,103	2,103	2,103	2,098	MO
	419	419	419	419	419	419	413	MO
	1,525	1,525	1,525	1,525	1,525	1,525	1,525	MO
	852	852	852	852	852	852	852	MO
	8	8	8	8	8	8	8	MO
	14	14	14	14	14	14	10	MO
	42	42	42	42	42	42	38	MO
	10,861	10,861	10,861	10,861	10,861	10,861	10,857	MO
	38	38	38	38	38	38	32	MO
	55	55	55	55	55	55	49	MO
	4,223	4,223	4,223	4,223	4,223	4,223	4,219	MO
	1,100	1,100	1,100	1,100	1,100	1,100	1,100	MO
	51	51	51	51	51	51	49	MO
	489	489	489	489	489	489	485	MO
	4,208	4,208	4,208	4,208	4,208	4,208	4,210	MO
	52	52	52	52	52	52	53	MO
	72	72	72	72	72	72	68	MO
	192	192	192	192	192	192	197	MO

(continued)

TABLE 18.1 BUDGET FOR 2017: SUPPLIES AND EXPENSES *(continued)*

Description	Account	Total	January	February	March	April	May
Outside services	2,855	66,120	5,510	5,510	5,510	5,510	5,510
Freight and delivery	2,860	1,202	100	100	100	100	100
Rental photo-copy machine	2,890	5,391	449	449	449	449	449
Rental building space	2,900	465,744	38,812	38,812	38,812	38,812	38,812
Meals	2,945	2,900	242	242	242	242	242
Miscellaneous	2,960	2,292	191	191	191	191	191
Real estate taxes	2,970	39,480	3,290	3,290	3,290	3,290	3,290
Capital equipment/ instrumentation	2,990	900	75	75	75	75	75
Total supplies	***	**953,896**	**79,496**	**79,496**	**79,496**	**79,496**	**79,496**

Prepared by	2017 supply target	Approved by
BRIAN	**859,929**	
Extension	**Variance to target**	
57270	(93,967)	

	June	July	August	September	October	November	December	Spread
	5,510	5,510	5,510	5,510	5,510	5,510	5,510	*MO*
	100	100	100	100	100	100	102	*MO*
	449	449	449	449	449	449	452	*MO*
	38,812	38,812	38,812	38,812	38,812	38,812	38,812	*MO*
	242	242	242	242	242	242	238	*MO*
	191	191	191	191	191	191	191	*MO*
	3,290	3,290	3,290	3,290	3,290	3,290	3,290	*MO*
	75	75	75	75	75	75	75	*MO*
	79,496	**79,496**	**79,496**	**79,496**	**79,496**	**79,496**	**79,440**	
				VP approval				

Personnel budgets are used to estimate the direct labor costs needed for the organization to effectively run. This budget is used to determine the costs for "productive" and "nonproductive" time. Productive time is often defined as hours worked. Nonproductive time is often referred to the time when an employee is being paid but is not actually working. This generally includes break time, benefit time (vacation, holiday, bereavement, jury duty, and sick time), as well as time spent in orientation, training, or education. It is usually calculated at a percentage of the worked hours or productive time. In addition, both time and money need to be set aside in the budget to account for the expense attributed to recruitment, hiring or turnover, orientation, education, and other personnel or human resource issues. The organization needs to make a determination of the number of staff needed to efficiently and effectively run the identified department by planning and calculating the cost for both productive and nonproductive time. When calculating an annual budget, it is important to consider the tenure of staff as that may impact the amount of vacation time or personal time off that staff will require and what the replacement factor will be to cover this time. Personal time off for staff or nonproductive time can vary depending on labor relations or collective bargaining agreements or contracts. For example, the nurse manager wants to figure out the nursing needs for the unit's patient population. How many registered nurses, nursing assistants, licensed practical nurses, front desk staff, or other personnel are needed each shift to safely take care of the patients on the unit? This is determined by the current staffing patterns, staff vacancies, and past patient volume. Employee turnover, recruitment, and orientation costs must be taken into account when planning this budget.

COST CENTER

A "cost center" is a specific area of assigned responsibility for expenses. Your unit is a cost center with an allocated budget for *direct* and *indirect expenses*. When you provide a service such as patient care, the costs associated with providing care such as staff, personnel, supplies, and equipment are considered a *direct expense*, whereas the costs of utilities, cleaning, and maintenance services are considered an *indirect expense* because they are needed to support the service of providing patient care. The nurse manager on your unit has responsibility for this cost center and for assuring that monthly expenditures and targets are met in keeping the budget balanced. The cost center is a financial unit or code from which wages are paid and costs identified and controlled by a specific administrator. There are two types of cost centers in the hospital setting: *revenue producing* (profit) or *nonrevenue producing* (service). "Revenue" is the money collected for providing a service. It is different than earnings. "Earnings" are what remain of your revenue after subtracting the cost of delivering the service. An example of revenue-producing cost centers might be radiology services where procedures are billed separately and patients may be coming to the center just for a diagnostic study. A surgery center is another example of a revenue center, where patients are coming in for a surgical procedure that is revenue for the institution. On the contrary, the supportive services in the hospital are nonrevenue producing. This would include the nursing cost centers, housekeeping, kitchen, and transport.

Healthcare can be paid for by state or federal governmental programs such as Medicaid and Medicare, commercial insurance plans, or individuals themselves. The rates for governmental reimbursement are usually a fixed payment per service, whereas commercial insurers can negotiate contracts and rates for services rendered to the patients who are covered in their plan. Revenue can be impacted by a variety of things such as increased patient length of stay, changes in volume or acuity, a change in reimbursement rates, and documentation that perhaps is not capturing the complexity or acuity of the patients.

FULL-TIME EQUIVALENT

A "full-time equivalent" (FTE) is used to describe personnel employed by the organization. An FTE is the number of worked hours that represents one full-time employee. FTEs help with work measurement by converting working load hours into the number of staff required to complete the work. FTE is often defined as the number of full-time employees needed or worked (hours or shifts) during a specific period. It is used when referring to all staff because the number of part-time and per diem employees are calculated as an equivalent of an FTE that equals 1.0; part time is usually 0.5 or 0.6 and per diem is 0.2. The FTEs of a unit are usually less than the number of required full-time and part-time employees (Waxman, 2015).

SELF-ASSESSMENT

The information that you have reviewed in this chapter prepares you to review unit-based healthcare budgets. We hope that this introductory information will help you develop your competence and confidence in budgeting and managing fiscal resources. Assess your current comfort with the information by reflecting on the following questions: Are you able to see similarities between managing your work budgets and managing your own personal budget for items such as household, vacation, and tuition expenses? Are you able to relate this information to either your current or past work/clinical experience? Are you now more familiar with the expenses and associated cost of staffing a unit or able to determine where the funds will be applied to cover the expense of new equipment? If your supervisor asked you tomorrow to help with the budgeting process, would you accept the challenge? See the case scenario in Box 18.3 for an illustration of such a challenge.

BOX 18.3 THE CASE SCENARIO CONTINUES TO UNFOLD

As you continue reading this case scenario, reflect on how as a nurse leader you would advocate for your unit needs. How would you justify the need for additional positions? Would you provide any additional data to justify your request?

You sit with your nurse leader to discuss what the current staffing matrix is and the projected patient volume. To prepare for the next planning meeting, you discuss with your nurse manager the current staffing matrix and the projected patient volume. She explains the process of how to determine whether a unit is sufficiently staffed to handle the patient volume. The nurse manager of your unit begins to discuss justification for added nursing positions. Her justification needs to be strong because usually it is not easy to add additional nursing jobs. Nurse staffing costs are a high percentage of the labor budget in acute care settings and represent the largest segment of the overall organizational budget (Douglas, 2011).

You have come back from another meeting and they have asked your nurse manager to review her nursing budget from the past 3 years to forecast what the new unit's budget may look like. Your manager shares with you the budgets from prior years—2016 and 2017. She asks you to review the two budgets for your opinion and to help prepare the anticipated expenses for the upcoming expansion. You are not familiar with the spreadsheet so she explains how she monitors the budget on a monthly basis. You see that there has been a drastic change between the 2 years and now realize the impact of the increased patient volume that you were experiencing in the clinic. This has added expenses to the staffing/personnel budget and the other than personnel or *operational* budget. So, this explains the need for the additional exam rooms. Also, you see that the overtime for personnel is really high and this would explain and/or perhaps justify the need for additional staff to decrease the cost of the overtime. Clinics ran later than usual as there was lack of space to see the patients; therefore, staff stayed later than the time they were scheduled to work. This too impacted the budget as overtime dollars were needed to pay the staff members who stayed to accommodate the increased patient volume. This is all important data to have and will be necessary to justify the request to increase the budget. In addition, you can now justify the need for additional exam space to see patients to facilitate throughput and decrease the need for overtime. Meeting all of these needs will ultimately increase staff satisfaction and improve the patient experience, both important to keep costs down by potentially reducing staff turnover. Patient satisfaction should also be positively impacted by the new space and reduced wait time to see the physician. This increased volume could potentially also impact revenue.

QUALITY AND SAFETY EDUCATION FOR NURSES (QSEN) CONSIDERATIONS

The QSEN competency that focuses on "patient-centered care" can be related to budgeting and managing fiscal resources. As nurses, we need help to provide compassionate, coordinated patient-centered care. One essential aspect of patient-centered care has to do with obtaining the patient's feedback. We should be soliciting patient feedback in formal (i.e., patient satisfaction surveys) and informal (i.e., rounding) ways. That feedback will provide us valuable information for planning our budget and managing our fiscal resources. For example, patient comments that focus on the need to improve the physical environment can be used as valuable data to justify a capital expenditure to update the environment (e.g., new exam tables, new furniture).

CONCLUSIONS

This chapter has presented you with the basic understanding of the financial aspects and the responsibility of managing the budget. Good management skills are essential elements in leading a successful nursing team and a cost-efficient unit. Both to develop the skills to clinically manage your team and to have the financial acumen to stay on target and project needs are essential components in management. This knowledge will also provide you with the ability to advocate for a budget that meets the projected costs of your unit, to help support the mission and goals of the institution, and to maintain your department's ability to provide quality, safe, and compassionate care, all while meeting the needs of the institution.

CRITICAL THINKING QUESTIONS AND ACTIVITIES

- Ask your supervisor whether you can view the budget for the past fiscal year. What is the operating budget? How many FTEs are budgeted for your practice area? Were any capital requests made? Determine the process at your organization for getting capital requests approved. How does your organization define capital requests (i.e., does the organization consider over a certain dollar amount a capital request)?
- Think about needed resources at your place of work. Are the needed resources personnel or equipment? If personnel, how many FTEs would you request and why? If equipment, what is the cost of the equipment? What is the maintenance for the equipment? What is the depreciation of the equipment? What data would you present to justify your case for obtaining these resources?

REFERENCES

DiNapoli, J. M., Garcia-Dia, M. J., & O'Flaherty, D. (2014). Theory of empowerment. In J. J. Fitzpatrick & G. McCarthy (Eds.), *Theories guiding nursing research and practice: Making nursing knowledge development explicit*, (pp. 303–322). New York, NY: Springer Publishing.

DiNapoli, J. M., O'Flaherty, D., Musil, C., Clavelle, J. T., & Fitzpatrick, J. J. (2016). The relationship of clinical nurses' perceptions of structural and psychological empowerment and engagement on their unit. *Journal of Nursing Administration, 46*(2), 95–100. doi:10.1097/NNA.0000000000000302

Douglas, M. R. (2011). Opportunities and challenges facing the future global nursing and midwifery workforce. *Journal of Nursing Management, 19*, 695–699. doi:10.1111/j.1365-2834.2011.01302.x

Finkler, S. A., & Jones, B. C. (2013). *Financial management for nurse managers and executives* (4th ed.). St. Louis, MO: Elsevier Saunders.

Hegwer, L. R. (2016). Capital planning for a new era. *Healthcare Financial Management, 70*(5), 60–63.

Tomey, A. M. (2009). *Guide to nursing management and leadership* (8th ed.). St. Louis, MO: Mosby, Elsevier.

Waxman, K. T. (2015). *Finance and budgeting made simple: Essential skills for nurses*. Brentwood, TN: HCPro.

19

SELECTION AND PROMOTION IN STAFF DEVELOPMENT

LISA M. REBESCHI

LEARNING OBJECTIVES

After completion of this chapter, the reader will be able to

- Describe the interviewing process used for selecting nursing staff.
- Relate motivational theories to the process of creating an effective practice environment.
- Discuss staff development strategies using performance appraisals.
- Apply principles of coaching in relation to staff development.
- Outline the use of progressive discipline and termination for disruptive staff problems.

Nursing practice continues to evolve within a rapidly changing healthcare environment. It is imperative to recruit, develop, and retain nurses who are well equipped to meet the challenge to provide high-quality safe patient care. Furthermore, leaders have a mandate to create work environments that maximize job performance. Because motivation is a major determinant of productivity, nurse leaders must be able to use motivational techniques to maximize the nurses' performance. As a registered nurse, you have already experienced factors that create positive work environments. However, additional knowledge and skills in relation to selecting staff and promoting staff development will further enable you to construct practice environments leading to positive patient outcomes. This knowledge is also considered an essential Quality and Safety Education for Nurses (QSEN) competency for both undergraduate and graduate nurses, as outlined in Table 19.1.

TABLE 19.1 SELECTION AND PROMOTION IN STAFF DEVELOPMENT: RELEVANT QSEN COMPETENCIES
Describe own strengths, limitations, and values in functioning as a member of a team (Knowledge)
Analyze self and other team members' strengths, limitations, and values (Knowledge)
Describe scopes of practice and roles of healthcare team members (Knowledge)
Initiate plan for self-development as a team member (Skills)
Act with integrity, consistency, and respect for differing views (Skills)
Value the perspective and expertise of all health team members (Attitudes)
Respect the unique attributes that members bring to a team, including variations in professional orientations and accountabilities (Attitudes)
Continuously plan for improvement in self and others for effective team development and functioning (Skills)
Be open to continually assessing and improving own skills as a team member and leader (Attitudes)
Describe strategies for identifying and managing overlaps in team member roles and accountabilities (Knowledge)
Discuss effective strategies for communicating and resolving conflict (Knowledge)
Value teamwork and the relationships on which it is based (Attitudes)
Contribute to resolution of conflict and disagreement (Attitudes)
Elicit input from other team members to improve individual, as well as team, performance (Skills)
Explain how authority gradients influence teamwork and patient safety (Knowledge)
Identify system barriers and facilitators of effective team functioning (Knowledge)

QSEN, Quality and Safety Education for Nurses.

American Association of Colleges of Nursing. (2012). *Graduate-level QSEN competencies: Knowledge, skills and attitudes*. Washington, DC: Author. Retrieved from http://www.aacnnursing.org/Portals/42/AcademicNursing/CurriculumGuidelines/Graduate-QSEN-Competencies.pdf?ver=2017-07-15-135425-900; Quality and Safety Education for Nurses Institute. (2014). QSEN competencies. Retrieved from http://qsen.org/competencies/pre-licensure-ksas

A case scenario is presented in Box 19.1 to assist with application of knowledge regarding selecting and interviewing staff.

QUESTIONS TO CONSIDER BEFORE READING ON

Have you been involved in the selection and interview process of nurses at your organization? If so, what process was used? What were the strengths of the process used? What opportunities for improvement can you identify?

SELECTING AND INTERVIEWING STAFF

The nurse's role in selecting competent professional nursing staff cannot be underestimated. Coordinated efforts with human resource and recruitment colleagues are highly suggested to identify the most appropriate

BOX 19.1 CASE SCENARIO

As you read this case scenario, begin to think about your role as a leader in selecting new nursing staff. Professional nurses often collaborate to identify candidates who best meet the needs of the unit and organization as a whole. How can you contribute to the successful hiring of professional nurses within your organization? Nurse managers play a pivotal role in staffing the patient care unit. How have the nurse managers with whom you have worked been effective in selecting new staff?

Philip Ortiz, MSN, RN, is the nurse manager of the neurological intensive care unit (NICU) at a 350-bed suburban community hospital in the Northeast. The NICU has experienced a high degree of nurse turnover over the past 6 months. The manager is committed to careful selection of new nursing staff as the hospital searches for two new registered nurses (RNs). The search committee has identified six potential new RNs from resume reviews and plans to bring these candidates on the unit for an interview.

potential staff (Finkelman, 2016). Once potential staff have been identified, one of the major contributions of nursing staff members is to participate in the interview process. Although the interview process is often costly in terms of resources and time, it is a critical component in selecting the best staff to ensure the continued delivery of effective nursing care services.

Immediately following the identification of candidates for a nursing position, the interview process should be carefully planned. Planning includes specific activities such as determining the specific format of the interview (i.e., one-on-one vs. group interviews), selection of interview questions, and consideration of applicable laws in relation to employment processes. A structured interview guide containing the interview directions and questions specific to the position should be prepared and implemented to maximize comparability between candidates (Sullivan & Decker, 2009). Consistency with the interview process is needed for each candidate for the positions.

The format of the interview for selecting staff can vary. Candidates may be interviewed individually or as a group with other candidates for the same position. Sometimes, interviews may include practice-based experiences. For example, candidates might be asked to spend time shadowing another nurse on the unit. Similarly, interviews might include demonstrating competencies during a simulation while being rated by members of the healthcare team. Frequently, candidate interviews include conversations with several members of the nursing staff and nurse administrators (Strout, Nevers, Bachard, & Varney, 2016). The selection of interview questions is critical to the success of the interview.

According to Strout et al. (2016), interview questions can be conceptualized within five topic areas: teamwork, difficult patients, performance, evidence-based practice, and patient-centered care. On the basis of recommendations from the Institute of Medicine (2011), continued emphasis is placed on the ability of nurses to participate as key members of the interprofessional healthcare team. Therefore, specific interview questions should include experiences working on teams including collaborative relationships, conflict resolution, and delegation strategies. Because nurses often work with difficult patients, it is important to ask candidates about their approach in these situations to ensure that candidates are able to place patient needs at the forefront of care. Further interview questions in regards to performance might include questions about the candidate's perceived strengths and areas of needed continued growth. Nurses must use evidence-based practice to make clinically sound decisions. Therefore, the interview should include questions about the way the candidate integrates evidence into his or her practice. Finally, the interview should include discussion regarding how patient preferences guide decision-making. Examples of sample interview questions are presented in Table 19.2.

There are a variety of applicable laws that the nurse must consider when planning for the hiring interview. Staff selection processes are subject to substantial surveillance in relation to equal employment opportunity and discrimination. The Civil Rights Act of 1964 (Title VII) prohibits employers from personnel discrimination on the basis of race, color, religion, gender,

TABLE 19.2 SELECTING STAFF: SAMPLE INTERVIEW QUESTIONS

Teamwork
- Do you prefer to work alone or as part of a team?
- What strategies do you use to resolve conflict?
- Describe how you make decisions about delegation.
- Give an example of when you worked effectively as part of a team.

Difficult patients
- What approaches have you used when working with difficult patients?
- Describe a situation when you did more than required for a patient.
- Describe a situation when you had a conflict with the patient over his or her plan of care and how you resolved the conflict.

Performance
- Describe your strengths as a professional nurse.
- What areas of your practice do you consider most challenging?
- How would your peers describe you as a nurse?

Evidence-based practice
- How have you used evidence-based practice in your nursing care?
- What barriers have you experienced when trying to incorporate evidence-based practice?

Patient-centered care
- What does patient-centered care mean to you?
- Describe specific strategies that you use to build relationships with patients.
- How do you demonstrate caring to patients and families?

or nationality (U.S. Equal Employment Opportunity Commission, n.d.). Therefore, it is inappropriate to include interview questions asking candidates about religious affiliation, ethnicity, number of children, or place of birth. Additional statutes relevant to the staff selection and interview process include the Age Discrimination Act of 1967 and Title I of the Americans With Disabilities Act (ADA) of 1990. Thus, interview questions or employment decisions with regards to age and/or disability are prohibited.

QUESTIONS TO CONSIDER BEFORE READING ON

- What communication skills will you use during the interview process?
- On the basis of your previous professional experiences, what aspects of the interview process have you found particularly effective? Particularly ineffective?

CREATING A MOTIVATING CLIMATE

Nurse leaders must create work environments that empower professional practice to ensure nursing excellence. Motivation is an essential concept to understand to ensure effectiveness and success (Toode, Routasalo, & Suominen, 2011). The concept of motivation must be viewed from the individual staff nurse's perspective in addition to the perspectives of teams and organizations.

MOTIVATIONAL THEORIES

In addition to necessary nursing knowledge, skills, and competencies, it is equally essential that nurses have the drive and desire to perform at their best. As described by Huber (2013), a primary characteristic of motivation is the drive, energy, or desire to act in a certain way to accomplish a task. Motivation creates a sense of enthusiasm and ability to establish clear achievement goals. It is imperative to understand nurses' motivations to create a motivating work climate so that specific strategies can be designed and implemented to increase motivation. There is no one accepted theory of motivation; rather, nurses draw upon a variety of motivation theories to create effective practice environments.

Maslow Hierarchy of Needs Theory

Maslow (1943, 1954) is one of the early theorists who used his Hierarchy of Needs Model to explain motivation (Figure 19.1). He claimed that individuals need to have their basic physiological and safety needs such as food,

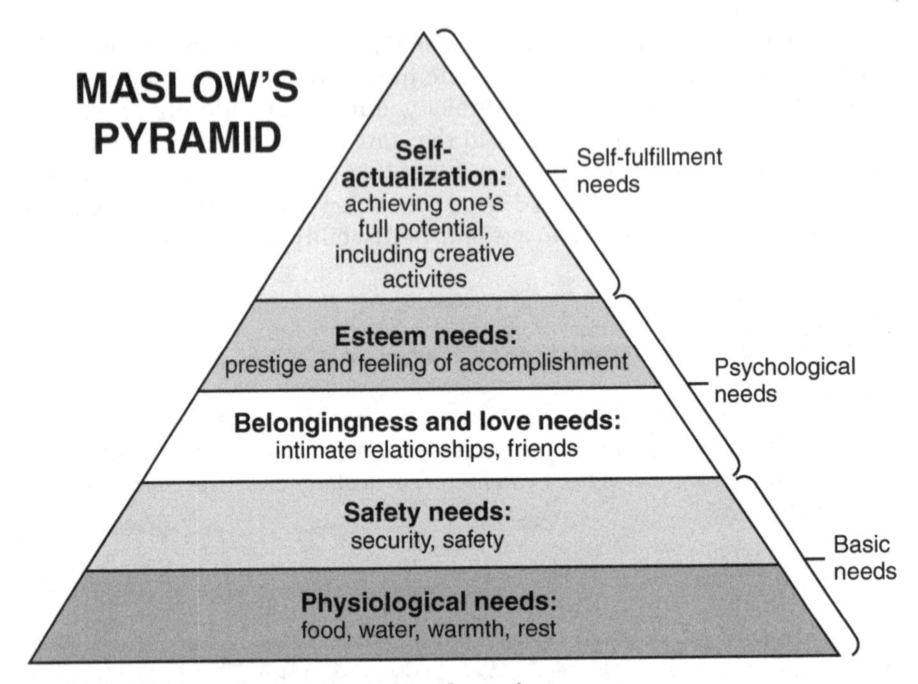

FIGURE 19.1 Maslow's hierarchy of needs.

Source: Retreived from https://simplypsychology.org/maslow.html

water, warmth, rest, and safety met first. Next, psychological needs, such as a sense of belonging and feeling of accomplishment, would need to be met before moving to the next stage, and finally of achieving one's full potential as the last priority. According to Maslow, after a need has been met, it no longer serves to motivate the person. In addition, performance can be affected when needs are not met because that causes a sense of stress, conflict, and frustration. Maslow's theory was not specific to work motivation. However, his work has had a significant impact on the development of other theories of motivation specific to the work environment.

Herzberg's Motivation–Hygiene Theory

One of the first motivation theories specifically focused on work motivation was developed by Herzberg, Mausner, and Snyderman (1959) who described a two-factor theory of motivation known as Motivation–Hygiene Theory (Figure 19.2). The theory includes two different categories of needs known as hygienes and motivators. Hygiene factors, such as status, money, working conditions, and supervision, are related to the work environment itself, whereas motivators relate to the work itself and include factors such as advancement, increased responsibility for work,

Hygiene Factors	Motivator Factors
• Salaries, wages & other benefits • Company policy & administration • Good inter-personal relationships • Quality of supervision • Job security • Working conditions • Work/life balance	• Sense of personal achievement • Status • Recognition • Challenging/stimulating work • Responsibility • Opportunity for advancement • Promotion • Growth
When in place, these factors result in...	When in place, these factors result in...
✓ General satisfaction ✓ Prevention of dissatisfaction	✓ High motivation ✓ High satisfaction ✓ Strong commitment

FIGURE 19.2 Motivation–Hygiene Theory.
Source: Herzberg-Motivation-Model-01-JPG.jpg [Image]. (2017). Retrieved from http://wiki.engageeducation.org.au/wp-content/uploads/2015/07/Herzberg-Motivation-Model-01-JPG.jpg

challenge, recognition, and achievement. On the basis of this theory, Herzberg et al. (1959) posit that factors that contribute to job satisfaction and motivation are distinct from factors that contribute to job dissatisfaction. Motivators are viewed to be more effective in terms of the positive impact on job satisfaction.

Reinforcement Theory/Behavior Modification

Skinner (1953) derived one of the earliest theories of motivation, known as Reinforcement Theory. According to reinforcement theory, behavior is learned by operant conditioning as the behavior becomes associated with a particular outcome. The connection between the behavior and the outcome becomes stronger over time. Outcomes may be classified as "positive reinforcement" or "negative reinforcement." Positive reinforcement includes providing praise and/or recognition, whereas negative reinforcement includes some form of punishment (Figure 19.3). According to Skinner (1953), positive reinforcement is the preferred strategy for changing behavior.

McClelland's Learned Needs Theory

Yet another theory of motivation, characterized as a Learned Needs Theory, focuses on socially acquired needs (McClelland, 1976). According to McClelland, there are three learned needs: (a) achievement, (b) affiliation, and (c) power. Individuals learn about these needs as they interact within the

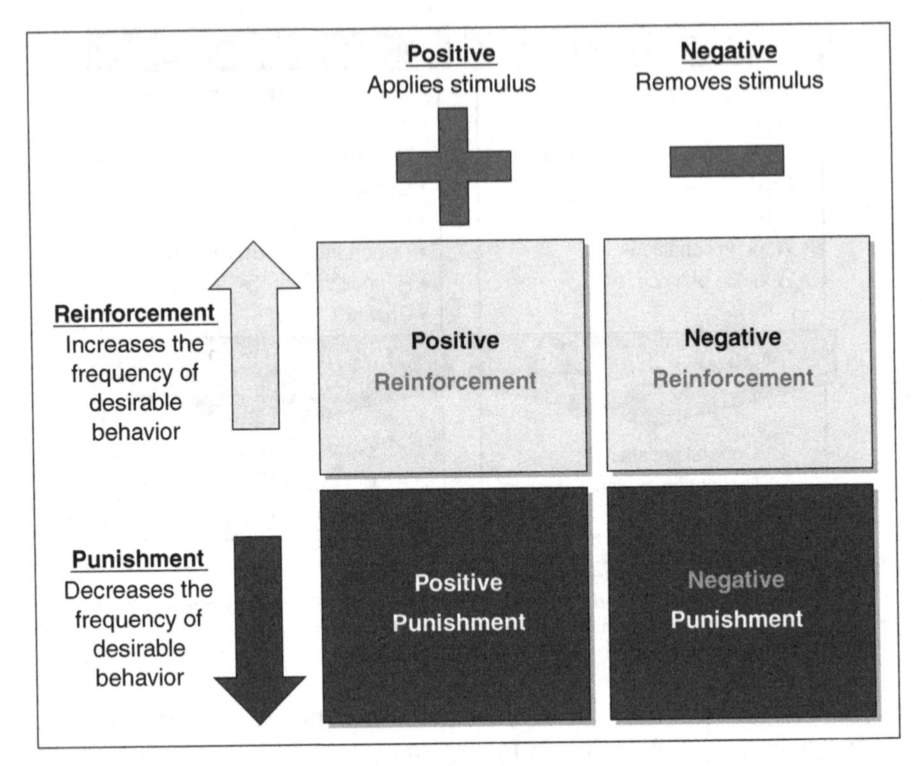

FIGURE 19.3 Reinforcement theory.

Source: From Redmond, B. F., & Johnson, V. M. (2016). Reinforcement theory. Retrieved from https://wikispaces.psu.edu/display/PSYCH484/3.%20Reinforcement%20Theory

environment and each person tends to have one central need. The need for achievement can best be described as having a strong desire to advance and grow. Those with a need for achievement desire responsibility and specific feedback. The need for affiliation involves the desire to develop pleasant, close relationships with other people. Finally, the need for power involves the desire to be in control and control other people and the environment. As these needs are learned, behavior that is rewarded will most likely increase (Figure 19.4).

McGregor's Theory X and Theory Y

McGregor (1960) describes two related theories of motivation on the basis of manager's beliefs, known as "Theory X and Theory Y." Beliefs consistent with Theory X include the assumption that people are lazy, do not want to be responsible, and are motivated by money and the fear of punishment. Therefore, it is necessary to impose close control. The challenging view is Theory Y, which is consistent with a view that people are complex, creative, and self-directed individuals. Management strategies consistent with Theory X are authoritarian in nature compared with participative management strategies consistent with Theory Y (Table 19.3).

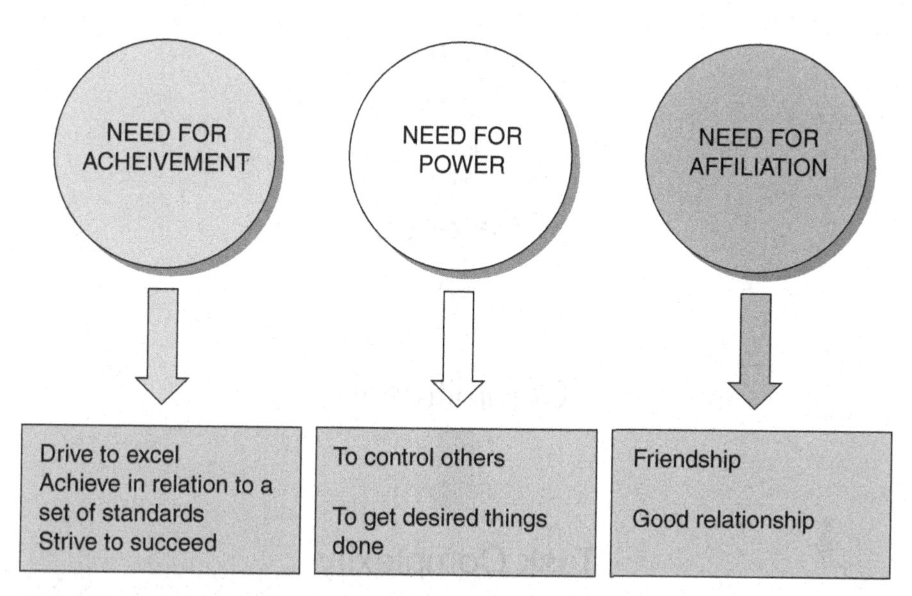

FIGURE 19.4 McClelland's Learned Needs Theory.

Source: mcclelland.jpg [Image]. (2015). Retrieved from https://mosaicprojects.files.wordpress.com/2015/05/mcclelland.jpg

TABLE 19.3 MANAGER BELIEFS: THEORY X VERSUS THEORY Y

Theory X	Theory Y
Managers believe employees: Dislike work Do not desire responsibilities Are motivated by fear and money Lack creativity	Managers believe employees: Take a great interest in their work Blossom with responsibilities Are motivated by self-direction Become highly creative with opportunities

Goal-Setting Theory

One of the most noteworthy motivation theories is Goal-Setting theory. Locke (1968) described a theory of task motivation and incentives. Specifically, he discussed how clear goals and feedback motivate employees and lead to improved performance. In fact, individuals tend to work harder when goals are both more specific and challenging. Having a goal that is not challenging enough will not produce motivation. Latham (2007) built upon the earlier work of Locke in studying the effects of goal setting in the workplace. Together, they have outlined elements for specific goal setting including clarity, challenge, commitment, feedback, and task complexity (Locke & Latham, 1990; Figure 19.5).

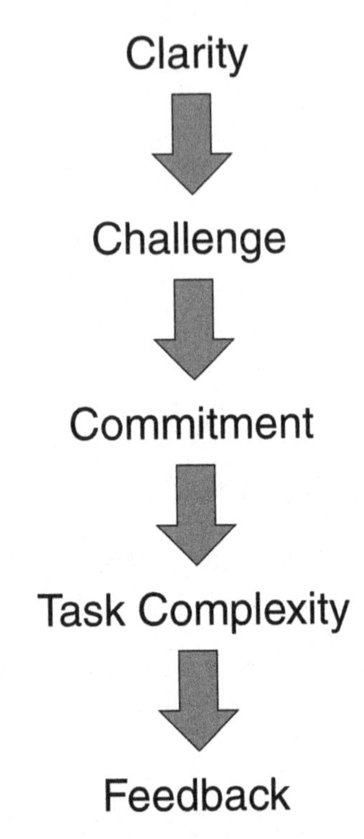

FIGURE 19.5 Elements for goal setting.

The development of clear and measurable goals assists individuals to identify what they are trying to achieve and serves as a strong motivator. Goals should be set at the appropriate level of challenge to be most effective. They should also be understood by members of the team to be most effective. In addition, it is imperative to listen to feedback to accurately gauge performance. Feedback also allows for adjustments to be made with goal setting. And finally, it is important to carefully consider task complexity. Because nurses often work in highly complex and demanding settings, it is critical to set goals that are not completely overwhelming (MindTools, n.d.).

QUESTIONS TO CONSIDER BEFORE READING ON

- What motivates you in your work as a registered nurse?
- What makes you want to improve your job performance?
- Why are some managers more effective in creating a better work climate?
- How can you motivate other professionals?

STRATEGIES TO PROMOTE POSITIVE MOTIVATIONAL CLIMATE

There is little doubt that nurse leaders and managers must create a positive motivational climate to foster safe, high-quality healthcare environments. As described by Latham and Ernst (2006), "employee motivation is inextricably tied to an organization's leadership" (p. 191). Furthermore, nurse leaders are well positioned to influence outcome variations such as employee and patient satisfaction, employee productivity, nurse retention, lower absenteeism, and improved patient safety (Macauley, 2015). Creating a positive motivational climate requires well-thought-out, creative strategies that empower nurses to feel energized about their practice. Nurse leaders and managers must be cognizant of the unique talents of all members of the healthcare team. Although no one theory on motivation is possible for all situations, nurses must draw upon a variety of motivational theories to create positive work environments.

Creating a positive motivational climate results in an engaged nursing workforce made up of those committed to the organization. "Engaged employees are emotionally and cognitively immersed in their job allowing a sense of meaningfulness and value in the work leading to higher sensitivity to the organization's mission and to organizational change" (Macauley, 2015, p. 298). Specific elements having an impact on employee engagement have been identified.

First, workload does matter. The nurse's workload needs to be reasonable and sustainable; this leads to opportunities for professional growth and facilitation of engagement. On the contrary, when the nurse's workload is beyond his or her capability in terms of time and skill, there is a risk for job dissatisfaction and eventual burnout. Therefore, as a nurse leader, it is imperative to design a nurse's assignments in a sensible manner.

Another effective strategy to enhance engagement is providing recognition/reward in relation to job performance. This includes meaningful and consistent feedback for employees to identify how they are doing and on what else they may need to focus. Because not all nurses are motivated by the same reward (monetary and nonmonetary rewards), to be most effective it is necessary to invest time in identifying individual differences and preferences. Examples of rewards include salary, benefits, positive feedback, promotion/clinical advancement, and position titles. Similarly, to maximize an employee's sense of self-worth and respect, it is paramount to strive for equity and fairness in relation to salary, workload, and professional responsibilities. Finally, nurse leaders need to foster a sense of community within the workplace, including opportunities for social interaction.

As you read the continuing case scenario in Box 19.2, think about what motivational theories Philip could use to address this situation. What strategies might he consider for creating a positive motivational climate?

BOX 19.2 THE CASE SCENARIO CONTINUES TO UNFOLD

Returning to the case scenario, nurse manager Philip Ortiz, MSN, RN begins to strategize on improving retention of current nursing staff. The acuity of patients in NICU continues to increase at the same time the unit is experiencing a staffing shortage resulting from the turnover. Some of the RNs are working overtime; they have expressed concern with their inability to manage the workload.

QUESTIONS TO CONSIDER BEFORE READING ON

Does your organization and nurse leader/manager provide you with opportunities for staff development to enhance your performance? Reflect upon your last performance evaluation. Were you given an opportunity to provide a self-assessment? Did you consider the process accurate and fair? Did you meet individually with your nurse leader/manager? If you met with your nurse leader/manager, what was positive about the process and what could have been improved with the process?

DEVELOPING STAFF

Staff development refers to activities designed to enhance staff performance. It is a major responsibility for nurse leaders and managers and contributes to the continuous quality improvement initiatives of the healthcare organization. The overarching goal for staff development involves providing quality educational opportunities to improve and/or maintain the necessary knowledge, skills, and attitudes consistent with nursing practice. Performance appraisals are implemented with fairness and accuracy to ensure ongoing competencies.

PERFORMANCE APPRAISALS

Nurse leaders and managers are charged with the professional responsibility of managing the performance of employees. This includes establishing professional standards of performance so that employees are able to set specific performance goals that may serve to motivate the employee. Job performance is a function of both ability and motivation.

Performance appraisals are conducted on an established schedule with periodic reassessment occurring at least every 3 years to evaluate nursing practice (Huber, 2013). In the practice setting, reassessments often occur on an annual basis. Albrecht (1972) defined the "performance appraisal" as a systematic and standardized evaluation of an employee conducted by the supervisor. The aim of the performance appraisal is to judge the contribution of the employee's work against established standards while providing constructive feedback; the employee's work is often rated as superior, excellent, average, or unacceptable. Further components of the performance appraisal may include peer review from other staff members and self-evaluation. Contemporary performance appraisals also include a shift from performance evaluation conducted solely by the supervisor to performance demonstration by the nurse via a professional portfolio (Porter-O'Grady & Malloch, 2013).

Strategies for Accuracy and Fairness

Laws with regard to fair employment practice must be considered when conducting performance appraisals. Nurse managers must ensure that performance appraisals are accurate to prevent claims of unfairness and discrimination. Specific strategies to ensure accuracy and fairness include a regular schedule for appraisals, written documentation shared with the employee, opportunity for the employee to respond and/or appeal, adequate time for the manager to directly observe the employee's practice, proper training of the manager, and a focus on the employee's behaviors rather than on personal traits such as gender, sexual orientation, age, and race (Finkelman, 2016; Huber, 2013; Sullivan & Decker, 2009). The focus of the performance appraisal must remain on job performance while providing specific example to substantiate the results.

The Appraisal Interview

One of the initial steps in staff development is the appraisal interview. On completion of the performance appraisal, the nurse manager should arrange a mutually convenient time for the appraisal interview. Attention to privacy, nondisruption, and sufficient meeting time must be considered to maximize the effectiveness of the process. The most successful appraisal interviews result from a process characterized by the sharing of feedback throughout the period of evaluation. In this way, the employee has a preconceived idea on how he or she will be rated and what factors were considered in determining the performance rating. During the interview, it is important for the nurse manager to provide specific performance examples as data to substantiate the judgments made about the nurse's practice performance. Typical items included within the performance appraisal are application of the nursing process, collaboration with the interprofessional team, effective communication and documentation, competency with clinical skills, mentoring of new employees, customer service/patient focus, attention to safety and quality initiatives, accountability, and commitment to the organization's mission, values, and integrity.

The overarching goal of the appraisal interview is for the manager and the employee to work collaboratively to improve practice in the subsequent evaluation period. The purpose of the appraisal interview in terms of improving practice should be made clear at the start of the interview. The manager should facilitate open, two-way communication to conduct the most successful appraisal interviews. Specifically asking the employee to comment about the ratings is important to facilitate open communication and collaboration. It is also imperative to provide the employee with time to communicate his or her own self-evaluation throughout the interview. Providing both positive and negative examples to substantiate ratings is suggested. Overfocusing on negative aspects of the performance appraisal is counterproductive because this often causes the employee to assume a defensive posture during the appraisal interview. As suggested by Sullivan (2013), discussion of behaviors requiring immediate improvement should be limited to no more than two areas. Toward the end of the interview, the conversation should shift toward the future in terms of improved performance and goal setting. In fact, a plan of action may be developed to include specific timelines for follow-up. The nurse manager documents the completion of the performance appraisal interview and maintains these records within the personnel file.

Coaching

Nurse leaders and managers often act in a coaching role. According to Walker-Reed (2016), "coaching" is defined as "enabling personal and professional growth leading to service improvement" (p. 42). As a formal relationship, coaching is much akin to a partnership designed to meet the learning needs of a colleague for the purpose of improving performance. Coaching is accomplished over a prolonged period of time and in a nonjudgmental manner in which performance is discussed on a regular basis.

The main goal of coaching is to improve performance. It begins with the mutual development of goals that map a plan for maximizing strengths and monitoring progress with performance. According to Batson and Yoder (2012), effective coaching influences improved self-efficacy (i.e., how a person views his or her ability to carry out an action) and performance.

Coaching follows three stages: preplanning and assessment, active coaching, and follow-up (Batson & Yoder, 2012). The steps of the coaching process are similar to the steps of the nursing process and are depicted in Figure 19.6. During the initial stage, an *assessment* is completed to determine competencies and a beginning relationship is established between the coach and the coachee. Then during the *active stage*, the coach's role is to use techniques to generate insight from the coachee. These techniques involve skills such as role-modeling, active listening, and questioning. As the coachee gains further insight, less frequent coaching is needed and the relationship begins to come to a close. During the stage of *follow-up*, activity shifts to monitoring progress and identifying an end to the relationship.

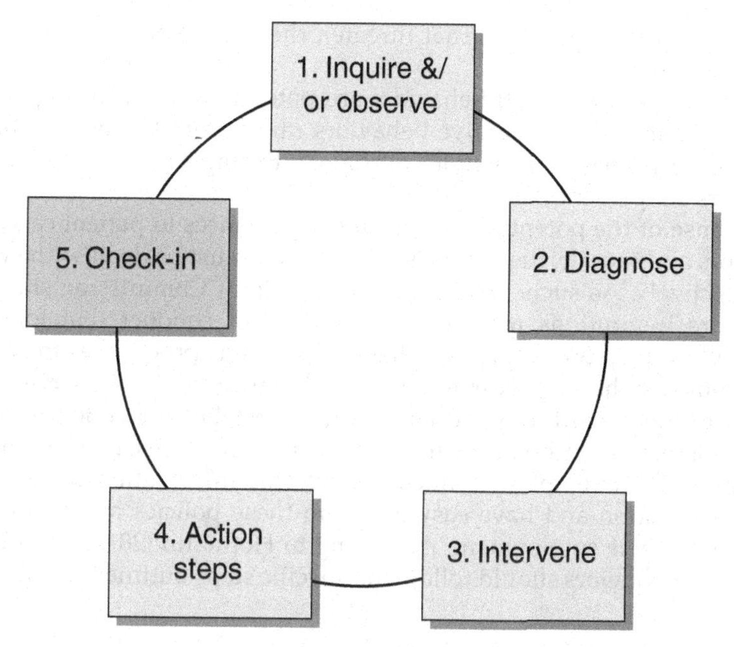

FIGURE 19.6 The five-step coaching process.

Source: Dore, K. (2011). Coaching: Moving from control to growth [PowerPoint presentation]. Retrieved from https://www.slideshare.net/kristendore/coaching-101-8883277

ACCOUNTABILITY AND STAFF MANAGEMENT ISSUES

Nursing professionals in leadership and management positions are both responsible and accountable for their own practice as well as the practice of those with whom they work. As a manager and leader, the nurse has responsibility and accountability for accomplishing a variety of tasks including selecting staff, retaining staff, and addressing staff problems. It is imperative that nurse managers are aware of policies and procedures for addressing problems such as disruptive behaviors.

DISRUPTIVE STAFF PROBLEMS

Disruptive staff behaviors are in stark contrast to behaviors congruent with a culture of safety. Therefore, in 2008, The Joint Commission established a standard for healthcare institutions requiring a code of conduct as well as a process to manage disruptive and inappropriate behaviors. According to The Joint Commission (2008), disruptive behavior includes both overt and passive actions that include verbal outbursts, physical threats, uncooperative attitude, and refusal to perform assigned tasks because these are behaviors that threaten the overall performance of the healthcare team.

Again, disruptive staff behaviors are potentially harmful to patients. Specific examples of disruptive behaviors range from the use of abusive language to refusing to mentor colleagues. Examples of disruptive staff behaviors are presented in Table 19.4.

Because of the potentially harmful consequences to patient care, staff retention, and morale, disruptive staff behavior must be dealt with swiftly and effectively. As such, on the basis of The Joint Commission standard, healthcare institutions must develop a code of conduct that identifies acceptable versus unacceptable behavior as well as procedures to address unacceptable behaviors. Nurse leaders and managers should serve as role models for demonstrating and enforcing the established code of conduct while responding to breaches in conduct in a fair, consistent manner. In addition, all new employees must receive this information during their initial orientation and have easy access to these policies and procedures throughout their employment. According to Hofmann (2010), response to disruptive behaviors should follow the specific steps outlined in Table 19.5.

Progressive Discipline and Termination

Nurse managers use progressive discipline strategies to correct and/or prevent employee behaviors that are potentially detrimental to a healthcare organization. Progressive discipline refers to a process that addresses behaviors that do not meet expected performance standards. The central purpose of progressive discipline is not punitive in nature. Rather, it is to facilitate employee understanding of the performance issue and/or provide an opportunity for improvement. A reasonable amount of time should be provided for the employee to correct deficiencies except in cases where there are immediate threats to the employee or to others.

Disciplinary situations often pose a number of challenges for nurse managers including learning how to effectively use discipline strategies. A clear

TABLE 19.4 EXAMPLES OF DISRUPTIVE STAFF BEHAVIORS
• Threats toward others • Use of abusive language • Attempts to humiliate colleagues • Sending inappropriate email messages • Refusal to mentor new colleagues • Refusal to assist colleagues • Intimidating behaviors • Bullying

Source: Longo, J. (2010). Combating disruptive behaviors: Strategies to promote a healthy work environment. *Online Journal of Issues in Nursing, 15*(1), Manuscript 5. doi:10.3912/OJIN.Vol15No01Man05

TABLE 19.5 RESPONDING TO DISRUPTIVE BEHAVIORS: STEPS TO FOLLOW
• Inform all members of the healthcare team about the policies and procedures regarding disruptive behavior in the work setting • Follow the established policies and procedures without variations • Collaborate with other members of the leadership team • Consult with the organization's legal resources • Ensure respect and confidentiality with the process • Provide an opportunity for the employee to respond to the complaints of disruptive behavior • Maintain documentation of all meetings • Inform the leadership team about the process

Hofmann, P. B. (2010). Fulfilling disruptive-behavior policy objectives. Leaders must promptly address improper clinician behavior. *Healthcare Executive, 25*(3), 60–63.

knowledge and understanding of processes are necessary to prevent outcomes such as grievances, arbitration, and charges of unfair labor practice. Throughout the process of disciplining staff, it is imperative for the manager to collaborate with the human resources department of the organization to maintain due process, fairness, and legal expectations.

Nurse managers should follow a methodical process to address issues related to poor job performance. To begin with, references to the job description and expected performance should be used as a framework for discussion. Discussion should include specific examples from the employee's practice that do not meet expected standards. Documentation should be objective in nature and focused on developing an action plan for improvement. In fact, the first step of the progressive disciplinary process is counseling regarding areas in need of improvement. If performances issues have not been adequately addressed and corrected within the stipulated time identified in the action plan, discipline progresses to a written warning, also known as "written reprimand." The written warning serves as notice that the employee's performance must improve to prevent further action such as suspension and/or termination (Heathfield, 2017; Young, 2014).

Although many instances of progressive discipline will lead to improved performance, there are situations in which employees may continue to fail in meeting expected performance outcomes despite efforts such as coaching and counseling. With clear communication during the progressive disciplinary process, termination should not be a surprise to the employee (Heathfield, 2017). Actions to terminate an employee should be coordinated with other administrators including one's own immediate supervisor and those in the human resources department. When meeting with an employee who is being terminated, the manager describes the reason(s) for termination.

As you read the case scenario given in Box 19.3, think about how the nurse manager should address this situation.

BOX 19.3 THE CASE SCENARIO CONTINUES TO UNFOLD

Returning to the case scenario, nurse manager Philip Ortiz, MSN, RN has been providing coaching to Terri Gleason, BSN, RN, who began her nursing position about 8 months ago. Despite coaching, Terri has continued to demonstrate performance below expectations in the areas of interprofessional communication, teamwork, and clinical skills.

CONCLUSION

This chapter presented various strategies used in the selection and promotion in staff development. The importance of recruiting, developing, and retaining nurses able to meet the demands within a rapidly changing practice environment cannot be understated. Nurse leaders must draw upon theoretical knowledge of motivation to create high-functioning work environments. Leaders must also demonstrate professional accountability and responsibility in developing staff through performance appraisals and coaching. Knowledge of progressive discipline and termination is also required to effectively address staff performance in need of improvement.

CRITICAL THINKING QUESTIONS AND EXERCISES

- Think about the last interview for a nursing position in which you participated. What about the interview made it a positive experience? In what aspects of the interview would you suggest improvement?
- On the basis of your professional nursing experiences, describe how leaders on the unit and/or organization created a positive motivational climate.
- Locate the published code of conduct and established procedures to address unacceptable behaviors from your place of employment.
- Access the following documents from a healthcare organization: job description, expected performance outcomes, and performance appraisal tool. On the basis of your review of the documents, evaluate the congruency between these documents. Can you identify areas in need of improvement?

REFERENCES

Albrecht, S. (1972). Reappraisal of conventional performance appraisal systems. *Journal of Nursing Administration*, 2(2), 29–35. doi:10.1097/00005110-197203000-00011

American Association of Colleges of Nursing. (2012). *Graduate-level QSEN competencies: Knowledge, skills and attitudes.* Washington, DC: Author. Retrieved from http://www.aacnnursing.org/Portals/42/AcademicNursing/CurriculumGuidelines/Graduate-QSEN-Competencies.pdf?ver=2017-07-15-135425-900

Batson, V. D., & Yoder, L. H. (2012). Managerial coaching: A concept analysis. *Journal of Advanced Nursing, 68*(7), 1658–1669. doi:10.1111/j.1365-2648.2011.05840.x

Dore, K. (2011). Coaching: Moving from control to growth [PowerPoint presentation]. Retrieved from https://www.slideshare.net/kristendore/coaching-101-8883277

Finkelman, A. (2016). *Leadership and management for nurses: Core competencies for quality care* (3rd ed.). Boston, MA: Pearson.

Heathfield, S. M. (2017). Learn what progressive discipline is in the workplace. *The Balance Careers.* Retrieved from https://www.thebalance.com/what-progressive-discipline-1918092

Herzberg, F., Mausner, B., & Snyderman, B. B. (1959). *The motivation to work.* New York, NY: John Wiley & Sons.

Hofmann, P. B. (2010). Fulfilling disruptive-behavior policy objectives: Leaders must promptly address improper clinician behavior. *Healthcare Executive, 25*(3), 60–63.

Huber, D. L. (2013). *Leadership and nursing care management* (5th ed.). St. Louis, MO: Elsevier Health Sciences.

Institute of Medicine. (2011). *The future of nursing: Leading change, advancing health.* Washington, DC: National Academies Press.

The Joint Commission. (2008, July 9). Behaviors that undermine a culture of safety. *Sentinel Event Alert Issue 40.* Oakbrook Terrace, IL: Author. Retrieved from https://www.jointcommission.org/assets/1/18/SEA_40.PDF

Latham, G. P. (2007). *Work motivation: History, theory, research, and practice.* Thousand Oaks, CA: Sage.

Latham, G. P., & Ernst, C. T. (2006). Keys to motivating tomorrow's workforce. *Human Resource Management Review, 16*(2), 181–198. doi:10.1016/j.hrmr.2006.03.014

Locke, E. A. (1968). Toward a theory of task motivation and incentives. *Organizational Behavior and Human Performance, 3*(2), 157–189. doi:10.1016/0030-5073(68)90004-4

Locke, E. A., & Latham, G. P. (1990). *A theory of goal setting & task performance.* Upper Saddle River, NJ: Prentice Hall College Division.

Longo, J. (2010). Combating disruptive behaviors: Strategies to promote a healthy work environment. *Online Journal of Issues in Nursing, 15*(1), Manuscript 5. doi:10.3912/OJIN.Vol15No01Man05

Macauley, K. (2015). Employee engagement: How to motivate your team? *Journal of Trauma Nursing, 22*(6), 298–300. doi:10.1097/JTN.0000000000000161

Maslow, A. H. (1943). A theory of human motivation. *Psychological Review, 50*(4), 370–396. doi:10.1037/h0054346

Maslow, A. H. (1954). *Motivation and personality.* New York, NY: Harper.

McClelland, D. (1976). Power is the great motivation. *Harvard Business Review, 54*(2), 100–110.

McGregor, D. (1960). *The human side of enterprise.* New York, NY: McGraw-Hill.

MindTools. (n.d.). Locke's goal-setting theory: Setting meaningful, challenging goals. Retrieved from https://www.mindtools.com/pages/article/newHTE_87.htm

Porter-O'Grady, T., & Malloch, K. (2013). *Leadership in nursing practice: Changing the landscape of health care.* Burlington, MA: Jones & Bartlett.

Quality and Safety Education for Nurses Institute. (2014). QSEN competencies. Retrieved from http://qsen.org/competencies/pre-licensure-ksas

Redmond, B. F., & Johnson, V. M. (2016), 3. Reinforcement theory. Retrieved from https://wikispaces.psu.edu/display/PSYCH484/3.%20Reinforcement%20Theory

Skinner, B. F. (1953). *Science and human behavior.* New York, NY: Free Press.

Strout, K., Nevers, J., Bachard, D., & Varney, S. P. (2016). Evidence-based interview strategy for new nurses. *American Nurse Today, 11*(9), 45–46. Retrieved from https://www.americannursetoday.com/evidence-based-interview-strategy-for-new-nurses/

Sullivan, E. J. (2013). *Effective leadership and management in nursing* (8th ed.). Upper Saddle River, NJ: Pearson.

Sullivan, E. J., & Decker, P. J. (2009). *Effective leadership and management in nursing* (7th ed.). Upper Saddle River, NJ: Pearson.

Toode, K., Routasalo, P., & Suominen, T. (2011). Work motivation of nurses: A literature review . *International Journal of Nursing Studies, 48*, 246–257. doi:10.1016/j.ijnurstu.2010.09.013

U.S. Equal Employment Opportunity Commission. (n.d.). Title VII of the Civil Rights Act of 1964. Retrieved from https://www.eeoc.gov/laws/statutes/titlevii.cfm

Walker-Reed, C. A. (2016). Clinical coaching: The means to achieving a legacy of leadership and professional development in nursing practice. *Journal of Nursing Education and Practice, 6*(6), 41–47. doi:10.5430/jnep.v6n6p41

Young, M. O. (2014). Constructive feedback and disciplinary action. *American Nurse Today, 9*(4). Retrieved from https://www.americannursetoday.com/constructive-feedback-and-disciplinary-action

V

INTEGRATING LEADERSHIP AND MANAGEMENT COMPETENCIES INTO NURSING PRACTICE—YOUR EVOLUTION AS A PROFESSIONAL

20

ENVISIONING AND DEVELOPING YOUR CAREER: WHERE AM I GOING?

LINDA RONEY

LEARNING OBJECTIVES

After completion of this chapter, the reader will be able to

- Discuss the role of career *envisioning* as part of the career planning process.
- Identify Quality and Safety Education for Nurses (QSEN) competencies that relate to career development skills.
- Explain the role of a career coach in successful professional development.
- Use the CHAMP process to select a professional mentor for career development.
- Apply the Nursing Professional Networking (NPN) model to develop one's personal career.

Many nurses encounter challenges in envisioning and developing their careers. Although some nurses pursue their bachelor of science in nursing (BSN) degree with a specific career opportunity in mind, for many, the path is not as clear. The steps for professional development following graduation may present opportunities to develop new skills and ideas. Although you may have some thoughts from colleagues at your workplace, who may have motivated you to complete your bachelor's degree, you will continue to gain additional knowledge and tools to plan for the next phase in your career.

This chapter will help you understand the process of thoughtful envisioning as part of this next step in your career planning process. Thoughtful envisioning is based on the Quality and Safety Education for Nurses (QSEN) competencies (QSEN Institute, 2014) that relate to career development. The role of the career coach is described as it relates to your role development as a BSN-prepared registered nurse. You will learn how to use the CHAMP model to select a professional mentor to assist you with your career development.

BOX 20.1 CASE SCENARIO

Tamika is a registered nurse (RN) who earned her associate's degree in nursing at an area community college 3 years ago. After taking the National Council licensure examination (NCLEX®; NCBSN, n. d.), Tamika started her nursing career as a staff nurse on a musculoskeletal unit at an American Nurses Credentialing Center (ANCC) Magnet®-accredited medical center (ANCC, n. d.). At the same time, Tamika enrolled in an RN-to-BSN program at a state university near her home. This spring, she will graduate with her BSN degree. Many of her coworkers have completed their BSN degrees and continue to work on the musculoskeletal unit; however, Tamika has aspirations of doing something different with her career. Although both her manager and unit educator have their master's degrees in nursing, they do not seem to be able to provide Tamika any support related to developing her career in a new direction. As a first-generation American and the first in her family to graduate from college, Tamika does not know to whom to turn for advice as she envisions her career. At the end of one particularly busy shift, Tamika begins to think that she would like to explore options for her next phase in her professional development as she asks herself: Where am I going?

In Box 20.1, you will consider a case scenario of an associate's degree–prepared registered nurse who begins to consider the next phase in her professional development journey. Finally, the significance of developing a lifelong professional network is described using the Nursing Professional Networking (NPN) model.

ENVISIONING AND DEVELOPING YOUR CAREER

Until this point in your career, much of the career planning that you have done might have been linked to finding and securing a job as an RN. Now that you have taken this important step in your nursing career to earn your BSN degree, you have the opportunity to consider new opportunities this degree will open for you. An important step in this reflective process is visualization. Visualization, or envisioning, is a form of mental rehearsal that has been found to have a positive effect on the brain, which enhances one's motivation, confidence, and self-efficacy (Neason, 2012).

In the 1970s and 1980s, researchers began to study the influence of visualization on athletic performance. Ungerleider and Golding (1991) explored the effect of visualization on the performance of elite track and field athletes before the 1988 Olympic trials and after the Olympic games in Seoul, Korea. Findings support that visualization has a positive effect on performance. Over three decades since this original study and in preparing for the 2016 Summer Olympics in Rio, Olympic gold medalist Kayla Harrison spent 10 minutes every night before bed visualizing her performance at the Olympics (Maese, 2016). By the time she made it to the Olympics, she had already envisioned the moment thousands of times in her mind and reported that when she stood on the podium to receive her medal, she felt she had been there before.

Although most of us never will become elite Olympic athletes, you can take these findings and use them to aid in *envisioning* and developing your career. Much in the way an athlete trains for a high-profile game or competition, you need to deliberate in planning your nursing career. There are times that you may have long-term career goals in mind, such as wanting to return to school to pursue a graduate degree to become an advanced practice registered nurse (APRN). Other times, the path may not be as clear and you will need more time, direction, and focus to determine how you envision your career development.

QSEN COMPETENCIES SUPPORT PROFESSIONAL CAREER DEVELOPMENT

QSEN (2014) offers competencies that will help you develop skills in your own professional career development (Table 20.1). Consider each of these QSEN competencies and reflect on actions that you can take related to these competencies in your current or future practice area. The competencies are divided into three domains: knowledge, skills, and attitudes.

QUESTIONS TO CONSIDER BEFORE READING ON

- Which of these competencies do you believe you meet?
- Toward which competencies are you now working?
- With which competencies do you need assistance to understand and pursue?

Perhaps you are returning to school for your BSN degree because your employer requires that you return to school as a condition of your employment. If the choice to return to school is not your own, it might seem like a burdensome task. Before you started taking classes for your BSN degreee, you might have felt that you already have the clinical skills to effectively care for patients in your work setting. Yet the skills that you are developing as part of your BSN program will enhance your professional performance as well as broaden your career trajectory. Table 20.1 presents each of the QSEN competencies that you can consider and reflect upon relating to your own professional career development. QSEN Institute (2014) competencies that relate to developing knowledge in career development are a great example. Perhaps when you first started working on your unit, you learned about standards, such as national patient safety resources and clinical practice guidelines you need to integrate into your daily nursing practice. With

TABLE 20.1 DEVELOPING SKILLS IN CAREER DEVELOPMENT: RELEVANT QSEN COMPETENCIES

Knowledge	Skills	Attitudes
Discuss potential and actual impact of national patient safety resources, initiatives, and regulations	Evaluate research and evidence reports related to patient safety	Explain the importance of regularly reading relevant professional journals
Delineate the reliable sources for locating evidence reports and clinical practice guidelines	Use national patient safety resources for own professional development and to focus attention on safety in care settings	Acknowledge own potential to contribute to effective team functioning
Describe own strengths, limitations, and values in functioning as a member of a team	Demonstrate awareness of own strengths and limitations as a team member	Value relationship between national safety campaigns and implementation in local practices and practice settings

Source: Adapted from Marchi, N., & Sweeney, M. (2013). Using QSEN Competencies to foster professional development among baccalaureate nursing students. Retrieved from http://qsen.org/using-qsen-competencies-to-foster-professional-development-among-baccalaureate-nursing-students; Quality and Safety Education for Nurses Institute. (2014). QSEN competencies. Retrieved from http://qsen.org/competencies/pre-licensure-ksas

your enhanced knowledge as a bachelor's-prepared nurse, you may soon be ready to take a leadership role seeking out new national patient care standards to integrate into nursing practice on your unit. Instead of relying on the information others tell you to integrate into your practice, you will learn new skills to evaluate research and evidence to develop a culture of safety at work. Perhaps your attitude about reading professional journals related directly to your nursing practice has changed since you have returned to school as you now see how this information can improve patient outcomes.

APPLYING WHAT YOU LEARNED

Building on these ideas generated from the QSEN competencies (QSEN Institute, 2014), there are specific strategies to help you envision and develop your career. These include developing a professional vision board, creating a career map, finding a career coach, selecting mentors, and developing a professional network. Each of these is described in detail. Make time to pursue and complete each of these skills with the guidelines and directions provided as follows.

VISION BOARDS

A professional vision board is a collage of artifacts, images, and other important items that an individual can collect and display in one area to remind him or her of a goal or to be kept inspired (Figure 20.1). Developing a professional vision board may help bring you closer to identifying your goals (Rider, 2015).

Identify a box or a folder in your home where you can collect artifacts for your professional vision board. These items might include an ad for your "dream job" from a professional journal, a picture of the newly built medical center in a location where you hope to move when you graduate, the text from your professional organization's website identifying a professional certification you hope to achieve, or a motivational quote that you print from the Internet. Create a collage on a wall or corkboard in an area where you regularly work, which will keep these visions in the forefront of your mind. You can add to or change artifacts as your ideas regarding your professional development evolve. Place this board in a location where you can regularly see it so you can easily incorporate envisioning your career into your daily routine. As the case scenario continues in Box 20.2, Tamika begins to envision her career and creates a professional vision board.

CAREER MAPPING

Taking this identified vision to the next and more concrete level, career mapping is a process in which an individual describes his or her career destination and goals and then identifies a specific career goal and strategic career plan to meet his or her career destination. The career map and career goal are routinely revisited and revised until the career goal is met (Feetham & Doering, 2015).

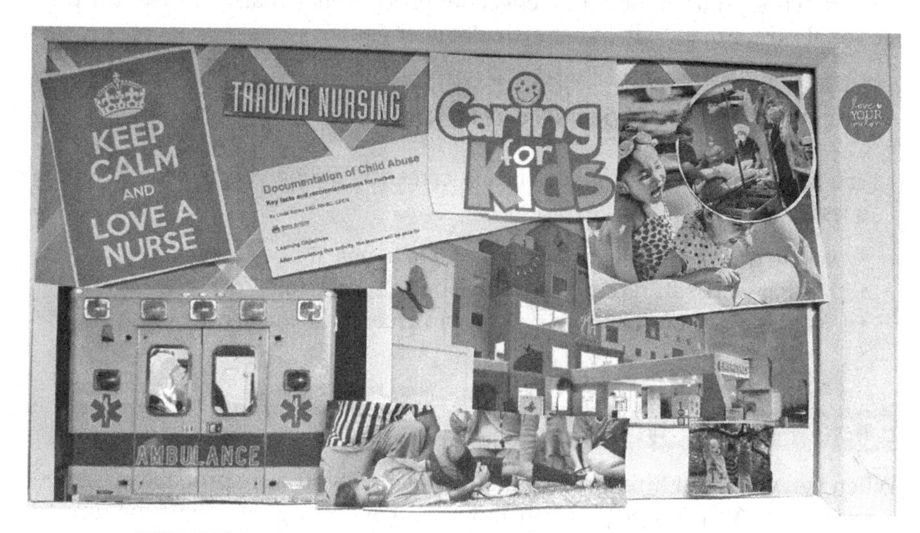

FIGURE 20.1 Example of a professional vision board.

BOX 20.2 THE CASE SCENARIO CONTINUES TO UNFOLD

Although Tamika enjoys her job on the musculoskeletal unit, she feels that her eyes have opened to exciting new possibilities about which she has been learning as a student in the RN-to-BSN program. She decides to designate a file folder for the process of career envisioning. Every time she sees something (e.g., a newspaper article, an ad in a professional journal, or a picture that inspires her to reach her goals), she puts it in this folder. When she has time on one of her days off from work, she sorts through the items in the folder and carefully organizes them on corkboard over her desk. This vision board inspires her to keep studying when she starts to get distracted while finishing her homework. She quickly learns that she receives more inspiration taking a break from studying to walk her dog, Bruno, and come back and focus on her vision board than she did from the hours she had spent earlier scrolling through the Facebook posts of friends and near acquaintances.

Career mapping can assist you to create your lifelong learning and professional goals, provide service to your community and profession, and achieve your specific goals. We all have strengths and talents that can lead to success. This can be achieved by using a career map to promote self-discovery in one's professional life. To start your career map, consider where you are currently in your professional career and where you aspire to be in the future (Inglis, 2014). Webb, Diamond-Wells, and Jeffs (2017) created the Professional Career Map (Figure 20.2) that you can use to articulate the plan for your career vision. This tool provides you with the opportunity to consider the intermediate goals that you will need to achieve to reach your major career goal. It also prompts you to identify strategies to reach those goals. In Box 20.3, Tamika reflects on the artifacts she has gathered to reflect her professional goals. She uses the professional career map to help her articulate her goals.

QUESTIONS TO CONSIDER BEFORE READING ON

You can begin envisioning your future career by asking yourself the following questions:

- Where do I see myself professionally in 5/10 years?
- In what work setting can I see myself being successful?
- What is one professional goal that I can accomplish in the next year?

CAREER COACHING

When you were first hired into a nursing position, you were probably assigned a preceptor. A "preceptor" is an individual who is given the time-limited responsibility of helping the new nurse develop the clinical skills and

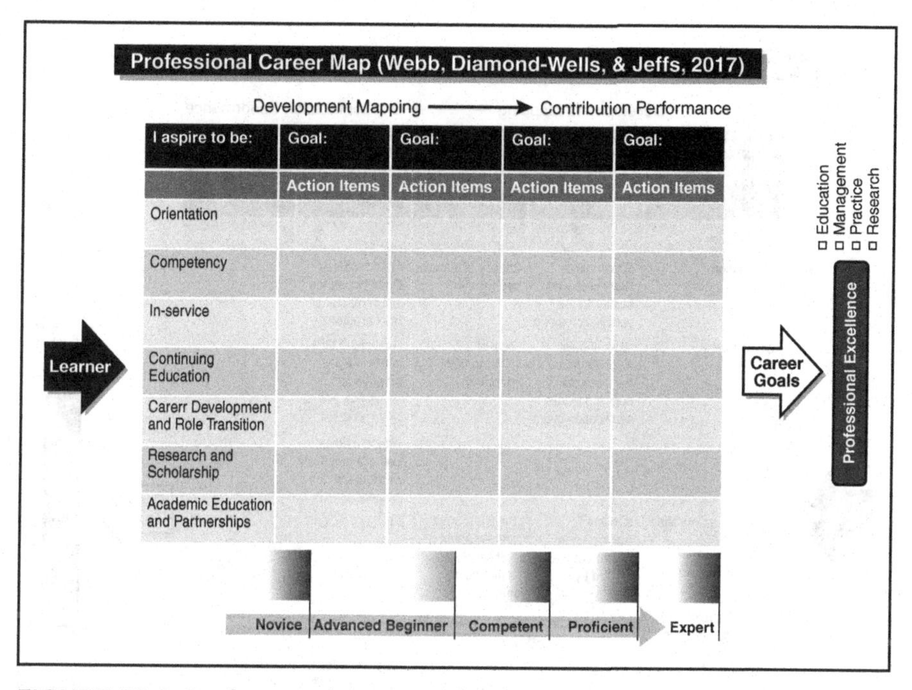

FIGURE 20.2 Professional Career Map.

Source: Webb, T. R., Diamond-Wells, T., & Jeffs, D. (2017). Career mapping for professional development and succession planning. *Journal for Nurses in Professional Development, 33*(1), 25–32. doi:10.1097/NND.0000000000000317. (Used with author permission.)

BOX 20.3 THE CASE SCENARIO CONTINUES TO UNFOLD

While in her leadership class, Tamika reads about the Professional Career Map (Webb, Diamond-Wells, & Jeffs, 2017) and decides to use this tool as she begins to plan her professional goals. In reviewing the professional vision board, she notices that she has many "artifacts" related to unit-based orthopedic nursing education. After some reflection, Tamika begins to realize that this goal is a natural fit for her. She uses the Professional Career Map (2017) as a model to create her own professional career map in her journal (Figure 20.3).

orientation necessary to work on a specific unit (Paton, 2010). Similar to this, a "career coach" is someone who interacts with a client in a specific, purposeful, and result-oriented way to help a person reach higher effectiveness (Fowler, 2014). There are times that this person might be a peer, as in the case of a colleague who has completed his or her portfolio for advancement on the clinical ladder and shares his or her experience with you and helps you learn from his or her perspective as you prepare to apply for promotion. A career coach is

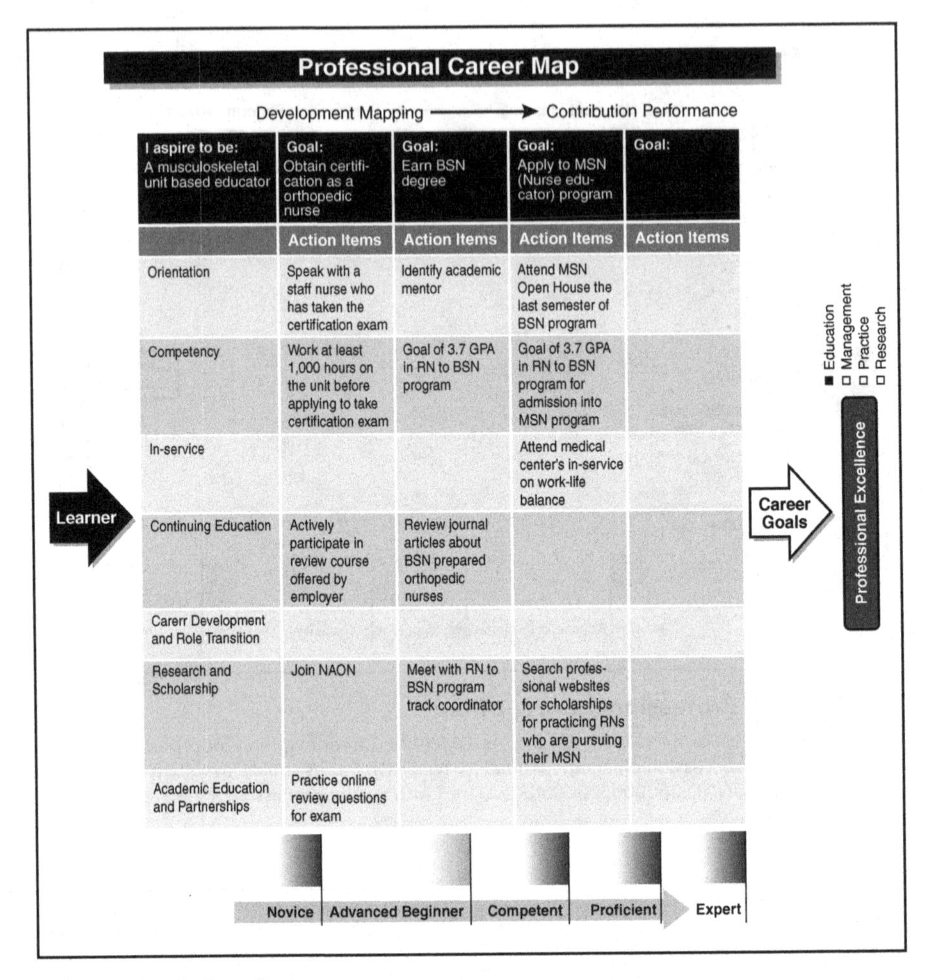

FIGURE 20.3 Tamika's career map.

Source: Based on the Professional Career Map, Webb, T. R., Diamond-Wells, T., & Jeffs, D. (2017). Career mapping for professional development and succession planning. *Journal for Nurses in Professional Development, 33*(1), 25–32. doi:10.1097/NND.0000000000000317. (Used with author permission.)

someone who may or may not be paid to help you identify solution-oriented steps to achieve your career goals (Cheek, Walsh Dotson, & Ogilvie, 2016).

CHAMP PROCESS OF PROFESSIONAL DEVELOPMENT: FINDING YOUR MENTORS

A "mentor" is a more experienced professional in your field (or one that you aspire to pursue) who offers career advice, guidance, and support from a real-world point of view (Scivicque, 2011). Mentors address mentees' attainment of professional goals (Cheek, Walsh Dotson, & Ogilvie, 2016). There is a five-step process, "CHAMP" (Figure 20.4), that can help you select professional mentors. (Box 20.4 describes Tamika's exciting experience attending her first professional conference. While there, she uses the CHAMP model for selecting a professional mentor.)

Choose mentors you admire. Take a moment to think about individuals in either your personal or professional life whom you admire. Maybe you admire one of your former coworkers who has left to work in another department after finishing a BSN degree. Perhaps you have attended a professional nursing conference and one of the speakers left a significant impression on you. I have chosen several mentors who had a national reputation for being the best at their careers.

Have the courage to ask. Many mentoring relationships develop informally through professional working relationships. For many nurses who are looking for new opportunities or career mobility, this might not meet their needs. Once you have identified a mentor(s) you admire, do not be afraid to ask them directly. For example, after hearing a presentation at a professional nursing conference on a topic about which you are passionate, you might approach the speaker during a break and introduce yourself. After a brief conversation, ask if it would be okay to meet for coffee or to set up a time to talk by telephone if he or she does not live close to you. In one of your first meetings, say what you admire about him or her and ask if he or she would be willing to be your professional mentor. While the first time you do this, it might feel quite awkward but, with practice, it will become less uncomfortable as you realize how flattering it is to be asked to be a mentor.

A good mentor should have a perspective different than your own. Although it might feel more comfortable to ask a friend at work to be your mentor, there is limited value in seeking mentorship from a person whose perspective is

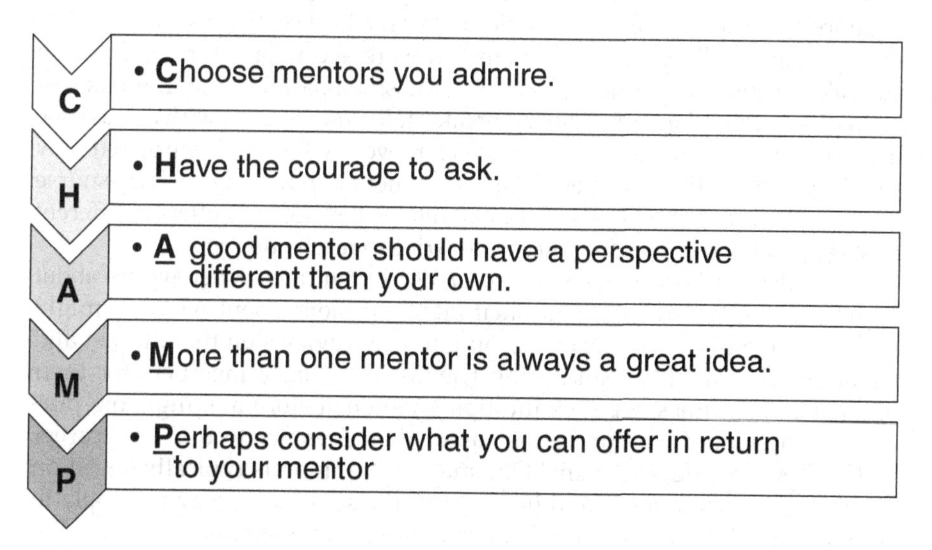

FIGURE 20.4 How to be a CHAMP when selecting professional mentors.

BOX 20.4 THE CASE SCENARIO CONTINUES TO UNFOLD

Tamika decides to take her professional development to the next step and attend the National Association of Orthopedic Nurses annual conference. While on the airplane to travel to the conference, she reads about the CHAMP model for selecting professional mentors. During the conference, she attends a focus session about innovations in pain management for postoperative joint replacement patients. She is captivated by the speaker (Dr. Michaels) and despite sweaty palms and a racing heart, Tamika approaches the podium to introduce herself to the speaker. They quickly greet one another, and Tamika is thrilled when Dr. Michaels offers her email address so they can connect with one another in the future.

Tamika emails Dr. Michaels on the last day of the conference and they set up a time to speak by telephone the following week. Inspired by her career path, Tamika asks Dr. Michaels if she would be willing to be her mentor. Dr. Michaels works as a clinical nurse specialist for the musculoskeletal service line at a major medical center almost 2,000 miles away from where Tamika works. The stories that she shares with Tamika on the basis of her experience are so interesting and her medical center is so different from where Tamika works. Their discussions open Tamika's eyes to a new perspective and new ideas to consider in her own professional development. Although Tamika has mentors at her own workplace, she enjoys her conversations with Dr. Michaels because the focus is less on hospital politics and more on improving patient outcomes.

exactly the same as yours. Instead, if there is someone who has a skill set that you aspire to develop, you might want to reach out to that person. For example, if you have a strong desire to work as a charge nurse, you might want to seek out opportunities to meet new people at your medical center. Instead of sitting with the same colleagues with whom you work every day on the unit when you take a continuing education course or hospital-based training, find a seat in another part of the room. During breaks, talk and network with at least one new person. If you have not done this before, you will be very surprised how easy this is to do. You may meet your future mentor in the role of charge nurse who works on a unit other than yours. This fresh set of eyes offers a different vantage point and advice for you as you strive to reach your goals.

More than one mentor is always a great idea. Oftentimes, when we are about to make a major purchase, we solicit many opinions about what we might buy. For some of us that means turning to user reviews on the Internet and for others that might mean asking friends and family members for their opinions. Most times, we seek multiple opinions before making a big purchase. Why would we not do the same when it comes to our own career and professional development? One mentor's opinion is typically based on his or her own experience and in all cases, the suggestion may not apply to your specific situation. You might speak with one mentor about the types of educational opportunities that might help you reach your goals. You might have another mentor with whom you discuss activities to build your resume. Perhaps another mentor works at another institution and he or she offers you practical advice about developing a clinical practice guideline for your unit. One person may not be able to help you accomplish all of your goals but having relationships with multiple mentors might help you do just that.

Perhaps consider what you can offer in return to your mentor. Although you may be adjusting to the idea of asking someone to be your mentor, did you ever think about what you can offer him or her in return? It is extremely generous for anyone to take the time to share his or her ideas with someone who is either just starting out or looking for new opportunities. In some of these relationships, you might offer to meet your mentor at a coffee shop at a time and location that is convenient for him or her (and then treating to coffee!). In other relationships, the exchange might be more reciprocal. Perhaps you used to work on a cardiac unit before transferring to work on a surgical unit. Your mentor may wish to develop skills in reading electrocardiograms (ECGs; something that you are very good at!). You offer to help your mentor learn ECG interpretation in exchange for his or her mentoring you in the area of professional development.

QUESTIONS TO CONSIDER BEFORE READING ON

- Who would be a great mentor for you in your current work setting?
- Who would be a great mentor for you outside of your current work setting but within your profession?
- How can you connect with a great mentor outside of your current work setting (e.g., through a professional organization, alumni organization professional meeting, seminar, or conference)?

NPN MODEL

WHAT IS NETWORKING?

Networking is the development of using contacts for purposes outside the original reason for the contact (Entrepreneur staff, 2017). For example, after completing a master's degree in nursing administration, a coworker leaves the hospital at which you work to take a promotion as a nurse manager on a medical surgical unit at another medical center in your state. To network with this former colleague, you reach out to meet for lunch and discuss potential job opportunities at the person's new place of work. Sometimes networking has a specific focus (e.g., looking for a new job) and sometimes it just involves a social exchange, either online or in person to broaden your thinking about your professional development. Professional networks lead to more job opportunities, deeper knowledge about your field, faster professional career advancement, and improvement in the quality of work (Casciaro, Gino, & Kouchaki, 2016).

START NETWORKING NOW

Networking is a proactive practice that should continuously take place before one decides to make a career move. Perhaps you are considering what will be your next steps following graduation with your BSN degree. Inviting a colleague who graduated a few years before you to meet you for coffee to discuss the steps he or she took to advance his or her career might be a great initial step. Perhaps you are at a nursing conference and you meet a nurse who works in the same clinical specialty at a hospital 30 minutes away from you. Discussing your clinical and professional interests might be a great first step in networking.

PLAN WHAT DO YOU WANT AND WHAT YOU CAN OFFER

Using tools presented earlier in this chapter, such as the career vision board and the professional career map, you have had the opportunity to consider what you want. The CHAMP model guided you in considering what you can offer a mentor. These same considerations apply when you meet with others as you try to broaden your professional network. Figure 20.5 presents the NPN model, a tool to help you get started with professional networking.

Start networking now
Plan- What do you want & what you can offer
Develop a positive online presence
Professional involvement & activites
Show appreciation toward your network

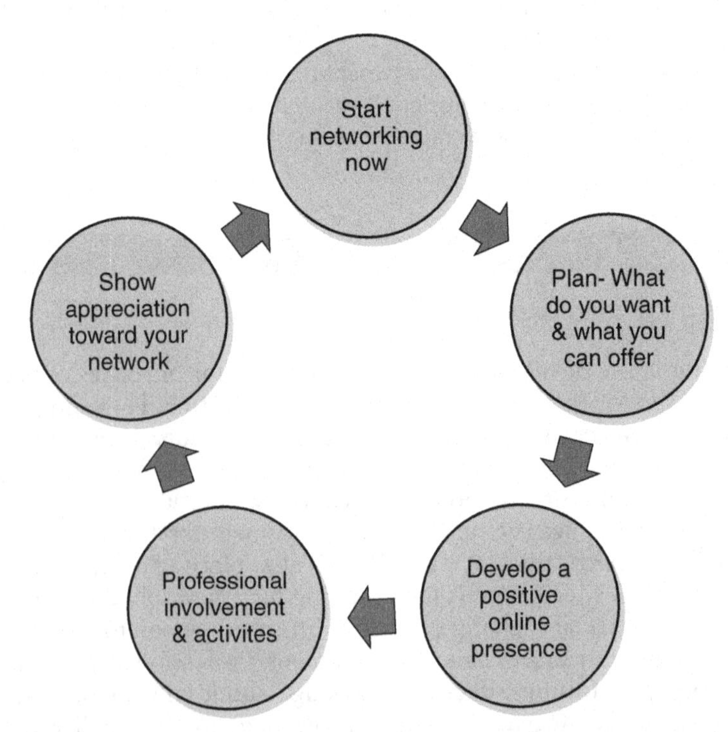

FIGURE 20.5 Nursing Professional Networking (NPN) model.

DEVELOPING A POSITIVE ONLINE PRESENCE

Going online is so much easier now that many of us have access to the Internet from a smartphone; nearly two-thirds of Americans own one. Having a smartphone has made it easier for people to go online to receive and post information. In a recent study, 43% of participants have used their smartphones to look up information about a job and 18% of people have used their smartphones to apply for a job online (Smith, 2015).

This increased access to going online also includes searching and posting on social media. Kung and Oh (2014) studied social media use among nurses and describe that 94% of nurses use social media with over 90% of nurses using social networking sites such as Facebook and Instagram. These activities can support professional development, such as "Liking" a professional nursing organization's Facebook page or following a governmental organization's Instagram page. Professional social media platforms, such as LinkedIn, can help nurses build and engage with a professional network online. Nurses can build a professional profile and virtually connect with a professional network. Best practices with LinkedIn include joining professional groups, sharing professional articles, and making networking connections with those who are in your specialty area of practice (University of Arizona with Duquesne University, n.d.). Most employers do maintain policies about social media use by employees, which includes activities both inside and outside of work, so be sure to familiarize yourself with their guidelines before posting any information that identifies your place of work or your role as an employee at your organization. Never post anything online that might look unprofessional or breach patient confidentiality (Smith, 2016). Box 20.5 describes how Tamika's engagement with her professional organization continues to grow after the conference.

BOX 20.5 THE CASE SCENARIO CONTINUES TO UNFOLD

Tamika enjoys attending the National Association of Orthopedic Nurses annual conference so much that she decides to join the educational committee. Her commitment to the committee is participation in every other month conference calls. During these meetings, she is able to share and receive information from other orthopedic nurses from across the country. She creates a LinkedIn profile that is linked to her professional organization's online community. The committee collaboratively develops a quarterly continuing education webinar series for orthopedic nurses across the country. Tamika really enjoys working on the committee and looks forward to the regular communication that she has with her new network.

PROFESSIONAL INVOLVEMENT AND ACTIVITIES

If you have not already done so, join a professional organization. After you do that, take the next step and determine the steps to join a committee or special interest group (SIG) for that professional organization. This will provide you with close interactions and the opportunity to work with others whose interests are similar to your own.

SHOW APPRECIATION TOWARD YOUR NETWORK

Whether it is by sending holiday cards or posting professional, inspirational quotes on platforms, such as LinkedIn and tagging your network, it is important to show your appreciation. If someone has been particularly helpful to you, a handwritten note or a small token gift goes a long way in our fast-paced lives.

HELPFUL HINT

Many professional organizations offer discounted memberships to students. If you are considering joining a professional organization, do not wait until you graduate. There might be opportunities that might apply to your career goals. Once you join a professional organization, consider attending the annual state or national conference. This is a great way to get involved in the organization and to find out how to join a committee or other work group. Some employers do offer financial assistance to employees for conference travel. If you are thinking about attending a conference, check in with your employer early as there might be a stipulation for the financial assistance (e.g., you must present a poster for them to support your travel expenses). If your employer does not offer financial assistance to attend a conference, you still should consider attending. Career development expenses may be tax deductible. Discuss this with your professional tax preparer.

SELF-ASSESSMENT

Do you effectively manage your career? Answer "true" or "false" to the following statements to determine your level of competency with regard to career development:

- I understand the strengths I offer to work.
- I know my areas for professional growth.
- I have a long-term vision for my career.
- I set goals consistent with performance feedback.
- I take my department's goals into account when setting my career goals.
- I effectively balance my career goals and personal priorities.
- I remain current on the skills that are relevant to my nursing specialty.

- I participate in training/educational activities each year to develop my skills.
- I have a mentor for my professional and career development.
- I have developed a professional network to help develop my personal career.

Reviewing the results of these statements, what competencies have you met? What competencies can you continue to develop? What strategies presented in this chapter can you use to further develop these competencies?

CONCLUSIONS

In this chapter, you have had the opportunity to consider specific strategies to envision and develop your career. After reading this chapter, you have seen that none of these strategies are particularly challenging or demanding. They do require time and planning on your part. Time spent planning is time well spent. Take time after completing this chapter to consider ways that you can use these new tools to help you with your own professional development. It takes time to achieve your goals but with an organized and systematic approach, career development should be a natural progression of your goals that you develop over time.

CRITICAL THINKING QUESTIONS AND EXERCISES

- After using the tools presented in this chapter, what is clearer about your career goals? What needs more thought? Privately journal your thoughts or discuss with your mentor.
- Use your calendar to set up a monthly appointment for 30 minutes with yourself to review your plans for career development. Use this time to reach out to mentors to meet for coffee or update your online professional profile on a site such as LinkedIn. If something comes up, you should commit to reschedule this appointment within 1 week.
- Identify one professional article about a topic of interest to you. Use an Internet search engine (e.g., Google) to find out more about the author of this article. Do they have a professional online presence? If they do, make an attempt to join their professional network or reach out to them by email to share comments of appreciation of their work.

REFERENCES

American Nurses Credentialing Center. (n.d.). ANCC Magnet recognition program. Retrieved from https://www.nursingworld.org/organizational-programs/magnet

Casciaro, T., Gino, F., & Kouchaki, M. (2016, May). Learn to love networking. *Harvard Business Review*. Retrieved from https://hbr.org/2016/05/learn-to-love-networking

Cheek, R. E., Walsh Dotson, J. A., & Ogilvie, L. A. (2016). Continuing education for mentors and a mentoring program for RN-to-BSN students. *Journal of Continuing Education in Nursing, 47*(6), 272–277. doi:10.3928/00220124-20160518-09

Cheeks, D. (2013, July 9). 10 Things you should know about career coaching. *Forbes Magazine*. Retrieved from https://www.forbes.com/sites/learnvest/2013/07/09/10-things-you-should-know-about-career-coaching/#3a85ca947d5e

Duquesne University (n.d.) Nurses using LinkedIn for professional advancement. Retrieved from https://onlinenursing.duq.edu/blog/nurses-using-linkedin-professional-advancement

Entrepreneur staff. (2017). Networking. Small business encyclopedia. *Entrepreneur*. Retrieved from https://www.entrepreneur.com/encyclopedia/networking

Feetham, S., & Doering, J. J. (2015). Career cartography: A conceptualization of career development to advance health and policy. *Journal of Nursing Scholarship, 47*(1), 70–77. doi:10.1111/jnu.12103

Fowler, D. L. (2014). Career coaching: Innovative academic-practice partnership for professional development. *Journal of Continuing Education in Nursing, 45*(5), 205–209. doi:10.3928/00220124-20140417-02

Inglis, N. (2014). How to map your career path. *U.S. News and World Report*. Retrieved from http://money.usnews.com/money/blogs/outside-voices-careers/2014/01/23/how-to-map-your-career-path

Kung, Y. M., & Oh, S. (2014). Characteristics of nurses who use social media. *Computers, Informatics, and Nursing, 32*(2), 64–72. doi:10.1097/CIN.0000000000000033.

Maese, R. (2016, July 28). For Olympians, seeing (in their minds) is believing (it can happen). *Washington Post*. Retrieved from https://www.washingtonpost.com/sports/olympics/for-olympians-seeing-in-their-minds-is-believing-it-can-happen/2016/07/28/6966709c-532e-11e6-bbf5-957ad17b4385_story.html?utm_term=.c3b3c4ff018e

Marchi, N., & Sweeney, M. (2013). Using QSEN competencies to foster professional development among baccalaureate nursing students. Retrieved from http://qsen.org/using-qsen-competencies-to-foster-professional-development-among-baccalaureate-nursing-students

National Council of State Boards of Nursing. (n.d.). NCLEX & other exams. Retrieved from https://www.ncsbn.org/nclex.htm

Neason, M. (2012, August 8). The power of visualization. *Sports Psychology Today*. Retrieved from http://www.sportpsychologytoday.com/sport-psychology-for-coaches/the-power-of-visualization/

Paton B. I. (2010). The professional practice knowledge of nurse preceptors. *Journal of Nursing Education, 49*(3), 143–149. doi:10.3928/01484834-20091118-02

Quality and Safety Education for Nurses Institute. (2014). QSEN competencies. Retrieved from http://qsen.org/competencies/pre-licensure-ksas

Rider, E. (2015, March 14). The reason vision boards work and how to make one. *The Huffington Post*. Retrieved from http://www.huffingtonpost.com/elizabeth-rider/the-scientific-reason-why_b_6392274.html

Scivicque, C. (2011, June). How to start a mentorship relationship. *Forbes Magazine*. Retrieved from https://www.forbes.com/sites/work-in-progress/2011/06/18/how-to-start-a-mentorship-relationship/#57e73da74a27

Smith, A. (2015). Chapter Two: Usage and attitudes toward smartphones. *Pew Research Institute*. Retrieved from http://www.pewinternet.org/2015/04/01/chapter-two-usage-and-attitudes-toward-smartphones/

Smith, L. S. (2016). Changing course: Midcareer nurses and the job search. *Nursing, 46*(1), 51–52. doi:10.1097/01.NURSE.0000475484.28632.a5

Ungerleider, S., & Golding, J. M. (1991). Mental practice among olympic athletes. *Perceptual and Motor Skills, 72*(3), 1007–1017. doi:10.2466/pms.1991.72.3.1007.

Webb, T. R., Diamond-Wells, T., & Jeffs, D. (2017). Career mapping for professional development and succession planning. *Journal for Nurses in Professional Development, 33*(1), 25–32. doi:10.1097/NND.0000000000000317

21

PREPARING FOR PROFESSIONAL OPPORTUNITIES

KARRI DAVIS ● DAVID M. DEPUKAT

LEARNING OBJECTIVES

After completion of this chapter, the reader will be able to

- Distinguish between a résumé and a curriculum vitae.
- Compose a curriculum vitae.
- Demonstrate the value of specialty certification.
- Construct a nursing portfolio.
- Determine promotional opportunities within nursing.
- Devise a plan to secure a promotion.
- Prepare for a behavior-based interview.
- Devise a plan to negotiate a job offer.
- Evaluate the commitment to professional development and lifelong learning.

The time surrounding graduation from a nursing program, completing the National Council Licensure Examination (NCLEX®) for registered nurses, and transitioning to the professional nurse role is filled with many emotions ranging from anxiety to excitement of what the future holds. The same emotions are experienced when preparing, applying, interviewing, and accepting a new position. Academic preparation at the baccalaureate level in conjunction with the commitment to lifelong learning is the foundation that leads to a wealth of professional leadership opportunities in healthcare.

This chapter is framed to showcase the preparation phases necessary to apply for and accept different nursing leadership positions. The

BOX 21.1 CASE SCENARIO

Lori graduated from a community college with her associate's degree in nursing 5 years ago. Her ideal future was to be a flight nurse. She began by creating a résumé and applying for, and subsequently working in, an emergency department to meet her goal of becoming a flight nurse. Later this year, Lori will be graduating from her registered nurse to bachelor of science in nursing (RN-to-BSN) program. Lori had the opportunity during her coursework to implement an evidence-based practice project that decreased the use of indwelling urinary catheters in her emergency department. After the development and implementation of this project, Lori realized that her new focus is nursing leadership. The assistant nurse manager position in the emergency department was recently posted as an open position. Lori decided to review her résumé.

components of lifelong learning are explored that are needed to foster new career endeavors. As a registered nurse (RN), you may already have experience with going through these processes to apply for a nursing position and accepting it. However, this chapter provides you with additional, more in-depth skills to enhance this application process as you continue to move forward in your nursing career. An evolving case scenario (see Box 21.1) is used to exemplify the critical components of preparation including building a résumé or curriculum vitae (CV), creating a professional portfolio, interviewing, and negotiating.

RESUMES AND CURRICULUM VITAES

Your résumé or CV is the first impression an employer will have of you as an applicant. A "résumé" is a clear, concise, one- to two-page document that lists your past education, work experiences, qualifications, and accomplishments. It is, in essence, a short personal success story in which the creator decides what details to share, what to leave out, and how to present each element. A "CV" is longer than a résumé as it also includes your presentations, publications, projects, and committee work. Employers use the content of a résumé or CV for screening purposes to obtain a first impression. The employer may receive hundreds of résumés or CVs for one available position. Therefore, a résumé or CV that does not describe the applicant as meeting or exceeding expectations may be discarded and the applicant will not get a call, despite being extremely qualified for the position. Most applications, including employment or continued education, will not be complete without either a résumé or a CV. There are significant differences, which are discussed in the subsequent text, to determine which option will be the most advantageous for you as a nurse to capture the eyes of the employer.

RÉSUMÉ

There are two types of résumés, a "general résumé" and an "application-specific résumé. "The *general résumé* will include all headings that are discussed in the following text. It is used as a repository from which to pull when creating an application-specific résumé. The *application-specific résumé* should be customized based on the focus of each position in which you choose to apply. A résumé for a management position will look different than one for an educator position. The résumé used for a new graduate nurse will look much different than the résumé of an experienced nurse. In Figure 21.1, the résumé is tailored to demonstrate that the applicant is ready for an entry-level leadership position such as an assistant nurse manager. The following headings are recommended to be included to build an effective résumé: contact information, license, objective statement, education, and employment in reverse chronological order. Other headings to consider if there is meaningful information to support the topic include achievements or professional affiliations, key qualifications, and volunteerism. As an experienced nurse, clinical rotations are removed from the résumé that may have been used when applying for a new graduate nurse position.

Organization

Although different suggestions for organizing one's résumé exist, what is consistent is that employers are most likely to read the top third of the page known as the "visual center" (Whitcomb, 2007). This location is where the most important information must be located to "hook" the reader or potential employer. A résumé should begin with *name, credentials, and contact information*. According to the American Nurses Credentialing Center (ANCC, 2013), *credentials* listed with the highest earned degree first, followed by license, state requirements, honors, and lastly other recognitions. If relocation is an issue in *contact information*, there are options to consider including: listing a current address with the understanding that some employers may not look at out-of-state applicants; not putting an address; or in the address section putting relocation to city, state in month, year. Next is a *qualifications summary statement* that quickly highlights, in two or three lines, experience and accomplishments that will capture the employer's attention. Next, list *education*, beginning with a degree in progress (as applicable), followed by most recent education, and continue in reverse chronological order. Include the full name and location of all schools attended to fulfill degree requirements, years attended, and degree obtained. Keep in mind any honors or awards received during a program as they can be listed here or placed in an achievement section. The award should include the title, organization from which the award was received, significance, and date. Some may argue that work history should be prior to education. The general rule is that education should be first if an applicant has graduated in the past 3 years or if it is a big selling point (Whitcomb, 2007). Many hospitals are

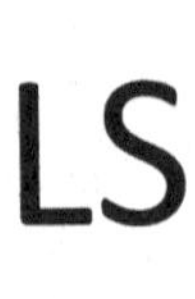

Lori Smith BSN, RN, CEN

SUMMARY

Compassionate Registered Nurse with five years' experience. Skilled in providing exceptional care to diverse patient populations with a passion for emergency medicine. Collaborative team player seeking leadership position

CERTIFICATIONS

- **2015-Present:** Certified in Emergency Nursing
- **2012-Present:** Registered Nurse, State of Connecticut
- **2011-Present:** BLS and ACLS Certifications, American Heart Association

EDUCATION

BSN • 2015-2017 • Anytown University, Anytown, CT

- Bachelor of Science in Nursing
- Cum Laude

ADN • 2010-2012 • ABC University, Sometown, CT

- Associate Degree in Nursing
- Student Leadership Award, ABC University Department of Nursing, Recognized by peers for leadership ability during nursing program, April 2012

EXPERIENCE

Registered Nurse – Adult Emergency Department; Level I Trauma • Best Hospital, New Haven, CT • 2012-Present

- Charge Nurse, Triage Coordinator; utilize global approach to facilitate patient placement and throughput based on patient acuity, safety, and available resources
- Managed, continuously changing patient assignments; Triage, interview, asses, plan, implement, evaluate, and document nursing interventions for patients experiencing emergency alterations of holistic integrity
- Developed a nursing peer mentor program which improved retention in the emergency department by 12% over 2 years
- Chair-elect of the hospital professional development nursing shared governance council

PROFESSIONAL AFFILIATIONS

Sigma Theta Tau International Nursing Honor Society
ABC Chapter at ABC University (Anytown, CT) Inducted in April 2012 for achievement and commitment to nursing excellence.
Emergency Nurses Association
Member: 2014-Present

FIGURE 21.1 Sample résumé.

seeking applicants with bachelor's-in-nursing preparation in alignment with the Institute of Medicine's (2011) goal of 80% of nurses being bachelor's-prepared by 2020; thus, this important success should be highlighted.

Employment history will consume a large section of the résumé. In the general résumé, list every position you have held including as much information as possible about the position. Each employer should be listed in reverse chronological order beginning with the most recent. This will facilitate forming an application-specific résumé easier. When an application-specific résumé is created, the applicant will determine the critical employment information to use from his or her general résumé. It is essential in the employment history section that the applicant balance being succinct and brief, but highlight the knowledge and skills to demonstrate that the applicant is the best candidate for the position.

Lastly, consider adding any *professional affiliations*, conferences, volunteerism, special skills, and/or *certifications*. Professional affiliations exhibit commitment and dedication to the profession. Skills that may be highlighted are languages, phlebotomy, telemetry, and computer documentation system proficiency. If there are other specialty certifications such as advanced cardiac life support (ACLS), they can be listed here. If there are multiple certifications, they should have their own section. Volunteer activities should include responsibilities and hours volunteered. Conferences, as well as professional affiliations, validate the commitment to lifelong learning.

Every application will require a different résumé, thus having one general résumé that can be used for pulling information will make each application easier. In other words, one's résumé should be adapted to the opportunity for which the individual is applying. Résumés may be used for more than just employment applications; they can be used for admission to graduate school, speaking engagements, and conferences. The order of topics within each résumé is based on the purpose of the document. For example, if it is a school application, education may be highlighted, even if it was years ago. Employers can receive many résumés for just one job, so taking the extra time to create a professional résumé will be beneficial. Résumés should be updated at minimum yearly, but more frequently as accomplishments, awards, or significant events occur.

CURRICULUM VITAE

The CV is more than a résumé as it encompasses one's entire nursing journey. The term CV used to be reserved for faculty within a college or university setting. More recently, nurses in formal and informal leadership positions have also started to use a CV because they can use it to list their publications, presentations, and committee work. Remember that nurses at the bedside are also leaders within their assignments and within the interdisciplinary team. It takes a leader to coordinate patient care among the multidisciplinary healthcare team members and healthcare providers. According to White and Castaldi (2017), all nurses need to promote themselves as leaders and create a CV to showcase their work. After all, a CV allows a nurse to capture ongoing data about his or her professional nursing practice, areas of expertise, and education over time, creating a total picture of one's nursing career.

Akin to a résumé, a general CV is created and then modified depending on the application or purpose. All of the topics discussed in the résumé section are included on the CV in addition to other topics. A CV provides a pathway to showcase publications, presentations, and other leadership development success not included in a résumé. See Table 21.1 to determine what to include within a CV and the order of topics, which can be used as a guide. Not every nurse, particularly those early in their careers, will have data for every section heading in the CV. In that case, the nurse should present future goals for those sections. For example, the nurse may not have served on a committee but is striving to become more active in decreasing the catheter-associated urinary tract infection (CAUTI) rate on the unit and thus has requested to be the unit representative on the CAUTI prevention committee for the hospital. If the nurse has a research proposal or quality improvement project in process, this proposal or project should be included under research-in-progress section. At first, novice nurses will develop a short CV but will continue to update over time with their professional career development. Therefore, a CV is considered a living documentary of a nurse's individualized and personal, professional career.

QUESTIONS TO CONSIDER BEFORE READING ON

- Consider your future in nursing. What are your professional nursing career goals? Include both formal and informal roles and opportunities that you desire to obtain.
- What competencies in an RN-to-BSN program would be important for an assistant nurse manager such as Lori?
- How often should Lori update her résumé or CV?
- Should all nurses create a CV to apply for a nursing position or acceptance into an advanced educational degree program? Why or why not?

PROFESSIONAL SPECIALTY CERTIFICATION

Nurses who pass the NCLEX-RN are considered to have met the basic minimum requirements for practice as a registered nurse. As nurses continue with professional development and lifelong learning, certification can validate a nurse's expertise in and commitment to a particular specialty. "As healthcare becomes increasingly complex and challenging, the value of certification as a mark of excellence is more important than ever. Achieving certification demonstrates to patients, employers and the public that a nurse's knowledge, skills and abilities meet rigorous national standards – and reflects a deep commitment to patient safety" (American Association of Critical-Care Nurses, 2017a, "Board Certification"). In Box 21.2, the evolving

TABLE 21.1 MODEL FOR CURRICULUM VITAE

Suggested Headings	Examples
Name and credentials	Lori Smith, BSN, RN, CEN
Contact information	Lori.Smith@email.com 800-111-1111
Education	ADN: ABC University BSN: Anytown University
Work experience	Short summary of work responsibilities from past and present jobs Example: Cared for high-acuity trauma patients in a level-one trauma center; charge nurse and preceptor experience; created the schedule, shift assignments, staffing, and patient concerns
Certifications	• National: Certified in emergency nursing • Work related: Basic life support; advanced cardiac life support • Educational: End-of-life nursing education consortium trainer
Honors and awards	• DAISY Award: Nominee • Great Catch Award
Professional membership	• Emergency Nurses Association • Sigma Theta Tau International
Continuing education	• End-of-Life Nursing Education Course • Include name, title of conference, location, number of contact hours
Professional presentations	• Unit council meetings • Conferences
Local publications	• Article within a hospital newsletter
National or international publications	• Peer-reviewed journal article
Committee appointments	• Unit quality committee • Hospital committee • Specialty organization
Community/volunteer activities	• Boy/girl scout leader • Fundraising relay team

Source: Adapted from White, K. A., & Castaldi, C. L. (2017). Creating and developing a professional CV. *American Nurse Today, 12*(9), 58–60. Retrieved from https://www.americannursetoday.com/creating-professional-cv

BOX 21.2 THE CASE SCENARIO CONTINUES TO UNFOLD

During Lori's final semester in her RN-to-BSN program, her class was learning about professional nursing certification. Lori realized that this was critical if she wanted to continue with her passion of nursing leadership. She was working full time in the emergency department and discovered that she qualified to take the Certified Emergency Nurse (CEN) examination on the basis of education and experience. Lori knew that to be a leader, she needed to set herself apart from her peers and demonstrate her expertise and commitment to emergency nursing. After a few hours of studying and a preparatory course, Lori passed her CEN examination.

case scenario highlights certification as demonstrating expertise and commitment to a specialty area of nursing.

Certification is a formal process of validating knowledge, skills, and abilities in a particular specialty. The certification exam is based on established standards of nursing care in a practice specialty area, such as critical care, or an advanced role, such as a clinical nurse leader. There are educational and experience requirements for a nurse to qualify to take the exam. "Certification is a profession's official recognition of achievement, expertise, and clinical judgment. It is a mark of excellence that requires continued learning and skill development to maintain" (ANCC, 2010). Certification provides the nurse with a mark of distinction among one's peers and demonstrates to the public a commitment to his or her patients. After a nurse successfully completes certification, it is considered active for a specified number of years depending on the certification. Nurses who have committed to lifelong learning will be able to recertify easily if they have met the ongoing continuing educational and practice requirements necessary to complete the recertification process.

In today's highly complex healthcare system, which cares for patients across the lifespan and in all healthcare settings, the benefits of nursing certification are clear for patients, families, employers, and the nurses themselves. "Americans prefer hospitals that employ nurses with specialty certification. Approximately three in four (73%) said that, given a choice, they are much more likely to select a hospital that employs a high percentage of nurses with specialty certification" (American Association of Critical-Care Nurses, 2017b). Employers are concerned with assuring ongoing competency of staff, retention of highly qualified nurses, and patient safety; nursing certification validates these essential components. There is also a significant benefit for the nurse. Certification demonstrates excellence in nursing and provides a vehicle for professional recognition, promotion, confidence, career development, dedication, and personal achievement. "Certification empowers nurses with pride and professional satisfaction" (ANCC, 2018). As a nurse, it is a professional obligation to obtain certification to provide the best opportunity for professional advancement.

QUESTIONS TO CONSIDER BEFORE READING ON

- If you are not already certified, what certification would you be interested in pursuing? Do you foresee any barriers to becoming certified? Consider how to overcome those obstacles. How is certification viewed by your organization's leadership and your colleagues?
- If you are already certified, are there other certifications you are seeking to obtain? What drove you to become certified? How has this certification been recognized by your employer? Your peers?
- Do you think Lori's CEN certification will make her more credible in her specialty of emergency nursing?

PROFESSIONAL PORTFOLIO

A "portfolio" is more than a CV in that it visually represents through physical evidence a nurse's progress and expertise developed throughout his or her professional career (Alfred, 2016). Portfolios and profiles are often used interchangeably; however, they are two different entities. Brown (1992) states, "A personal portfolio is a private collection of evidence which demonstrates the continuing acquisition of skills, knowledge, attitudes, understanding and achievement. It is both retrospective and prospective as well as reflecting the current stage of development and activity of the individual" (p. 53). Although this definition is 25 years old at the time of publication, it has stood the test of time as new research still reflects this description (Peate, 2006). As nurses move through their careers, it is imperative to keep up-to-date records for professional development, certifications, and accomplishments; thus, an all-inclusive portfolio is the best vehicle. The professional portfolio should be developed and structured in an organized method, electronically, in a hardcopy form (such as a binder), or both. The individual decides the actual layout. A portfolio is used to market one's competencies and accomplishments. A "profile" on the other hand is selected elements from the portfolio (Table 21.2) depending on the audience at hand. If the portfolio is used for a job interview, graduate application, or performance appraisal, the nurse can determine which documents to select for the occasion or "the profile" to showcase his or her professional pathway of nursing expertise and keep the rest aside for use with future opportunities.

Box 21.3 highlights Lori's decision to select a portfolio to showcase the evidence-based practice project.

TABLE 21.2 COMPARISON OF RÉSUMÉ, CURRICULUM VITAE, PORTFOLIO CONTENTS

Suggested Headings	Résumé	CV—Summary of Evidence	Portfolio—Actual Evidence
Name and credentials	X	X	X
Contact information	X	X	X
Education	X	X	X
Work experience	X	X	X
Certifications	X	X	X
Honors and awards	X	X	X
Professional membership	X	X	X
Continuing education		X	X
Professional presentations		X	X
Local publications		X	X
National or international publications		X	X
Committee appointments		X	X
Community/volunteer activities	X	X	X

BOX 21.3 THE CASE SCENARIO CONTINUES TO UNFOLD

Now that Lori has graduated with her BSN degreee and attained certification in her specialty, she wanted to consider options to showcase her work from both her RN-to-BSN program and her professional career. Lori created a CV instead of a résumé so she could highlight her evidence-based practice project that decreased the use of indwelling urinary catheters in her emergency department. However, Lori needed a place to display the presentation of the project and decided to create a portfolio.

PURPOSE

Portfolios are beneficial to the nurses in a variety of different ways. Hespenheide, Cottingham, and Mueller (2011) and Anderson, Gardner, Ramsbotham, and Tones (2009) identified the following purposes or ways for nurses to use a portfolio:

- Career planning/achievements
- Professional development opportunities

- Graduate admissions
- Interviews
- Clinical ladder advancement
- Speaking engagements
- Marketing/networking
- Goal development both educationally and employment
- Competency assessment
- Performance appraisals
- Self-reflection

CONTENTS

Nurses should start collecting the contents as early as possible and update the portfolio regularly. If a portfolio is going to be used for an interview, make copies and assure that original documents are maintained at home. The potential employer could ask to keep the portfolio during the decision process. The recommended contents as adapted from Alfred (2016) and Chamblee, Conkin, Drews, Spahis, and Hardin (2015) are as follows, but the nurse may include other documents as appropriate for the purpose of the portfolio:

- Nursing philosophy or personal statement
- CV
- Summary of education—include transcripts and diplomas
- Licenses
- Employment—include performance appraisals and current job description
- Professional nursing certifications: Board Certification (RN-BC) and Critical Care Registered Nurse (CCRN), among others
- Patient-care certifications such as basic life support (BLS) and ACLS
- Contact hour certificates
- Committee membership or project work at both the employer and the professional organization level
    - Examples: Policy, protocol, procedure, or clinical pathway development
- Awards
- Preceptors and/or mentors—maintain a list of nurses taught and how their professional development was impacted by you as the preceptor/mentor
- Presentations and publications—include the abstract, brochure, a picture of the presentation, evaluations, and complete citation if applicable
- Immunizations
- Letters of recommendation, appreciation, or thank-you letters/notes from patients or colleagues
- Any documents that demonstrate expertise in a specialty area of practice

QUESTIONS TO CONSIDER BEFORE READING ON

- What components of Lori's professional nursing journey should she showcase in her portfolio?
- List five accomplishments in your nursing career that make you proud.
- What elements of your professional nursing career would you showcase in your portfolio?

PROMOTIONS

Nursing careers today are more like a maze to the end goal and less of a ladder to the top. Each new nursing opportunity provides experience and expertise in the clinical, educational, or management arena. In the clinical arena, nurses have the opportunity to advance by being preceptors and charge nurses, and climbing the clinical ladder when available. Many organizations have a clinical ladder that has three or more tiers. Many of the clinical ladders require nurses to attend in-services, read journals, mentor new nurses, and implement evidence-based projects. Nurses can also continue with education to become an advanced practice registered nurse, clinical nurse specialist, or a variety of other advanced clinical roles. There are also new roles being developed on the horizon such as a clinical nurse leader. Nursing continues to evolve its role in shaping how care is delivered across the healthcare continuum. The bedside possibilities are ever changing.

In education, nurses in formal educational roles can teach in a variety of clinical settings including acute care, long-term care, home care, and physician offices. Training is usually designed for the direct bedside caregivers. In the hospital setting, these nurses are often referred to as "education specialists" or "clinical nurse educators" and have obtained a master's degree in nursing. Staff education has the potential for manager- and director-level promotions within the organization. Nurses who aspire to teach in the academic setting are encouraged to obtain a doctoral degree. In academia, there are multiple promotional levels within a university setting including adjunct professor, associate professor, dean, provost, and up through university president.

The management sector of nursing is a very traditional trajectory for promotions. (See Box 21.4 highlighting the next step of the management ladder for a staff nurse such as Lori.) The general roles include assistant nurse manager, manager, associate director, executive director, and vice president of nursing. Each role listed earlier may have different designations, but for purposes of explanation, a manager's span of control involves operational, financial, personal, and regulatory oversight of one or more clinical areas. The assistant nurse manager of a unit assists the manager with the aforementioned functions as appropriate. A director oversees multiple clinical units and programs. A vice president of nursing has oversight of the entire nursing body. Beyond a nursing vice president, a select group of nurses has climbed the ladder into the "C-suite."

BOX 21.4 THE CASE SCENARIO CONTINUES TO UNFOLD

Lori has put together her CV and her professional portfolio. In her portfolio, she highlighted the success of her RN-to-BSN project: Decreasing Unnecessary Indwelling Urinary Catheter Insertions in Adult Patients. The outcome of this project resulted in decreased indwelling urinary catheter insertions in the emergency department. Lori feels prepared for the next step of her leadership career and feels ready for the promotion to assistant nurse manager.

It was stated that nursing is more of a maze rather than a ladder. There are now a plethora of nursing leadership opportunities that are considered promotions including, but not limited to, performance improvement coordinators, risk managers, case managers, utilization reviewers, and patient safety nurses. Each of these roles usually requires nurses to have a baccalaureate degree and clinical expertise within a specialty, which can be demonstrated by professional certification.

SECURING A PROMOTION

Each year, employees will receive a performance evaluation that provides an opportunity to sit down with their manager and discuss performance over the past year and set new goals for the upcoming year. The conversation provides an opportunity to discuss the potential for current or future promotional opportunities. The reason an employee who is deserving of a promotion does not get one may simply be that the right people are not aware of one's desire or intent. Individuals such as the manager should be aware so that feedback can be directed at facilitating growth and development to that next level. If an employee wants a promotion but does not feel confident at the time, there are four recommendations to prepare for future opportunities that include the following: find a mentor, be visible where it counts, always keep learning, and reflect back on the CV and portfolio to determine on what pieces may be beneficial to work. If you as a staff nurse aspire to be an assistant nurse manager, implementing an evidence-based practice project would strengthen your CV and portfolio and joining a hospital committee would be an option to increase your visibility.

QUESTIONS TO CONSIDER BEFORE READING ON

- Have you considered a promotion? If not, what has stopped you?
- What type of leadership opportunities interest you? How would you describe your ideal nursing role, which may include a component of patient care?

INTERVIEWING

Many nurses are anxious about participating in their first interview for a leadership position. If you are applying for a position in a different agency, you should research the healthcare agency before the formal interview. Examine the mission statement, vision statement, clinical and nonclinical specialties, and awards. If possible, determine what interview process or model the agency uses by networking, social media, or calling human resources. Interview types include phone, team interviews, informational, competency based, behavioral, and others. Many healthcare organizations and Fortune 500 companies are using behavior-based interviewing, making it one of the most common interview styles (LaMaster & Larsen, 2010). The "behavioral interview" can best be defined as an analysis of an applicant's ability by assessing skills used in past performance (Strasser, 2005). After determining the style of interview, explore what types of questions may be asked in that type of interview. Behavior-based interviews ask questions that are open-ended and allow the candidate to tell a story.

- "Tell me about a time you advocated for a patient."
- "Tell me about a time you helped a coworker."
- "Tell me about a time you went above and beyond for a patient."
- "Tell me about your biggest accomplishment." (See Box 21.5—Lori could select her project, certification, or promotion to a clinical nurse II.)

The hallmark indication of behavior-based interviewing is "Tell me about a time you ...." Take time to reflect on different nursing scenarios to answer the questions. Outside of the patient care arena, consider committee work, accomplishments, and education when answering the interview questions, especially when applying for nursing leadership positions. Behavior-based interviewing predicts future behavior (Strasser, 2005). The answers to the different questions should demonstrate accountability, respect, teamwork, conflict resolution, compassion, integrity, and patient-centered care. During your cognitive rehearsals, think about

BOX 21.5 THE CASE SCENARIO CONTINUES TO UNFOLD

Lori discussed with her manager that she would like a promotional opportunity and thus has applied for the assistant nurse manager position within her unit. She is awaiting her upcoming interview. Lori prepared her CV and portfolio. In her portfolio, she included her project, contact hours, certification, and her promotion to a level II on the clinical ladder.

different answers to the same question to determine which will be the best (Table 21.3).

Researching different types of questions and reflecting on your past and future professional nursing career are very effective ways to determine what answers to provide during the interview. The "SHARE" model, as shown in Table 21.4, provides a comprehensive, consistent response and demonstrates

TABLE 21.3 BEHAVIORAL INTERVIEW QUESTIONS

1	Tell me about what made you who you are, why you got into this line of work, and why you want to do this job.
2	Tell me about a time when you advocated for a patient.
3	Tell me about a time when you helped a coworker.
4	Tell me about a time when you went above and beyond for a patient.
5	Tell me about a situation in which you had to adjust to changes over which you had no control. How did you handle it?
6	Describe a work situation that required you to really listen and display compassion to a coworker or patient who was telling you about a personal/sensitive situation.
7	When have you had to work with conflicting, delayed, or unclear information? Tell me exactly what you did.
8	Give me an example of a time when you tried to accomplish something and failed. Did this discourage you? What did you do about it?
9	Describe a time when something you said was not understood in the manner you meant. How did you interpret the miscommunication? What did you do about the situation and what was the outcome?
10	Tell me about a time you discovered a mistake someone else made. What was it and how did you deal with it?
11	Tell me about a time you went against a policy or procedure (bent the rules) to accomplish something.
12	Tell me about some things you have done for other people without being asked.

TABLE 21.4 SHARE MODEL

S	Describe a specific situation
H	Identify hindrances or challenges
A	Explain the action that you took
R	Discuss the results or outcome
E	Evaluate or summarize what you learned

Source: LaMaster, M. A., & Larsen, R. A. (2010). Prepare for a behavioral interview, then ace it. *American Journal of Nursing, 110*(Suppl. 1), 8–10. doi:10.1097/01.NAJ.0000366152.10576.00

preparation (LaMaster & Larsen, 2010). Interviewers typically score candidates on different scales, but in the end, they want to assure that a candidate is prepared for the role on the basis of his or her knowledge, skills, and attitudes.

Aside from the questions, there are other indicators of professionalism at which employers are looking. If you are being interviewed, arrive early, dress professionally, and have copies of your résumé, CV, or portfolio. Demonstrate continued interest in the job by having questions for the interviewer, for example: "What objectives would a successful employee be completing in the first 3 to 6 months?" This question highlights the expectations an employee would need to meet and facilitates information gathering for a negotiation process later. At the end of the interview, send a follow-up thank-you letter. There is only one opportunity to make a first impression, so make it count.

QUESTIONS TO CONSIDER BEFORE READING ON

- What are some examples of behavior-based interviewing questions you would ask Lori?
- Reflect on your first interview as an RN. What was the most challenging question that you were asked? If you had to answer it again, how would you answer it? What feedback would you give yourself about that first interview?

NEGOTIATING

Negotiating may be difficult at first as one does not want to give an impression of being overconfident, yet many nurses do not realize their full worth. Potential employees are afraid they will lose the job opportunity if they negotiate. According to a recent survey, 84% of employers expect candidates to ask for a higher compensation, yet only 13% of employers have rescinded a job offer as a result of negotiations (Salary.com, n.d.). A candidate should be aware of the job market and the salary of comparable positions within the area. A candidate, however, needs to be self-aware of the lowest salary he or she is willing to accept; negotiating includes much more than just salary. Other options a candidate can negotiate include extra vacation time, tuition reimbursement, flexible scheduling, or weekend options. Candidates need to consider the entire package surrounding the promotion including the title, pay, nonsalary benefits, and any future opportunities the position may present for future career growth and advancement. Box 21.6 highlights a multitude of factors Lori must consider in making her final decision to accept the assistant nurse manager position.

BOX 21.6 THE CASE SCENARIO CONTINUES TO UNFOLD

Lori just completed her interview for the assistant nurse manager. She is expected to hear about her potential promotion today. Lori is concerned that she will take a pay cut because the assistant nurse manager position is full-time days. Lori has been working full-time nights and weekends and will lose her differential. She also knows that there are more benefits to the position than money. She will have more paid time off, greater flexibility with scheduling, and all holidays off. Lori certainly may feel uncomfortable asking other assistant nurse managers in the organization what their salary is; however, it is perfectly acceptable to ask what the salary range of an assistant nurse manager would be.

INDIVIDUAL RESPONSIBILITY FOR PROFESSIONAL DEVELOPMENT

The healthcare landscape is ever changing and nurses need the knowledge, skills, and attitudes to keep up with the patient care demands. At the national level, certification exams require continuing education to be eligible for obtaining certification and maintaining competency. Passing the NCLEX is the minimum requirement to be a nurse; many states require continuing education to maintain licensure. "The nursing profession must adopt a framework of continuous lifelong learning that includes basic education, academic progression, and continuing competencies" (Institute of Medicine, 2011). Although the nursing profession must support lifelong learning, the nurse is responsible for individual professional development. (See Box 21.7, in which Lori just started as the assistant nurse manager and is already considering professional development opportunities.)

Professional development is the cornerstone of preparing for professional opportunities. New graduates and experienced nurses alike should use their CV and portfolio to determine the direction to take

BOX 21.7 THE CASE SCENARIO CONTINUES TO UNFOLD

Lori has begun her career as the assistant nurse manager of the emergency department. She is aware that this is a stepping stone up the career ladder. Lori is already thinking about her professional development within her current role and to prepare for what is to come.

for professional development. If a nurse has a lot of projects relating to education in his or her portfolio, he or she may look into joining committees that will facilitate development of management skills. Some will argue that the employer is responsible for providing professional development opportunities, which may be true in some instances. For example, if the position requires ACLS certification, the employer may be responsible for providing this learning opportunity. However, in the end, the employee is also held accountable for his or her own professional career competencies.

Newly required nursing competencies and/or skills often arise such as knowledge of healthcare policy and clinical informatics. The nurses are then responsible for educating themselves to remain competitive in higher leadership positions. It is also essential for nurses to take responsibility for their own learning to position themselves as the best candidates for future employment opportunities. Employees look to careers that match their strengths, support their development, and challenge them to learn new skills. Agencies seek employees who have developed the competencies themselves to meet their organizational needs. Employees view competencies as defining responsibilities for successful performance, identifying strengths and gaps within their personal competency profiles, developing opportunities to close the gaps, and effectively managing their own career growth. Organizations benefit from competencies as they are used for assessment of employee performance, coaching, mentoring, and developing structured educational programs.

There are both formal and informal options for nurses to continue their education at all levels of experience. Despite the level of expertise, what remains constant is that nurses want professional development opportunities that are timely, convenient, and relevant. Employers want professional development courses that they cultivate to be data driven on the basis of the organization's and employees' strengths and vulnerabilities (Spitzer & Miranda, 2017). It is imperative that organizations leverage the right data to determine competency gaps.

Leadership within the organization is responsible for ensuring competency of its staff to ensure the safety of the patient. Increasing the nurse's competency level through professional development is critical to promote patient safety and optimal outcomes (Stobinski, 2015). Nurse leaders have built expertise through professional development that allows them to provide guidance to staff and make critical decisions. Nurses in leadership roles usually have demonstrated a commitment to learning new roles beyond bedside care that were not taught in a nursing program. Nurses who are leaders within an educational role are required to be clinical experts within their specialty, have a business sense, and be familiar with policy development. Managers and directors who oversee units require a combination of high-level clinical oversight and superior customer service skills for staff, patients, and families, along with being business savvy including the day-to-day operations, budgeting, policies, and strategic planning. It is a change in thinking for nursing leaders to be responsible for developing strategic goals to produce high-quality patient care outcomes while decreasing cost. Most nurse leaders have an intrinsic drive for excellence that allows success.

Education does not end just because an individual is no longer in school. Learning is continuous throughout one's life in many professions. It is not limited to nursing or the medical field. Lifelong learning goes hand in hand with professional development. It is not limited to pursuing a degree, but can be obtained through in-services, attending conferences, reading journals, and joining committees that use evidence-based practice. It allows nurses of all experience levels to continue to strive toward excellence in their professional nursing practices.

QUESTIONS TO CONSIDER BEFORE READING ON

- Do you think Lori or her employer is responsible for professional development? What possibilities should Lori consider to build her leadership development? How should Lori measure the outcomes of learning opportunities?
- Reflect on your own journey of lifelong learning. What motivated you to return to school for your BSN degree? How is that impacting your work in your organization? In your future trajectory, what learning opportunities and competencies are important for you to consider?

SELF-ASSESSMENT

There are a lot of factors to consider when preparing for professional opportunities in the nursing profession. Consider the following questions when thinking about applying to a position, preparing for an interview, and accepting a promotion:

- Are you on the lookout for opportunities for advancement?
- Do you seek out professional development opportunities to improve your knowledge, skills, and potential?
- Do you professionally network?
- Do you thrive on change?
- Are you ready for a new challenge?
- Are you ready for more responsibility?
- Are you willing to accept that advancement may come with potential stress?
- Do you consistently strive to do your best and become more efficient?

CONCLUSION

Reflecting back on the chapter promotes the opportunity for critical thinking and self-understanding. Nurses have so many opportunities within healthcare, but it is up to each individual to best position himself or herself for those opportunities. Nurses have the opportunity to showcase their journeys and accomplishments using a résumé, CV, or a professional portfolio. Nurses who take ownership of their professional development will be able to reevaluate their careers at different points to determine where there may be gaps in professional development. Nurses who address an identified gap in their professional development will position themselves in the best possible light for future potential promotional opportunities.

CRITICAL THINKING ACTIVITIES

- Review your last résumé. Using a format such as the templates in most word processing programs, update your résumé. What is different? What is being added?
- Use a template such as the one available at www.visualcv.com/examples/nursing. Document your own nursing journey by creating a CV. As you reflect on the accomplishments that you have had, including committee work, of what are you most proud?
- Consider a leadership or other professional opportunity for which you would want to apply. This opportunity can be hypothetical or real. Respond to the following questions:
  - Would you use a résumé or CV? Why?
  - What elements and experiences would be important for you to include?
  - How would you prepare for an interview for such an opportunity?

REFERENCES

Alfred, L. (2016). Polishing your professional portfolio. *Radiation Therapist, 25*(1), 87–88.

American Association of Critical-Care Nurses. (2017a). Board certification. Retrieved from https://www.aacn.org/certification?tab=First-Time%20Certification

American Association of Critical-Care Nurses. (2017b). Certification benefits patients, employers and nurses. Retrieved from https://www.aacn.org/certification/value-of-certification-resource-center/nurse-certification-benefits-patients-employers-and-nurses

American Nurses Credentialing Center. (2010). Certification. Retrieved from http://www.nursecredentialing.org/Certification

American Nurses Credentialing Center. (2013). How to display your credentials [Brochure]. Retrieved from https://www.nursingworld.org/~4abf5a/globalassets/certification/renewals/DisplayCredentials-Brochure

American Nurses Credentialing Center. (2018). About ANCC. Retrieved from https://www.nursingworld.org/ancc/about-ancc

Anderson, D. J., Gardner, G. E., Ramsbotham, J., & Tones, M. J. (2009). E-portfolios: Developing nurse practitioner competence and capability. *Australian Journal of Advanced Nursing, 26*(4), 70–76. Retrieved from https://eprints.qut.edu.au/47211/1/AJN_nurse_practitioner_paper_26-4_Anderson.pdf

Brown, R. A. (1992). *Portfolio development and profiling for nurses.* Lancaster, PA: Quay Books.
Chamblee, T. B., Dale, J. C., Drews, B., Spahis, J., & Hardin, T. (2015). Implementation of a professional portfolio: A tool to demonstrate professional development for advanced practice. *Journal of Pediatric Health Care, 29*(1), 113–117. doi:10.1016/j.pedhc.2014.06.003
Hespenheide, M., Cottingham, T., & Mueller, G. (2011). Portfolio use as a tool to demonstrate professional development in advanced nursing practice. *Clinical Nurse Specialist, 25*(6), 312–320. doi:10.1097/NUR.0b013e318233ea90
Institute of Medicine Committee on the Robert Wood Johnson Foundation Initiative on the Future of Nursing, at the Institute of Medicine. (2011). *The future of nursing: Leading change, advancing health.* Washington, DC: National Academies Press.
LaMaster, M. A., & Larsen, R. A. (2010). Prepare for a behavioral interview, then ace it. *American Journal of Nursing, 110*(Suppl. 1), 8–10. doi:10.1097/01.NAJ.0000366152.10576.00
Peate, I. (2006). *Becoming a nurse in the 21st century.* Hoboken, NJ: Wiley.
Salary.com. (n.d.). Negotiation. Retrieved from https://www.salary.com/articles/negotiation
Spitzer, R., & Miranda, E. (2017). Enhancing professional role competency through data analytics and evidence-based education. *Nurse Leader, 15*(3), 189–192. doi:10.1016/j.mnl.2017.03.009
Stobinski, J. X. (2015). Nursing's invisible architecture: Individual responsibility for professional development. *Association of periOperative Nurses Journal, 102*(4), 324–328. doi:10.1016/j.aorn.2015.08.014
Strasser, P. B. (2005). Improving applicant interviewing: Using a behavioral-based questioning approach. *American Association of Occupational Health Nurses Journal, 53*(4), 149–151. doi:10.1177/216507990505300401
Whitcomb, S. B. (2007). *Resume magic: Trade secrets of a professional resume writer* (3rd ed.). Indianapolis, IN: JIST Works.
White, K. A., & Castaldi, C. L. (2017). Creating and developing a professional CV. *American Nurse Today, 12*(9), 58–60. Retrieved from https://www.americannursetoday.com/creating-professional-cv

22

CONTRIBUTING TO THE PROFESSION—OUR RESPONSIBILITY AS A PROFESSIONAL NURSE

SUSAN A. GONCALVES

LEARNING OBJECTIVES

After completion of this chapter, the reader will be able to

- Discuss the importance of mentoring others in nursing.
- Discuss benefits of active involvement in professional nursing organizations.
- Describe the importance of actively engaging in evidence-based practice.
- Explore the possibilities that can arise when advocating for the nursing profession.
- Describe the role of the professional nurse for maintaining a healthy work environment.
- Discuss the role of nurse advocacy in nurturing a healthy work environment.
- Describe the importance of the nurse's role in civic, social, and volunteer activities.

Professional nursing is defined as "the protection, promotion, and optimization of health and abilities, prevention of illness and injury, alleviation of suffering through the diagnosis and treatment of human response, and advocacy in the care of individuals, families, communities, and populations" (American Nurses Association [ANA], 2010, p. 10). The ANA has noted that as of January 2016, there are approximately 3.6 million licensed registered nurses (RNs) in the United States (ANA, 2016). It based this estimate on historical data gathered from the last National Sample Survey of Registered Nurses (NSSRN) conducted by the U.S. Department of Health and Human Services (2008) as well as the RN employment data from the U.S. Department of Labor, Bureau of Labor Statistics. This figure is staggering and should be noted that this does not include retired nurses who are no longer actively practicing.

For decades, there exists the ongoing debate on whether a nursing shortage actually exists. Although these numbers may sound large, it is important to note that the American Association of Colleges of Nursing (AACN), the Institute of Medicine (IOM), and the Bureau of Labor Statistics all concur that the United States is currently experiencing a shortage of RNs and this shortage is expected to continue to grow and intensify in numbers as our baby boomers age and seek out healthcare. According to the "United States Registered Nurse Workforce Report Card and Shortage Forecast" published in the *American Journal of Medical Quality*, this shortage of RNs was projected to spread across the country between 2009 and far into 2030 and possibly beyond. This report card/forecast provides an analysis broken down by state and predicts the largest impact occurring in the south/west parts of the nation (Juraschek, Zhang, Ranganathan, & Lin, 2011).

In addition, although RNs are listed as a fast-growing profession, the Bureau of Labor Statistics (*Employment Projections for 2014–2024*) predicts a growth of approximately 440,000 nurses and a shortage of approximately 650,000 nurses to replace aging or retiring nurses, leaving a shortage of approximately 1.09 million nurses by 2024. Complete details and projections can be found by visiting www.bls.gov/news.release/pdf/ecopro.pdf.

The Future of Nursing report (2011) from the IOM is the result of an initiative, "The Future of Nursing," sponsored by the Robert Wood Johnson Foundation. In the report, the IOM calls on all nurses to stand up and take a greater role in America's increasingly complex healthcare system. The ANA highly commended the IOM for its report on the nursing profession and acknowledges the need for all nurses to take a leadership role in all settings to meet the ever-changing demands so evident in our evolving healthcare system.

This chapter explores several key concepts in regard to the nurse's role as a contributing member of the nursing profession as well as healthcare systems. Advocacy for the profession and promotion of a healthy workplace are explored. The influence of professional organizations is explained as well as ways in which you can engage in active involvement and benefit from being a member. Finally, mentoring and volunteerism are discussed challenging you to partake in opportunities to grow and develop personally as well as strengthen your own nursing profession and leave an everlasting legacy for future generations of the nursing profession.

To begin the discussion of advocacy and benefits of active involvement in professional organizations, we will begin with a case scenario Box 22.1.

QUESTIONS TO CONSIDER BEFORE READING ON

Imagine if all 3.6 million nurses played an active role in our healthcare system as the IOM urges.

- What would healthcare look like?
- What would the profession of nursing look like?
- What contributions to the profession do you currently make?

BOX 22.1 CASE SCENARIO

As you read the following case scenario, think about the reasons Danielle's mentor would suggest joining a professional organization and attending conferences.

A new nurse, Danielle, is working in the intensive critical care unit at a large urban hospital. As part of her first annual review, Danielle's mentor encouraged her to join the critical care professional organization (American Association of Critical-Care Nurses) and attend the annual conference with her. Prior to attending the conference, Danielle had become increasingly frustrated with the high mortality and morbidity rate of the patients on the unit who arrive from the medical-surgical floors after sustaining a cardiac arrest. Danielle looks forward to attending the conference to hear how others across the state and nation must deal with the same issue.

SELF-ASSESSMENT: CONTRIBUTIONS TO THE PROFESSION OF NURSING

As a professional nurse, it is important to contribute to the profession of nursing. As a baseline, reflect on your own current contributions to the profession of nursing.

The assessment given in Table 22.1 serves to be a reflective activity and provides you with a snapshot of your current contributions. Some of these activities may be familiar, whereas others are not but are of interest. Take a moment and examine where you are in regards to your participation and level of engagement. Are your contributions what you thought they were? Is it where you want to be? To which activities or contributions are you realistically willing and able to commit over the upcoming year?

QUESTIONS TO CONSIDER BEFORE READING ON

- What can I do to advocate for myself as a nurse?
- What can I do to advocate for my colleagues? The unit I work on? My organization?
- How can I advocate for the nursing profession?
- How do I go about it? How and where do I start?

Place an X for "yes" or "no" on which activities you are currently engaged.

TABLE 22.1 SELF-ASESSMENT OF CURRENT CONTRIBUTIONS AND ENGAGEMENT

Activities in Which I Am Currently Engaged and/or Involved	Yes	No
Mentor or tutor another nurse/student		
Committee member in my organization (unit level, organization level)		
Member of a professional nursing organization		
Community volunteer (parish nurse, Special Olympics, health fair, health screening)		
Medical mission—local or international		
Clinical research		
Professional certification		
Advanced nursing degree		
Member of professional or state nursing organization—participate		
Publication		
Preceptor/mentor		
Clinical inquiry—analyze/evaluate new processes/practices		
Clinical inquiry—conduct research that supports evidence-based practice (EBP)		
Professional journals		
Educational conferences, symposia, workshops		
Health-related presentation at nursing conference, workshop, etc.		
Certified in my area of expertise (e.g., medical/surgical, psychiatric, emergency department [ED], critical care)		
Participation in quality improvement initiatives		

ADVOCATING FOR THE NURSING PROFESSION AND HEALTHY WORK ENVIRONMENTS

As a professional nurse and leader, it is your responsibility to foster a healthy, positive work environment. Nurses are positioned in a perfect place to make a long-lasting, effective change in the work environment and the profession of nursing but it requires effort and advocacy for self and others.

Organizations and the leadership team must also be open to input from their employees. Nurses usually make up the majority of a healthcare organization's workforce. It is imperative that nurses' voices be heard from all levels (bedside to boardroom) in any decision-making process. Nurses need to communicate their passion and perspective as they advocate for themselves, colleagues, and the nursing profession.

Your professional responsibility to advocate for your patients, your colleagues, and the profession is highlighted in several key nursing documents. For example, Nursing's Social Policy Statement (ANA, 2010) is a landmark document that describes the profession of nursing and its professional framework and responsibility to society. In addition, the *Code of Ethics for Nurses With Interpretive Statements* (ANA, 2015) is an ideal example of how nurses contribute to and advocate for their profession. The *Code of Ethics* outlines the obligation of nurses to go through the proper processes to address issues and concerns found in the healthcare environment. There are a range of advocacy skills and activities that professional nurses should develop that are discussed in the *Code of Ethics*.

The *Code* is written with two main components: the provisions and the accompanied interpretive statements. There are currently nine provisions. The interpretive statements provide very specific direction and guidance regarding the obligation of current nursing practice, thus the reason why it has undergone periodic revisions. It is important to note that the *Code* is written by nurses, for nurses, and expresses and articulates what nursing means to them, translating their commitment to society. The *Code of Ethics* not only describes the nursing profession's values, duties, obligations, and professional ideals but also stresses that these interpretive statements reflect only broad expectations without articulating specific activities or behaviors (Epstein & Turner, 2015). The *Code of Ethics* has many legal implications; thus, many state nurse practice acts incorporate the *Code of Ethics* with slight variations as laws and jurisdictions vary state to state (Epstein & Turner, 2015). Over the years, the *Code of Ethics* has been revised (1976, 1985, 2001, and 2015) to be reflective of societal changes, education, legislative policies, and the advanced practice roles that have emerged and the obligations that go with this advancement and commitment to building and maintaining a healthy work environment (Epstein & Turner, 2015).

Take a moment and familiarize yourself with the current *Code of Ethics for Nurses With Interpretive Statements* that is available at: http://nursingworld.org/DocumentVault/Ethics-1/Code-of-Ethics-for-Nurses.html. Which interpretive statements do you feel are your strong suit? Which interpretive statements do you feel could benefit from some improvement in your current practice?

The Nursing's Social Policy Statement and the *Code of Ethics* emphasize the need for nurses to be advocates. What is advocacy? "Advocacy" is the process of supporting a cause or proposal. An advocate helps to defend or support the causes of another. Nurses need to identify needs and then develop a way to address them. Typically, nurses are very skilled at advocating for the patient's needs. However, as a professional nurse, you will be expected to not only advocate for your patients but also advocate for your colleagues and your profession. Can you think of for what you might advocate to promote the profession and a healthy work environment? Some potential ideas include advocating for appropriate staffing ratios, instituting a smoke-free workplace, developing a wellness program for employees, and establishing shared governance models.

It seems logical that we would want to advocate for healthy work environments. In fact, there are documented benefits of having a healthy work environment as well as risks/costs of unhealthy practice environments (International Centre for Human Resources in Nursing [ICHRN], 2007). According to the ICHRN (2007), the benefits and risks are as follows:

Benefits of healthy practice environments include the following:

- High nurse retention rates
- Improved teamwork
- A commitment to safety (both patient and employee) found in most high-reliability organizations (HROs)
- High job satisfaction
- Low absenteeism
- Decreased turnover
- Improved quality patient outcomes
- Increased organizational employee satisfaction rates

Costs/risks of unhealthy work environments include the following:

- Increased absenteeism
- Job dissatisfaction
- Increased turnover
- Increased overtime
- Increase in training costs of new employees (orientation hours)
- Operational inefficiencies
- Low morale
- Poor-quality patient outcomes
- Horizontal violence
- Workplace violence and/or conflict

How can you advocate for the profession of nursing and for a healthy work environment? The answer is simple—get involved. As an advocate, you should consider getting involved in the decision-making committees at your organization (e.g., shared governance committees, policies and procedure committees). You can also be involved in advocating for the profession of nursing outside of your organization. For example, you should consider getting involved in your state nurses association to learn what legislation is being proposed and how it might influence your nursing role and healthcare in general. For example, your state might be proposing that medical assistants can administer medication and that nurses teach them how to do so. How would you feel about this legislation? Is this something you would advocate for or against? How would it affect your practice? How would it affect patient care?

Once involved, you will need to make sure that you have the advocacy skills necessary to promote your success. The following advocacy skills should be honed to help you promote professional nursing practice and healthy work environments (Tomajan, 2012):

- Problem-solving:
  - Identify the problem/issue.
  - Develop a goal/strategy to address the concern.
  - Develop a plan of action with established time frames for completion.
  - Note: Most likely, you will need to bring your concerns to those with the power to make change (the decision makers). It is imperative that you develop a strong case and approach the appropriate person at the right time. You need to have patience as it often takes more than one attempt. Most likely, you will need to collaborate, negotiate, and compromise to achieve the desired outcome.
- Communication:
  - Clearly and concisely deliver a message that fits the situation and the intended audience.
  - Be factual and consistent.
  - Have data to support your argument.
  - Review the impact of the situation.
  - Present how the situation will affect individuals by using words that conjure images and that make the message more compelling.
  - Consider the 60-second speech: This is a concise, factual, practiced speech that introduces the issue as well as the proposed solution. Common elements included in a 60-second speech are as follows (Almidei, 2010; Tomajan, 2012):
    - Provide your name and title.
    - Explain the issue you are addressing.
    - Tell the story to help personalize the issue.
    - Identify what you would like the group to do (a well-defined action item or result that you desire).
    - Provide a brief fact sheet outlining the key facts and your request including your contact information.
- Influence:
  - Make sure that you have the ability to sway others' thoughts, beliefs, and actions.
  - Establish your competency.
  - Establish your trustworthiness and credibility. This can be done by keeping the best interests of those involved at heart.
  - Build a strong case for the needed change.
  - Base your case on facts and data.
  - Place a human face on the issue.

- Collaboration—working with others to achieve a common goal:
  - Establish positive relationships with others on the basis of trust, respect, and credibility.
  - Good communication skills are required; seek input and provide updates on the progress toward the established goals.
  - Work with stakeholders, those with expertise, and individuals in support departments (e.g., human resources, employee health, infection control, legislative aids).

QUESTIONS TO CONSIDER BEFORE READING ON

- What elements of a positive, healthy practice environment exist in your place of practice (e.g., occupational health, safety and wellness policies, fair and manageable workloads, healthy work–life balance, equal opportunity and treatment, opportunities for professional development, autonomy and control over practice, job security, decent pay and benefits)?
- What aspects of your work environment would you like to change?
- How might you collaborate and advocate for those changes?

FIVE OPPORTUNITIES AND CHALLENGES FOR WORKFORCE ADVOCACY PROGRAMS

There are five well-established areas of opportunities that exist for healthcare workforce advocacy programs. These include the following:

1. Identification of mechanisms within healthcare systems to provide RNs the opportunity to affect institutional policies and procedures
2. Development of conflict resolution models for use within organizations that address RNs' concerns about patient care and delivery issues
3. Legislative solutions for workplace problems by reviewing issues of concern to nurses in employment settings and introducing appropriate legislation
4. Development of legal centers for nurses that could provide legal support and decision-making advice as a last recourse to resolve workplace issues
5. Provision of self-advocacy and patient advocacy information to all RNs

A more detailed description of these five opportunities for Workforce Advocacy programs with specific resources on how to accomplish each one can be found at www.nursingworld.org/practice-policy/workforce/five-opportunities-and-challenges-for-workforce-advocacy-program (ANA, 2017).

ASSESSMENT ACTIVITY

Assess your healthcare agency/organization and evaluate which of these five opportunities exist. Place an X for "yes" or "no" for each opportunity (Table 22.2).

TABLE 22.2 ASSESSING A HEALTHCARE AGENCY/ORGANIZATION

Does This Opportunity Exist at My Organization?	Yes	No
Opportunity 1: Mechanisms that provide opportunities for RNs to affect institutional policies such as: • Organization on the Magnet journey • Shared governance established • Shared governance committees in place, (e.g., quality, research, education, staffing, and scheduling) • Participatory management models • Statewide staffing regulations		
Opportunity 2: Existence of conflict resolution models that address RNs' concerns about patient care and delivery issues such as the ability to: • Use an identified reporting loop • Appoint a final arbiter in disputes		
Opportunity 3: Seek legislative solutions for workplace problems by reviewing issues of concern to nurses in employment settings and introducing appropriate legislation, such as: • Whistle-blower protection • "Safe harbor" peer review • Support for rules outlining strong nursing practice standards		
Opportunity 4: Develop legal centers for nurses that could provide legal support and decision-making advice as a last recourse to resolve workplace issues such as: • Provision of fast and efficient legal assistance to nurses • Earmarking precedent-setting cases that could impact case law and healthcare policy		
Opportunity 5: Does your organization provide RNs with self-advocacy and patient advocacy information, such as: • Laws and regulations governing practice • Use of applicable nursing practice standards • Conflict resolution and negotiation techniques • Identification of state and national reporting mechanisms that allow RNs to report concerns about healthcare organizations and/or professionals • Internal "hotline" to report concerns, (e.g., corporate compliance number that is anonymous and confidential)		

RN, registered nurse.

The more categories scoring "yes" indicate that there are mechanisms in place at your healthcare organization that afford opportunities for nurses to engage in and have a positive effect on institutional policies.

Box 22.2 depicts relevant QSEN competencies nurses should possess and develop as contributing members to the nursing profression as well as collaboration in inter-disciplinary healthcare teams.

QUALITY AND SAFETY EDUCATION FOR NURSES (QSEN) CONSIDERATIONS

Two QSEN competencies closely aligned with "contributing to the profession—your responsibility as a professional nurse" are teamwork and collaboration. As you read the QSEN competencies in the subsequent text that relate to "contributing to the profession—your responsibility as a professional nurse," ask yourself the following:

- Which of these competencies do I meet and which competencies do I need to develop more fully?
- What plan of action can I take to enhance those competencies in which I am weak and to develop those that I lack at this time?

BOX 22.2 RELEVANT QUALITY AND SAFETY EDUCATION FOR NURSES (QSEN) COMPETENCIES

- Describe own strengths, limitations, and values in functioning as a member of a team (Knowledge).
- Act with integrity, consistency, and respect for differing views (Skills).
- Describe scopes of practice and roles of healthcare team members (Knowledge).
- Assume role of team member or leader on the basis of the situation (Skills).
- Follow communication practices that minimize risks associated with hand-offs among providers and across transitions in care (Skills).
- Describe strategies for identifying and managing overlaps in team member roles and accountabilities (Knowledge).
- Assert own position/perspective in discussions about patient care (Skills).
- Respect the unique attributes that members bring to a team, including variations in professional orientations and accountabilities (Attitudes).
- Function competently within own scope of practice as a member of the healthcare team (Skills).
- Explain how authority gradients influence teamwork and patient safety (Knowledge).
- Appreciate importance of intra- and interprofessional collaboration (Attitudes).

Source: Quality and Safety Education for Nurses Institute. (2014). QSEN competencies. Retrieved from http://qsen.org/competencies/pre-licensure-ksas

QUESTIONS TO CONSIDER BEFORE READING ON

- What are the advantages and disadvantages of being a mentor?
- Have you mentored another nurse? If so, how was this experience? How might you improve this experience?
- If not, might you consider being a mentor to a nurse in the near future? How might you go about this?

MENTORING

Mentorship is oftentimes viewed as a key competency and skill required of the nursing profession and leadership. There are numerous different definitions of mentoring; however, all commonalities include the fact that it is a positive, dynamic, one-on-one experience between an experienced and a less experienced professional in which great satisfaction and personal and professional growth result. Finkelman and Kenner (2016) define "mentoring" as a career development tool that is a mutually agreed-upon relationship and can be either short-term or long-term and further note in today's world can be in person or virtual.

Nursing is a nurturing profession so it would make sense that nurses should mentor nurses, thus giving back to the profession. Nurse leaders and educators should mentor the new nurse leaders to strengthen the profession and leave a legacy on the basis of our values, principles, and ethics of our nursing profession to the next generation (Grossman, 2007). Mentoring is important in the career development of both the novice and the experienced nurses. In addition, as mentioned earlier in the chapter, with the anticipated shortage in nursing continuing far into 2030, it is important to highlight mentoring as an important factor that can foster professional career satisfaction and intent to stay in the profession (Mariani, 2012).

In Chapter 20, we shared the importance of finding yourself a mentor to promote your professional growth. The focus in this chapter is on your professional obligation to give back to the profession and mentor others. Mentoring opportunities and the relationships that are fostered during mentoring are perceived as very fulfilling and empowering connections for both the mentor and the mentee. These connections offer a very dynamic experience for the promotion of growth and development both professionally and personally again for both parties (McCloughen, O'Brien, & Jackson, 2013). It is important to note that not only does the mentee benefit from the mentorship experience, but it facilitates feelings by the mentor also, and both benefit from feeling like valued members of the nursing profession and/or organization in which they work. The unfolding case scenario depicted in Box 22.3 is an example of the benefits received from a mentoring relationship and participation in a professional nursing organization.

BOX 22.3 THE CASE SCENARIO CONTINUES TO UNFOLD

Danielle was mentored in the intensive care unit (ICU). It was her mentor who encouraged her to join a professional nursing organization. Danielle joined the Critical Care Nurses association. Both mentee and mentor received great satisfaction from belonging to the Critical Care Nurses association.

In participating in a professional organization and attending a conference, Danielle was empowered to share evidence-based practice (EBP) knowledge and best practices acquired from networking at an annual conference back at her organization.

The positive relationship Danielle had with her mentor facilitated change at their organization with the development of a rapid response team resulting in positive patient outcomes, job satisfaction, and pride in the profession for both mentor and mentee.

Madison (2010) emphasizes the fact that as the nursing workforce ages, mentoring is an ideal mechanism to value the seasoned experts and allow them an opportunity to feel valued and share their knowledge and expertise with the new novice nurse.

Many healthcare organizations, especially high-reliability organizations (HROs) embracing safety, encourage nurses to both engage in and pursue opportunities to mentor others throughout their professional careers. It is, in fact, the organization's as well as the nurse leader's responsibility to create positive workplace environments and cultures that value and support mentoring (Madison, 2010).

Mentoring offers an opportunity for the nurturing and development of personal, professional, career, and intellectual development with the hope of igniting a spark in nurses tapping into leadership potential that may not be evident yet or been given the opportunity to flourish, and the hope of preparing future nurse leaders. If you are interested in mentoring, there are a variety of different ways to get started. Let your leadership team know that you are interested in being a mentor. Mentors can be official or unofficial. You can volunteer to serve as a mentor as an alumnus(a) to a student. You can join a planned mentoring program and mentor a new nurse on your floor. Join a professional organization or volunteer to sit on a board in your community. You can also serve as a mentor by being a role model each and every day on the floor on which you work, challenging old practices, being optimistic and energized when opportunities to pilot new projects come along, and being supportive to all team members with whom you work.

You will need to develop the following skills to be an effective mentor who is able to empower the mentee (Vance, 2009):

- Communication: Effective communication skills are essential whether they be verbal, nonverbal, written, electronic, or face-to-face. The message

needs to be encouraging and supporting while maintaining high expectations. As the mentor, it is your role to inspire the mentee to perform at his or her greatest potential.
- Feedback: Offer your mentee feedback on a planned and regular basis. The feedback should provide the mentee with an assessment that promotes continuous learning. The feedback should not only help the mentee to correct errors but also help to develop a sense of confidence and accomplishment when a job is well done. A key is to provide opportunities for reflection and discussion.
- Challenge: Encourage your mentee to reach for higher goals. Provide him or her with professional development opportunities and trust that he or she will accept and meet the challenge. Express that the work may be difficult but that you believe in his or her abilities to perform.
- Climate and culture: Create a safe and caring environment that demonstrates your interest and acceptance. Always treat the mentee with respect even when offering constructive feedback. Create a "we can do it" culture.
- Investment and advocacy: As a mentor, you need to be willing to offer your time as well as your emotional and physical presence. Support the mentee's growth by opening doors to new experiences. Introduce your mentee to others who may be able to offer additional opportunities.

QUESTIONS TO CONSIDER BEFORE READING ON

- What can a professional nurse organization do for you?
- Why are professional organizations important to continued learning?
- How can professional organizations benefit both the employee and the employer?

MEMBERSHIP IN PROFESSIONAL NURSE ORGANIZATIONS

As a professional nurse and leader, you are expected to participate in professional organizations. Such a membership will provide you with an opportunity to enhance your personal and professional growth. There are a number of professional nursing organizations, each with its own mission and benefits. There are general nursing groups as well as specialty nursing organizations. We begin by talking about the ANA but also mention other organizations in which you can get involved as well as the benefits.

AMERICAN NURSES ASSOCIATION

The ANA, which has been in existence since 1896, represents the interests of the nation's RNs through its constituent and individual state nurses associations and its specialty nursing/affiliate organizations. It has supported and navigated nursing practice through policy development, the establishment of the scope and standards of nursing practice, and the implementation of the nationally accepted *Code of Ethics for Nurses With Interpretive Statements* (ANA, 2015). The ANA official site can be accessed via http://nursingworld.org.

In addition to the ANA, and your own specific state nurses' association, there are numerous other professional organizations that you can join based on your interests or areas of specialty. It is important to note that there are three categories of professional nursing organizations: state organizations, national organizations, and international professional nursing organizations. A few examples for some national organizations include the following:

- Academy of Medical-Surgical Nurses
- Academy of Neonatal Nursing
- American College of Nurse Practitioners (ACNP)
- Alliance for Psychosocial Nursing
- Alliance of Nurses for Healthy Environments
- Alzheimer's Association
- American Academy of Ambulatory Care Nursing
- American Academy of Nurse Practitioners
- American Academy of Nursing
- American Assembly for Men in Nursing

A complete listing of all three categories of professional nursing organizations can be found at: http://nurse.org/orgs.shtml. Professional organizations have web-based information that one can access to gain information regarding their mission, local chapters, resources, events, and membership information. RNs join professional nurse organizations for a variety of reasons. A few examples may include the following: to enhance one's professional status, the desire to stay current in the nursing field or specialty area (e.g., Critical Care Nurses association or Emergency Nurses Association; Greggs-McQuilkin, 2005), as well as the ability to network with other nurses and make new friends. However, there are many other reasons why nurses join as well as benefits a professional nurse organization membership holds.

BENEFITS OF PROFESSIONAL NURSE ORGANIZATION MEMBERSHIP

Professional organizations serve and support nurses. In the case scenario presented in this chapter, Danielle found it gratifying to belong to the Critical Care Nurses association. Membership afforded her an opportunity to network with others and become involved in evidence-based practice (EBP) changes at her organization, and ultimately helped her to obtain certification in her specialty and clinical ladder advancement. Matthews (2012) emphasizes the benefit of participating in professional organizations and the importance of association advocacy. Professional nurse organizations provide many benefits to their members. In addition to the few mentioned earlier, benefits include the following:

- Self-gratification of belonging to a professional organization
- Networking opportunities
- Educational resources—as many organizations offer free continuing education units (CEUs)
- Ability to stay current on latest hot topics in profession or specialty area
- Annual conventions
- Free or discounted products or resources
- Career opportunities
- Standards of care
- Code of ethics
- Certifications
- Organizational websites with member-only access
- Public advocacy for the profession
- Advancement of profession through research
- Political policy and advocacy—legislative change opportunities

The public and society as a whole depend on professional organizations as a vehicle to reach members, learn about the profession, and learn about issues or concerns (Beyers, 2010). Joining a professional organization of interest provides you with an opportunity to benefit yourself, your colleagues, your profession, and society.

COMMITMENT TO LIFELONG LEARNING

As a professional nurse and leader, it is essential that you demonstrate a commitment to lifelong learning. Most likely, you already possess this characteristic. Every time you learn a new procedure or skill or you look up a new medication in a drug book and/or are open and listen to the suggestions of others, you are engaging in lifelong learning. However, there are more formal steps in lifelong learning. You are actively contributing and engaging in lifelong learning by the mere fact that you are reading this book and taking steps to pursue your degree. Congratulations!

The Institute of Medicine's (2011) *Future of Nursing* report noted that a commitment to lifelong learning is essential to nursing practice. Many believe that lifelong learning must consist of only the pursuit of a higher degree. Lifelong learning can consist of the formal process of a higher degree but can also consist of many other activities that you may not have considered. These include but are not limited to the following:

- Reading journal articles
- Participating in a journal club
- Continuing education sessions/credits (online or in-person)
- Advancing your degree (ASN–BSN–MSN–DNP–PhD–EdD)
- Obtaining an advance certificate (e.g., ACLS, PALS, dysrhythmia course)
- Obtaining certification in a specialty area (e.g., medical/surgical certification, certified nurse educator)
- Successfully attaining recertification of specialty certification
- Attendance at a local, national, or international conference
- Obtaining a level status change in your workplace
- Joining a unit-based or hospital-wide committee
- Joining a professional organization
- Volunteering to serve on a community taskforce (e.g., emergency preparedness, lead in homes awareness, drugs and alcohol prevention, and Internet safety)

The increasing complexity involved with our patient populations and the evolving healthcare environment today require nurses to engage in ongoing educational preparation. So, whether you decide to seek an additional degree, become certified, or join a committee at work, please do so. Our unfolding case scenario depicted in Box 22.4 reveals Danielle's growth and how she became a change agent. Lifelong learning is essential to the profession of nursing and the delivery of safe and effective care. Engage in lifelong learning for yourself, for the nursing profession, for the organization for which you work, and most importantly for the patients and families for whom you care.

BOX 22.4 THE CASE SCENARIO CONTINUES TO UNFOLD

It is important to remember that we ourselves as well as our family members could possibly be patients someday. As you read the case scenario, reflect on the following question: How is a nurse who is engaged in lifelong learning a benefit to the patient, the profession of nursing, and her organization? What happens to the profession of nursing and patient care when nurses are not committed to lifelong learning?

Through her commitment to lifelong learning, Danielle obtained her BSN degree, read monthly nursing journals, participated in shared governance committees, and joined a professional nurse organization. By doing so, she as well as other team members helped change policy and practice for patients and families in the ICU.

ENGAGEMENT IN EVIDENCE-BASED PRACTICE AND RESEARCH

Professional nursing practice should be grounded in the translation of current evidence. This statement is supported as EBP is noted in The Essentials of Baccalaureate Education (AACN, 2008) under essential III and in QSEN (QSEN Institute, 2014) as a core competency.

The ANA identifies research as being a critical component of professional nursing. The ANA's mission statement is the following: *"nurses advancing our profession to improve health for all"* (ANA, 2011). How does a nurse in today's healthcare environment advance our profession to improve health for all? It may seem like too daunting a task to consider. However, by focusing your efforts on improving quality outcomes, you will accomplish this vital mission.

Nurses work 24 hours a day, 7 days a week, 24/7 on the frontline of the healthcare system and have the unique opportunity more than any other discipline to improve patient care and outcomes through EBP (Hockenberry, Walaen, Brown, & Barrera, 2008). In fact, nurses cannot work in today's healthcare environment without engaging in EBP. Quality outcomes are reliant on the use of both research and EBP (ANA, 2011).

The term "sacred cow" refers to practices in which nurses engage despite evidence to the contrary. Nurses can sometimes be resistant to trying new strategies to achieve better patient outcomes. EBP improves the quality of care, patient outcomes, and financial outcomes. However, clinical practices can be so rooted in tradition that nurses are reluctant to examine their practice and the outcomes. Think about how many times you have heard the following statements: "We have always done it that way" or "That is the way it is done around here." EBP urges you to question whether these practices actually result in quality outcomes and if not why do we continue to engage in them? Being active at unit meetings, town meetings, and shared governance councils are some ways in which nurses can participate in crucial conversations that impact the delivery of care and practice concerns.

Challenging a long-established practice requires leadership skills as well as an evaluation of current literature and evidence (Hanrahan et al., 2015). By the same token, organizations must be willing to embrace EBP to improve outcomes. Boxes 22.5 and 22.6 start the conversation and depict how active participation in a professional organization, networking, and embracing EBP could possibly change practice at Danielle's organization. Some concrete suggestions of how you might engage in EBP include the following:

- Reading professional journal articles
- Joining a journal club
- Talking about EBP and evidence-based research (EBR) to colleagues and at staff meetings

- Brainstorming ideas on unit or alternate settings (e.g., physician's office, long-term care, urgent care, community nursing) to improve outcomes
- Hosting a "sacred cow" contest
- Joining a shared governance committee
- Volunteering to work on an EBP project
- Attending a local, national, or international conference

BOX 22.5 THE CASE SCENARIO CONTINUES TO UNFOLD

While Danielle was at the conference, a presentation was made on how critical care nurses participated in an interprofessional team that medical-surgical nurses were encouraged to call when they were concerned about their patients' conditions rather than wait for a life-threatening event to occur.

Today, the team is called Rapid Response Team or a similar name. Danielle became excited and thought this could be the answer for her hospital's issue.

When Danielle returned to work, she shared the information with her manager and, subsequently, with the critical care hospital committee. After discussion and review of statistics, the committee decided to pilot the program.

BOX 22.6 THE CASE SCENARIO CONTINUES TO UNFOLD

At her second annual evaluation, Danielle looked back at the pivotal moment of joining the professional organization and attending a national conference as a learning opportunity from others in her same specialty as invaluable to her practice. By challenging the status quo at her hospital, striving for excellence to improve patient quality outcomes, searching through current research and literature, and exploring evidence-based practice at other organizations, Danielle and the shared governance committee introduced rapid response teams at the organization. The program was a great success by having a critical care resource team support medical-surgical patients prior to sustaining a life-threatening event. Today, these teams have been widely implemented, changed practice, and improved patient outcomes.

QUESTIONS TO CONSIDER BEFORE READING ON

- What are the "sacred cows" in your practice setting?
- What actions can you take to examine and address the "sacred cows"?
- Consider hosting a contest for who can identify a "sacred cow" supported by the literature on a unit level or during Nurses Week.

TABLE 22.3 EXPLORING AND ENGAGING IN EBP: RELEVANT QSEN COMPETENCIES
Demonstrate knowledge of basic scientific methods and processes (Knowledge)
Read original research and evidence reports related to area of practice (Skills)
Describe EBP to include the components of research evidence, clinical expertise, and patient/family values (Knowledge)
Question rationale for routine approaches to care that result in less-than-desired outcomes or adverse events (Skills)
Value the need for continuous improvement in clinical practice on the basis of new knowledge (Attitudes)
Describe how the strength and relevance of available evidence influence the choice of interventions in provision of patient-centered care (Knowledge)
Participate in structuring the work environment to facilitate integration of new evidence into standards of practice (Skills)

EBP, evidence-based practice; QSEN, Quality and Safety Education for Nurses.

Source: Quality and Safety Education for Nurses Institute. (2014). QSEN competencies. Retrieved from http://qsen.org/competencies/pre-licensure-ksas

Table 22.3 displays the QSEN (QSEN Institute, 2014) competency of EBP as well as the knowledge, skills, and attitudes (KSAs) associated with the goal to integrate best current evidence into your clinical expertise taking into account patient/family preferences and values for the delivery of optimal care.

MAGNET® RECOGNITION PROGRAM

The Magnet Recognition Program developed by the American Nurses Credentialing Center (ANCC) is the most prestigious award or distinction a healthcare organization can achieve recognizing that organization's nursing excellence and quality patient outcomes. Hospitals need to meet specific criteria to obtain Magnet designation (ANCC, 2017).

These criteria include the following:

- High RN job satisfaction
- Excellent patient outcomes
- High patient/family satisfaction
- Culture of quality and safety

The category of RN job satisfaction is broad and encompasses the following factors:

- Nursing leadership values the staff nurses.
- Professional autonomy is promoted.
- Nursing practice is research based.
- Nursing is involved in decision-making in patient care delivery.
- Advancement in nursing practice is encouraged and rewarded.
- Professional education is provided.
- Teamwork and positive relationships among all departments and disciplines exist.

When these factors are present, the other criteria—excellent patient outcomes, high patient satisfaction, and a culture of quality and safety—are easily met.

SELF-ASSESSMENT

Consider your current practice environment and determine which of the criteria and factors are present (Table 22.4).

Does your practice environment meet the standards and factors noted earlier? What areas are strengths? Where are the opportunities for growth? How might you go about promoting such opportunities?

It is important to remember that Magnet designation is more than just an award—it is a framework for promoting and improving nursing excellence, thereby improving patient outcomes and the patient experience. Box 22.7 explores and provides an opportunity to discuss how EBP and/or Magnet Recognition could empower nurses to change policy and promote excellence in the delivery of nursing services to patients. Being on a Magnet journey refers to the process of creating and sustaining a culture of excellence (ANCC, 2017). Once an organization receives the initial designation, ongoing

TABLE 22.4 ASSESSING THE PRACTICE ENVIRONMENT

Criteria	Present	Not Present
High RN job satisfaction		
Excellent patient outcomes		
High patient/family satisfaction		
Culture of quality and safety		
Factor	**Present**	**Not Present**
Nursing leadership values the staff nurses		
Professional autonomy is promoted		
Nursing practice is research based		
Nursing is involved in decision-making in patient care delivery		
Advancement in nursing practice is encouraged and rewarded		
Professional education is provided		
Teamwork and positive relationships among all departments and disciplines exist		

RN, registered nurse.

BOX 22.7 THE CASE SCENARIO CONTINUES TO UNFOLD

As you read this case scenario, consider the following questions:

- Have you or a colleague experienced a similar situation?
- How would you have advocated for the family in this situation? Or would you?
- In your organization, what avenues do you have to change practice?

Ten years later, Danielle remains in the ICU and is one of the charge nurses and frequently mentors other nurses. One evening while in charge, Danielle is caring for a 24-year-old trauma patient named George. Throughout the course of the evening, he cardiac arrests or "codes." During the code, the resident and attending physician politely ask the family to wait outside the room. The family remains outside of the room the entire time. The code goes on for over an hour and unfortunately the patient expires.

George's family is irate and questions why, when it was apparent that George was slipping away, they were not called into the room to be a presence and be allowed to say goodbye. Danielle became very close to the family and is deeply disturbed by the events and the fact that the family was not afforded the opportunity to be with their son during his last moments before he died.

This scenario is not unusual for Danielle and she fears it will only happen again, sooner than later. Danielle brings up the topic during the code debriefing with members of the interdisciplinary healthcare team. Danielle finds that the issue of whether families should be allowed to be present during resuscitation efforts remains quite controversial. Many physicians as well as nurses feel that it is inappropriate to have the family members present. Furthermore, it is not uncommon for many organizations to have strict policies that restrict visitors in specialty areas and during resuscitation, emergent or invasive events, and procedures.

Danielle brings her concerns to her manager. The organization for which Danielle works is a Magnet-recognized organization.

- What does Magnet recognition mean?
- How does that help Danielle with her situation?

recertification occurs. This is an important factor to consider when looking at where you may want to work.

Employment in a Magnet facility has the following benefits:

- Professional autonomy
- Clinically competent staff
- Positive interdisciplinary relationships and collaboration
- Adequate staffing
- A culture that promotes safety and concern for the patient
- Educational support
- Nurse involvement in decision-making (committees, performance improvement, data collection, product evaluation)

- Professional growth and leadership opportunities
- Low staff turnover
- High patient satisfaction

There is also a financial benefit to the facility as there is recognition in the community for care excellence: low RN turnover/low RN vacancy rate equates to less expenditure for recruitment and orientation and improved outcomes (decreased falls, body substance isolations, urinary tract infections, ventilator-associated pneumonias) maintain revenues. Even if your organization is not a formal Magnet-designated facility, the Magnet standards can serve as a useful framework for nursing excellence for your organization. It is your obligation as a professional nurse and leader to continually strive for excellence. Box 22.8 depicts how participation in a profession organization, a sense of inquiry and application of EBP can promote nurse autonomy and change practice.

Your obligation as a nurse is to practice with an open mind and a sense of inquiry. You should not accept mediocrity or the status quo. You are essential to bringing evidence-based changes into clinical practice and transforming the healthcare system as the IOM urges us to do (IOM, 2011, 2013).

BOX 22.8 CASE SCENARIO CONCLUSION

At the next AACN conference, Danielle starts networking with colleagues and brings up the topic of family presence during resuscitation. She discovers that she is not alone nor is her organization alone, and there is currently an abundance of EBP literature supporting the fact that families should be allowed or given the option to be present during resuscitation and invasive procedures. Danielle discovers that one specialty organization, the Emergency Nurses Association, has issued an official statement that recommends that family should have an option of being present during such events.

Danielle does a literature search and brings her findings back to her organization that is Magnet designated. During the next Shared Governance Council meeting, Danielle shared her concerns observed in the ICU, the current review of literature, and recommendations from both the critical care association and the Emergency Room Associations.

Other nurses at the Council from various units concur that in the spirit of delivering patient-centered care, best practice should allow families to be present or given the option to be present during resuscitation efforts. Recommendations to change current policies and practice are brought to Operations Council and vetted through other disciplines in the organization such as physicians, pastoral care, case management, risk management, and security.

A few months later, the policy and procedure have changed at Danielle's organization. Family members are allowed in the resuscitation room not only in the ED and ICU but also house-wide in her organization on a case-by-case basis.

Best practice can occur only when you ask important questions such as the following:

- Why do we do it this way?
- Is there a better way?
- Is this practice a "sacred cow"?
- Is there recent literature/evidence to support this practice?

CIVIC AND SOCIAL RESPONSIBILITY AND VOLUNTEERISM

Historically, the concepts of volunteerism and nurses were synonymous. This spirit of volunteerism continues to be an integral part of the nursing profession today. Volunteerism appeals to nurses' fundamental commitment to help make a positive impact on individuals, communities, and society (Young & Rupert, 2009). The concept of volunteerism and commitment of nurses to their communities and society dates back to Florence Nightingale's and Clara Barton's efforts in regards to war and disaster management (Young & Rupert, 2009). Nurses continue to volunteer and are an integral visible part of health and wellness services, disaster management services, as well as humanitarian initiatives.

Many professional organizations today are almost totally dependent on volunteers for their mere existence and ongoing sustainment (Welch, 2009). In addition, many have a limited number of individuals in paid positions. Why do professionals like nurses volunteer their time and talent? As nurses, we are busy individuals. Many nurses are balancing work, family life, and educational pursuits. Something in nurses' altruistic nature may be calling them to volunteer. A study (Dignam & Gazley, 2008) examining associations and community volunteering found that both professionals and community volunteers did so as a result of altruistic or instrumental reasons translating into the desire to serve others as well as to reap self-rewards (Welch, 2009). It is this skill set of "prosocial" motivations that is indeed the cornerstone of volunteerism. Fraser (2014) asserts that nurses exemplify professionalism in our daily work. Volunteerism is part of this work, and in order to protect the role of nursing moving forward, nurses must ensure nursing is not just a job, but rather a cherished and valued profession.

Part of your professional obligation is to demonstrate civic and social responsibility. Nurses have an obligation to society to care for the health of its members. Through volunteer efforts, you can support the well-being of the community while forging a strong relationship with community partners. Some benefits of volunteering are the following:

- Provides learning opportunities for you as you serve others
- Builds new relationships with community
- Strengthens existing relationships with the community

- Improves health status of community members
- Promotes civic and social responsibility
- Provides networking opportunities
- Affords community leaders and members

Volunteer opportunities abound for nurses. For example, a pediatric office might help community children by hosting an event to get backpacks filled with supplies for children who otherwise could not afford them. An oncology center might engage in fundraising efforts to help pay for items/services that oncology patients might have difficulty affording (e.g., help pay for transportation to and from chemotherapy treatments, pay for wigs). You could get involved in parish nursing or medical mission trips. Professional organizations, schools, healthcare centers, and legislative venues would welcome your involvement in their leadership projects.

QUESTIONS TO CONSIDER REVISITED

Let us again ask that question posed earlier. Imagine if all 3.6 million nurses played an active role in our healthcare system as the IOM urges.

- What would healthcare look like?
- What would the profession of nursing look like?
- What contributions to the profession will you make?

It is up to each one of the 3.6 million nurses and *you* to contribute to the profession of nursing. One way to contribute is through leadership and service. A great example of this is an initiative that is underway to place nurses in boardroom positions. Although nurse leaders engage in many leadership roles within healthcare organizations, only approximately 6% of nurses hold board positions versus their physician counterparts at 20% (Hassmiller & Combes, 2012). This is an interesting statistic as nurses possess many of the core competencies desired for board leadership and in addition understand all the caveats of patient care with a focus on improved quality indicators and cost control (Hassmiller & Combes, 2012).

CONCLUSION

The IOM's landmark 2011 report, *The Future of Nursing: Leading Change, Advancing Health,* encouraged nurses to step up, advocate, and lead efforts in which to improve and redesign the U.S. healthcare system. If every nurse took an opportunity to contribute to the profession, then our collective efforts would have the potential to make a positive difference in healthcare. As an individual nurse, you have an opportunity to contribute to the profession and leave your own footprint on the nursing profession. You are graced to be part of a profession that has an opportunity to have significant valuable influence on our patients, our communities, and on society.

CRITICAL THINKING QUESTIONS AND ACTIVITIES

- Using the following website, explore a professional nursing organization of interest: state, national, or international organization: http://nurse.org/orgs.shtml.
  - Read the mission of the organization, and explore the benefits, costs, and opportunities it offers. If this organization meets your professional interests and goals, consider joining and getting actively involved.
- Explore the policy and advocacy section of the ANA website from the link provided: http://nursingworld.org.
  - Navigate to the **Join Us** field and enter your name and email address.
  - By doing so, you will be updated on the latest policy and legislative updates that affect *your* work.
  - Then visit the **Policy & Advocacy** tab of the AACN website in the link provided: www.aacnnursing.org.
  - Navigate to the **Get involved** field. Challenge yourself to step out of your comfort zone and get involved advocating for yourself, your workplace, and the profession of nursing. Join a committee, follow a legislative bill, and join a taskforce. It is not as hard as you think. This will be the first step to your ongoing contributions to the profession of *nursing*.
  - Every nurse's *voice matters*. How and where will you leave your footprint on the profession of nursing? What are your plans to accomplish this?

REFERENCES

Almidei, N. (2010). *So you want to make a difference: Advocacy is the key* (16th ed.). Washington DC: OMB Watch.

American Association of Colleges of Nursing. (2008). *The essentials of baccalaureate education for professional nursing practice*. Washington, DC: Author.

American Nurses Association. (2010). *Nursing's social policy statement: The essence of the profession*. Silver Spring, MD: Author.

American Nurses Association. (2011). ANA Annual Report. Retrieved from: https://www.nursingworld.org/~48db72/globalassets/docs/ana/2011-ana-annual-report.pdf

American Nurses Association. (2015). *Code of ethics for nurses with interpretive statements*. Silver Spring, MD: Author.

American Nurses Association. (2016). ANA's nurses by the numbers. Retrieved from http://assets.1440n.net/16-150

American Nurses Association. (2017). Five opportunities and challenges for workforce advocacy programs. Retrieved from https://www.nursingworld.org/practice-policy/workforce/five-opportunities-and-challenges-for-workforce-advocacy-program

American Nurses Credentialing Center. (2017). Magnet recognition program: Overview. Retrieved from http://www.nursecredentialing.org/Magnet/ProgramOverview

Beyers, M. (2010). Nursing's professional associations. In C. J. Huston (Ed.), *Professional issues in nursing: Challenges & opportunities* (2nd ed., pp. 403–430). Philadelphia, PA: Wolters Kluwer Health/Lippincott Williams & Wilkins.

Dignam, M., & Gazley, B. (2008). *The decision to volunteer: Why people give their time and how you can engage them.* Washington, DC: ASAE & The Center for Association Leadership.

Epstein, B., & Turner, M. (2015). The nursing code of ethics: Its value, its history. *Online Journal of Issues in Nursing, 20*(2), 4. doi:10.3912/OJIN.Vol20No02Man04

Finkelman, A., & Kenner, C. (2016). Success in your nursing education program In A. Finkelman & C. Kenner (Eds.). Professional nursing concepts: Competencies for quality leadership (p. 131). Burlington, MA: Jones & Bartlett.

Fraser, D. (2014). Volunteerism: What's in it for you? *Neonatal Network, 33*(1), 3–4. doi:10.1891/0730-0832.33.1.3

Greggs-McQuilkin, D. (2005). Why join a professional nursing organization? *Nursing, 35,* 19. doi:10.1097/00152193-200509001-00006

Grossman, S. C. (2007). *Mentoring in nursing: A dynamic and collaborative process.* New York, NY: Springer Publishing.

Hanrahan, K., Wagner, M., Matthews, G., Stewart, S., Dawson, C., Greiner, J., … Williamson, A. (2015). Sacred cow gone to pasture: A systematic evaluation and integration of evidence-based practice. *Worldviews on Evidence-Based Nursing, 12*(1), 3–11. doi:10.1111/wvn.12072

Hassmiller, S., & Combes, J. (2012). Nurse leaders in the boardroom: A fitting choice. *Journal of Healthcare Management, 57*(1), 8–11. doi:10.1097/00115514-201201000-00003

Hockenberry, M., Walaen, M., Brown, T., & Barrera, P. (2008). Creating an evidence-based practice environment: One hospital's journey. *Journal of Trauma Nursing, 15*(3), 136–142. doi:10.1097/01.JTN.0000337157.00841.cd

Institute of Medicine. (2011). *The future of nursing: Leading change, advancing health.* Washington, DC: National Academies Press.

Institute of Medicine. (2013). *Best care at lower cost: The path to continuously learning health care in America.* Washington, DC: National Academies Press.

International Centre for Human Resources in Nursing. (2007). *Positive practice environments: Fact sheet.* Geneva, Switzerland: International Council of Nursing. Retrieved from http://www.wpro.who.int/topics/nursing/ichrn_fact_sheet.pdf

Juraschek, S. P., Zhang, X., Ranganathan, V., & Lin, V. W. (2011). United States registered nurse workforce report card and shortage forecast. *American Journal of Medical Quality, 27*(3), 241–249. doi:10.1177/1062860611416634

Madison, J. (2010). Socialization and mentoring. In C. J. Huston (Ed.), *Professional issues in nursing: Challenges & opportunities* (2nd ed., pp. 4131–4144). Philadelphia, PA: Wolters Kluwer Health/Lippincott Williams & Wilkins.

Mariani, B. (2012). The effect of mentoring on career satisfaction of registered nurses and intent to stay in the nursing profession. *Nursing Research and Practice, 2012,* 168278. doi:10.1155/2012/168278

Matthews, J. H. (2012). Role of professional organizations in advocating for the nursing profession. *Online Journal of Issues in Nursing, 17*(1), Manuscript 3. doi:10.3912/OJIN.Vol17No01Man03

McCloughen, A., O'Brien, L., & Jackson, D. (2013). Journey to become a nurse leader mentor: Past, present and future influences. *Nursing Inquiry, 21*(4), 301–310. doi:10.1111/nin.12053

Quality and Safety Education for Nurses Institute. (2014). QSEN competencies. Retrieved from http://qsen.org/competencies/pre-licensure-ksas

Tomajan, K. (2012). Advocating for nurses and nursing. *Online Journal of Issues in Nursing, 17*(1), Manuscript 4. doi:10.3912/OJIN.Vol17No01Man04

U.S. Department of Health and Human Services. (2008). Nursing Workforce Survey data. Retrieved from https://data.hrsa.gov/topics/health-workforce/nursing-workforce-surveydata?tab=RegisteredNurses

Vance, C. (2009). *The mentor as pygmalion: Realizing potential through empowerment.* Las Vegas, NV: International Association of Mentoring.

Welch, V. (2009). Message from the board. Investing in the future - the value of volunteerism. *Urologic Nursing, 29*(4), 212–213.

Young, K., & Rupert, D. (2009). Volunteerism incorporated into nursing curriculum. *Online Journal of Rural Nursing & Health Care, 9*(2), 12–14.

INDEX

Printed in the United States
by Baker & Taylor Publisher Services